Wound Healing and Management

Wound Healing and Management

Editor: Connie Freeman

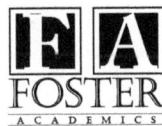

FA
FOSTER
ACADEMICS

www.fosteracademics.com

www.fosteracademics.com

FA
FOSTER
ACADEMICS

Cataloging-in-Publication Data

Wound healing and management / edited by Connie Freeman.
     p. cm.
Includes bibliographical references and index.
ISBN 978-1-63242-846-2
1. Wound healing. 2. Wounds and injuries. 3. Wounds and injuries--Treatment. I. Freeman, Connie.
RD94 .W68 2019
617.1--dc23

Foster Academics,
118-35 Queens Blvd., Suite 400,
Forest Hills, NY 11375, USA

ISBN 978-1-63242-846-2 (Hardback)

Contents

Preface

The main aim of this book is to educate learners and enhance their research focus by presenting diverse topics covering this vast field. This is an advanced book which compiles significant studies by distinguished experts in the area of analysis. This book addresses successive solutions to the challenges arising in the area of application, along with it; the book provides scope for future developments.

Any type of injury in which the skin gets cut, torn, punctured or results in a contusion is known as a wound. It can be either open or closed. The examples of open wounds are incisions, abrasions, avulsions and lacerations. Wounds caused by hematomas and crush injury are common examples of closed wounds. The process in which the skin and its tissues repair themselves after injury is called wound healing. Some of the main factors affecting it include moisture, edema, ischemia, low oxygen tension, smoking, alcohol, immunosuppression, etc. Blood clotting, inflammation, tissue growth and tissue remodeling are the main phases involved in the wound healing process. The topics included in this book on wound healing and management are of utmost significance and bound to provide incredible insights to readers. It explores all the important aspects of wound healing in the present day scenario. This book will serve as a reference to a broad spectrum of readers.

It was a great honour to edit this book, though there were challenges, as it involved a lot of communication and networking between me and the editorial team. However, the end result was this all-inclusive book covering diverse themes in the field.

Finally, it is important to acknowledge the efforts of the contributors for their excellent chapters, through which a wide variety of issues have been addressed. I would also like to thank my colleagues for their valuable feedback during the making of this book.

Editor

A Potential Mechanism for Diabetic Wound Healing: Cutaneous Environmental Disorders

Junna Ye, Ting Xie, Yiwen Niu, Liang Qiao,
Ming Tian, Chun Qing and Shuliang Lu

Abstract

Diabetes mellitus is a chronic multi-organ metabolic disorder caused by a combination of environmental and genetic factors. Diabetic complications are considered to be multifactorial with increasing evidence that one of the major pathways involved in the progression of both microvascular and macrovascular diseases is the biochemical process of advanced glycation.

We will combine in vitro and in vivo studies and other related literatures to discuss the role of advanced glycation end products (AGEs), which may exert deleterious effects in diabetes. Dr Shuliang Lu puts forward the theory of 'cutaneous environmental disorders' mediated by AGEs. The receptor for advanced glycation end products (RAGE) was first described as a signal transduction receptor for AGEs. Recent discoveries regarding AGEs-RAGE interactions expanded our understanding of the mechanisms by which RAGE evoked pathological consequences.

In this chapter, we report on the biology of AGEs, AGEs and wound healing, as well as address current strategies to interrupt the formation of AGEs and underscore strategies by which antagonism of RAGE and AGEs-RAGE crosslinks may be realized.

Keywords: diabetic wound healing, advanced glycated end products, RAGE, measurement, treatment

1. Introduction

Diabetes mellitus is characterized by chronic hyperglycemia and an altered cellular homeostasis, which lead to diffuse vascular damage and multi-organ dysfunction. Diabetic patients

risk both micro- and macro-vascular complications: the former result from damage to reti-
nal, renal, and neural tissues, which is the cause of blindness, end-stage renal failure, and
non-traumatic lower limb amputation, respectively [1]. Here, we will focus on diabetic
wound. Impaired wound healing is associated with increased morbidity and mortality in
diabetes mellitus. The majority of non-healing wounds often lead to amputation, increasing
the direct costs of their care, rehabilitation, and lost productivity [2].

According to a national survey, the prevalence of chronic cutaneous wounds among hospitalized patients was 1.7% in China. The leading causes were diabetes (31.3% men, 35.3% women)
and trauma (26.4% men, 19.2% women). Therefore, diabetes has recently become the leading
cause of chronic cutaneous wounds in China [3]. In Shuliang Lu's study, it was indicated that
new diabetic foot ulcers were already in poor condition when patients first visited the diabetic
foot clinic. Concomitantly, patients had worse health-related quality of life compared with the
general population [4].

Several mechanisms have played a role in this condition, such as neuropathy, peripheral
arterial disease, biomechanical factors, infection, and wound healing. Brownlee identifies the
production of reactive oxygen species (ROS) as the unifying mechanism behind the main
pathological pathways triggered by hyperglycemia, one of which leads to the formation of
heterogeneous moieties called advanced glycation end products (AGEs) via non-enzymatic
glycation and glycoxidation processes [5]. AGEs affect the wound healing process either
directly by their interference with various components involved or indirectly through their
association with diabetic neuropathy or angiopathy [6, 7]. In addition, RAGE was discovered
as a receptor for AGEs, such as carboxymethyl lysine (CML) [8]. RAGE has been postulated
to contribute to the development of diabetic complications [9]. The mechanism of RAGE has
also been widely discussed.

In this chapter, we will present data regarding the formation and the metabolism of AGEs, the
role of RAGE involved in diabetic conditions, evidence emerging from in vitro and in vivo
studies as well as studies using anti-AGEs and other related agents to support a pathogenic
role for AGEs in the impaired process of diabetic wound healing.

2. AGEs formation

It was not until 1980 that the pathophysiological significance of AGEs emerged in medical
science, particularly in relation to diabetic complications [10]. AGEs are a heterogeneous group
of molecules that form from the non-enzymatic addition of sugar moieties onto arginine and
lysine residues of proteins, free amino groups on lipids, or guanine nucleic acids [11]. Glycation
has to be distinguished from glycosylation, which is an enzymatic reaction. First described by
Louis Camille Maillard in the 1900s, non-enzymatic glycation involves condensation reaction
of the carbonyl group of sugar aldehydes with the N-terminus or free-amino groups of proteins
via a nucleophilic addition, resulting first in the rapid formation of a Schiff base. The physiological consequences of the Maillard reaction in the etiology of a range of important diabetic
complications have already been indicated [12]. The Schiff base then goes through rearrange-

ments to form the more stable Amadori products. Among most cellular and plasma proteins, Amadori products can change with glucose. That is to say, the levels of Amadori products will rise and fall depending on the levels of glucose. The most well-known example of an Amadori product is hemoglobin A1c (HbA1c), a naturally occurring modification to the N-terminal valine amino group of the β chain of hemoglobin [13]. Schiff bases and Amadori products are reversible reaction products. However, they can react irreversibly with amino acid residues of peptides or proteins to form protein adducts or protein crosslinks [14] (**Figure 1**).

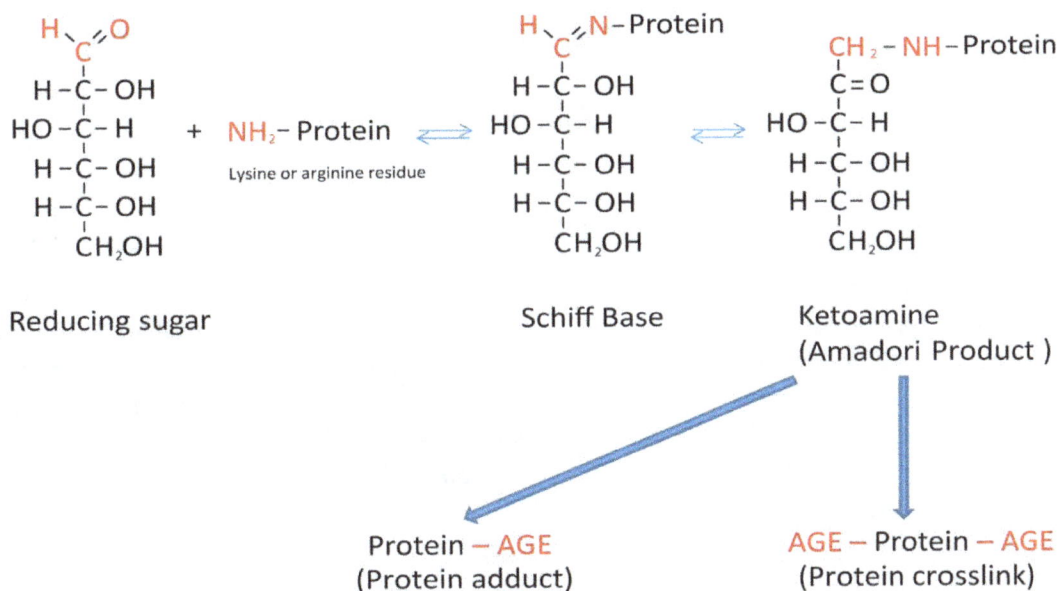

Figure 1. Schematic presentation of the Maillard reaction. Reactive carbonyl groups of a reducing sugar react with neutrophilic free amino groups of proteins to form a reversible Schiff base. Through rearrangement, a more stable Amadori product is formed. Depending on the nature of these early glycation end products, protein adducts or protein crosslinks are formed. (Illustrated from Ref. [54]).

In the context of intracellular glycation, it is important to note that glucose has the slowest rate in the glycation reaction of any sugar [15]. Because of the slow formation, it is believed that AGEs accumulate only on long-lived extracellular proteins. However, later a rapid extracellular AGEs formation on short-lived proteins and intracellular AGEs formation by reactive dicarbonyl compounds have attracted attention [16]. Thus, glycolytic intermediates such as dihydroxyacetone-phosphate, glyceraldehyde-3-phosphate and the dicarbonyl compounds glyoxal, methylglyoxal, and 3-deoxyglucosone are important for the intracellular Maillard reaction [17]. Among these compounds, methylglyoxal is regarded as the most potent glycating agent [18]. The transformation of glyceraldehyde-3-phosphate and dihydroxyacetone-phosphate formed methylglyoxal [19]. It could be detoxified by the conversion to S-Dlactoylglutathione and D-lactate, catalyzed in the cytosol of all cells by glyoxalase I and II. It has been reported that overexpression of glyoxalase I in endothelial cells completely prevented AGEs formation, thus indicating the importance of methylglyoxal to form AGEs [20]. Moreover, several studies on different animal models have established that dietary AGEs could play an important role in the pathogenesis of various pathologic conditions and their complications, such as type 1 diabetes mellitus in non-obese diabetic mice [21], atherosclerosis in apoE-deficient mice [22], type 2 diabetes, and impaired wound healing in db/db (+/+) mice [23]. It should be emphasized that a large portion of AGEs in the human body is derived from exogenous sources, e.g. from regular food, smoking, etc. [24]. Much attention has been paid to the so-called exogenous AGEs, harmful products of "browning" (or the Maillard reaction) in various foods. Together with endogenous AGEs, these compounds form the majority of glycation-free adducts. Among the various food processing methods, heating, sterilizing, and microwaves contribute to the generation of exogenous AGEs, all of which tend to accelerate the non-enzymatic addition of non-reducing sugars to free NH_2 groups of proteins and lipids [25].

3. RAGE

AGEs could exert their actions not only directly but also through a receptor system, which includes two types of cell surface AGEs receptors: first type is that binds AGEs and initiates cell activation and second type is that binds and degrades AGEs. Receptor for AGEs (RAGE) is one receptor of the first type; it recognizes AGEs and initiates oxidative stress. The second type of receptors consists of AGER1, AGER3, and CD36 [26, 27]. However, it is noteworthy that there are other AGE receptors, such as the macrophage scavenger receptor and the galectin-3 receptor, which might have similar deleterious effects to RAGE when they interact with AGEs [28].

RAGE is a multi-ligand receptor of the immunoglobulin superfamily of cell surface molecules acting as a receptor not only for several molecules including AGEs but also for S100/calgra-nulins and amyloid. Circulating isoforms of RAGE include soluble RAGE (sRAGE) that has been cleaved from the cell surface by matrix metalloproteinases and endogenous secretory RAGE (esRAGE), and a splice variant of RAGE that is secreted into blood. Both sRAGE and esRAGE protect body against the AGEs-elicited tissue damage by acting as a decoy receptor for AGEs [29, 30]. The ligands of RAGE have a common feature that they accumulate in tissues during aging, inflammation, and degenerative diseases. Engagement of RAGE results in intracellular signaling that leads to the activation of NF-kB, a pro-inflammatory transcription factor, which is then translocated to the nucleus and subsequently activates the transcription of target genes [31]. These include genes of cytokines, adhesion molecules, and prothrombotic and vasoconstrictive products. The activation of NF-kB results in upregulation of the receptors in return. In addition, cellular-signaling cascades such as the ERK signaling pathway and PI-3 kinases are activated by the binding of ligands with RAGE [32].

In the skin, RAGE expression was observed in both epidermis and dermis, and it was increased in sun-exposed compared with UV irradiation-protected areas [33]. Not only in vivo, but also in vitro, various skin cells types have been shown to express RAGE [34–36], such as keratino-cytes, fibroblasts, dendritic cells, and to a lesser extent endothelial cells and lymphocytes. Patients with diabetes also exhibit increased immunoreactivity for RAGE and AGEs. For example, in sural nerve biopsies, AGE-RAGE interaction was found which suggests it may have a clinical role in neuronal dysfunction that leads to neuropathy [37].

According to these reactions, researchers have put forward mechanisms by which AGEs lead to diabetic complications: (1) the accumulation of AGEs in the extracellular matrix causing aberrant crosslinking, resulting in a decrease of elasticity of vessels; (2) intracellular AGEs formation leading to quenching of nitric oxide and impaired function of growth factors [20]; (3) the binding of AGEs to AGE-receptors on different cell types and activation of key cell signaling pathways such as NF-kB activation with subsequent modulation of gene expression in vascular cells such as endothelial cells, smooth muscle cells, and macrophages [38].

4. AGEs and wound healing

It is generally believed that wound healing is impaired in diabetes. Wound healing is a complex process in which several pathophysiological processes are involved. They include inflammation, repair, and regeneration. Until now, there is evidence from experimental studies that glycation is involved in wound healing in diabetes.

4.1. AGEs and inflammation phase in a diabetic wound

In this part, the interaction between AGEs and RAGE could not be neglected. Data support that it negatively affects various aspects of inflammatory response in diabetic wound. Increased RAGE expression has been found in wound tissues from diabetic mice in parallel with increased AGEs accumulation and increased inflammation [39]. In Shuliang Lu's study [40], compared with the controls, enhanced expression of RAGE and accelerated cell apoptosis were observed in the burned skin of diabetic rats. The altered expression pattern of inflammatory cytokines and oxidative markers between diabetic and control groups revealed delayed neutrophil chemotaxis and respiratory burst. Furthermore, the results in vitro showed that exposure to AGEs inhibited the viability of neutrophils, promoted RAGE production and cell apoptosis, which was consistent with the findings in vivo. Besides, the mice fed with a rich AGEs diet demonstrated an increased and sustained inflammatory phase compared with those fed with a low AGEs diet [41]. In vitro, human neutrophils were isolated and treated with AGE-human serum albumin. Cell viability and reactive oxygen species levels were increased [42].

In keratinocytes, AGEs decrease cell viability and migration and induce the expression of proinflammatory mediators as well [43]. Various growth factors or proteins significant for cellular functions may be glycated inhibiting their functions [44]. Furthermore, treatment of murine macrophages with AGEs resulted in increased levels of iNOS, which has been found to be increased in diabetic wounds [45]. Macrophages play a critical role in wound healing and can be activated to two distinctive phenotypes in vitro: M1 and M2 [46]. It demonstrated insufficient M1 in the early stage but excessive M2 in the later proliferative phase. The macrophage activation markers were correlated with the instructive T helper cell type 1 (Th1)/

Th2 cytokines in both groups. Other studies suggested that RAGE expression has been strongly linked to the expression of matrix metalloproteinases (MMP)-1, MMP-3, MMP-9, mainly through RAGE engagement by AGEs [47]. In addition, AGEs induced the production of oxygen-reactive intermediates from inflammatory and endothelial cells via NADPH activation probably through their receptors, promoting further cellular activation and proinflammatory cytokine expression [48].

4.2. AGEs and proliferation phase in the diabetic wound

It has been reported that the presence of AGEs not only affected the interaction of the fibroblasts with the extracellular matrix but also reduced the amount of the extracellular matrix as well. This effect would influence almost all the cells involved in the proliferative process. In vitro incubation of human dermal fibroblasts with pentosidine or pyrraline resulted in reduction of the extracellular matrix content, which was collagen and proteoglycan [49]. In vitro study showed that type I collagen synthesis from fibroblasts was not affected in AGEs; however, the synthesis of hyaluronic acid was significantly reduced [50]. It also showed a direct effect of AGEs on fibroblast synthetic capacity and explained the decreased extracellular matrix in the diabetic wound. Because hyaluronic acid is associated with cellular locomotion, migration, and proliferation, decreased content in the matrix could result in disturbance of the proliferative phase of the healing process. Besides, histological evaluation of wound sections from diabetic rats demonstrated absence of actively migrating inflammatory cells toward the central region of the wound, reduced angiogenesis, a decrease in the secretion of extracellular matrix, and then poor granulation tissue formation [51].

AGEs may also change the action of the wound-associated cytokines and growth factors, by affecting the growth factors or their receptors. Glycation of bFGF, after its incubation with glucose-6-phosphate (G6P) or fructose, resulted in decreased heparin-binding capacity, which is necessary for the binding of bFGF to its receptor. A reduction in its mitogenic activity was also observed compared with the control bFGF group [45]. In addition, incubation of FGF2 with G6P resulted in glycation of FGF2. Bovine aortic endothelial cells incubated with the glycated FGF2 showed a reduction of proliferation, decreased mean capillary length and new blood vessel formation, a weaker increase in tyrosine-phosphorylated proteins, especially ERK-1 and ERK-2 [52] .While ECV304 cells were incubated with glyoxal proteins, a significant reduction in the free amino acid groups of the EGF receptors was found. It also showed that the EGF-induced recruitment and activation of the downstream effectors of the EGF receptor pathway PLCg1 and ERK1/2 was inhibited by AGEs [53]. Furthermore, an animal study using rats with subcutaneous implantation of sponge disks showed that pretreatment of animals with D-glucose resulted in a reduction in the angiogenesis measured by the hemoglobin content of the implanted disks and a reduction in the granulomatous response compared with control groups.

4.3. AGEs and remodeling phase in the diabetic wound

Every stage of normal wound healing appears to be disrupted in the diabetic patients. A derangement in wound contraction and remodeling is expectable. A large body of evidence supports the effects of AGEs on the phenotype, invasiveness, behavior, and survival of the cells and cell membrane interactions with extracellular matrix. Animal data showed that diabetic mice with lower circulating and tissue-bound AGEs as a result of exposure to a diet low in AGEs, showed improved reepithelialization, granulation tissue formation and angiogenesis compared with the group fed with a diet high in AGEs [54].

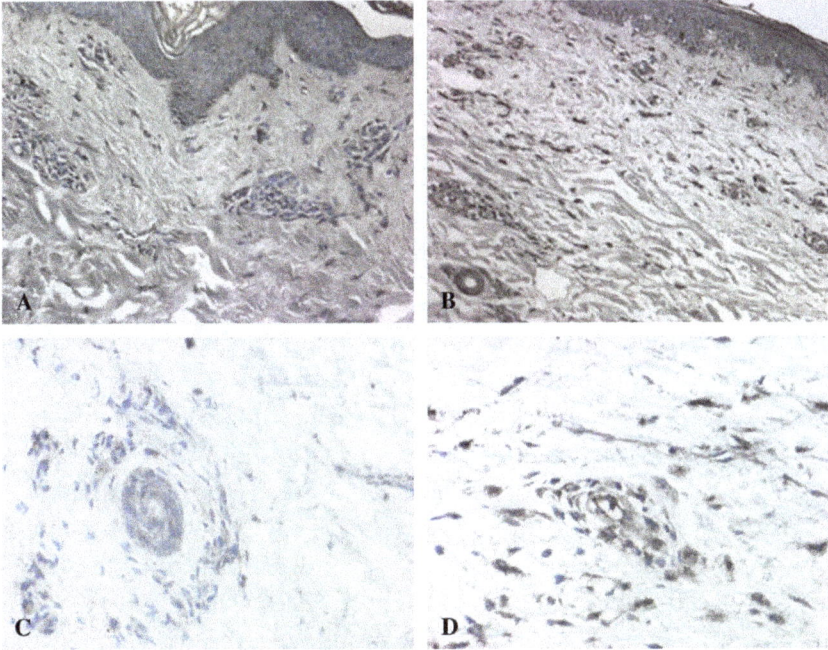

Figure 2. Immunohistochemical localization of AGE and RAGE proteins in dermis is shown. A, B, The distribution of AGE in normal skin tissue (A) and in diabetic skin tissue (B). AGE protein staining was expressed faintly at dermal matrices and cells in control skin but was prominent at the dermal matrices, cells, and basement membrane of vessels in the diabetic skin. C, D, The distribution of RAGE in normal skin tissue (C) and in diabetic skin tissue (D). RAGE-positive cells appear brown, and a light hematoxylin counter stain was used to visualize nuclei. More positive cells were detected in diabetic dermal layer than in control. [Original magnification, ×200 (A, B); original magnification, ×400 (C, D)]. (Illustrated from Ref. [55]).

The balance between proliferation and apoptosis of skin cells is responsible for the success of the wound healing process. Recent reports have shown that AGEs formation participates in dermatologic problems in diabetes. Shuliang Lu's group reported that effects of dermal micro-environment glycosylation. Histology and immunohistochemical staining were performed on type 2 diabetic and nondiabetic skin specimens to determine the distributions of proliferating cell nuclear antigen, apoptotic cells, AGEs and RAGE. Diabetic skin has degenerative, loosely arranged collagen and increased apoptotic cells compared with normal skin. Expression of AGEs and RAGE were increased in diabetic skin. Glycosylated matrix induced cell cycle arrest and apoptosis of cultured dermal fibroblasts, whereas application of RAGE-blocking antibodies redressed these changes [55] (**Figure 2**).

AGEs may alter the signaling of the wound cytokines and growth factors by disrupting the structure of either the growth factors or their receptors. Glycation of fibroblast growth factor (bFGF), after its incubation with intracellular sugars resulted in decreased heparin-binding capacity, which is essential for the ligation of bFGF to its receptor [56]. Bovine aortic endothelial cells incubated with the glycated FGF-2 showed a reduction in the proliferation, decreased mean capillary length and overall new blood vessel formation as well as a clearly weaker increase in tyrosine phosphorylated proteins, particularly ERK-1 and ERK-2 [57]. It has also been shown that the epidermal growth factor (EGF)-induced recruitment and activation of the downstream effectors of the EGF receptor pathway, the serine-threonine kinases ERK1/2, was inhibited by glyoxal and methylglyoxal [58]. Moreover, diabetic rats exhibited poor TGF-β1 expression in fibroblasts [20]. The effects of TGF-β1 on extracellular matrix synthesis and cellular phenotypes are crucial for the final stage of wound healing, suppression of MMP secretion, differentiation of fibroblasts into contractile myofibroblasts, and cellular programmed death. The increased levels of MMPs and proinflammatory cytokines in the context of a vicious self-perpetuating cycle of an inappropriately inflammatory response may be responsible for the derangement of the remodeling stage [42].

Literature data also support that in the presence of AGEs, not only the interaction of the fibroblasts with the extracellular matrix is affected, but also the amount of the extracellular matrix constituents normally secreted by cells is reduced. This effect would deprive almost all the cells involved in the proliferative process of the extracellular scaffold [59]. In vitro, studies showed a direct effect of AGEs on fibroblast survival and synthetic capacity, which might partially explain the decreased extracellular matrix density in the diabetic non-healing wounds. Human adult primary skin fibroblasts treated with CML-collagen (glycated collagen) showed a time- and dose-dependent apoptosis, which was threefold compared with that of control collagen-treated fibroblasts [60]. An insight has been gained into the mechanisms that underlie the AGEs-promoted cell apoptosis. The proapoptotic intracellular signaling consists of involving a chain of events, such as the generation of intracellular reactive oxygen species, which cause the activation of mitogen-activated protein kinase (MAPK) pathways and finally the induction of transcription factor FOXO1 and caspase-3. In addition, keratinocytes pretreated with glycoaldehyde and type I collagen exhibited reduced migration and an impaired adhesive capacity [61]. These effects were caused by conformational changes on the glycated collagen, which altered the effective receptor binding [62]. Furthermore, increased AGE/RAGE expression has been found in the diabetic skin. The apoptotic effects could be reversed by the application of RAGE antibodies, suggesting that AGEs and RAGE interaction played an important part in the cell dysfunction [40].

Another study of Shuliang Lu's group demonstrated that thickness of abdominal dermis from diabetic patients was reduced with obscured multilayer epithelium and disorganized collagen fibrils, as well as with chronic inflammatory cell infiltration. It was also shown that the prominent accumulation of AGEs in the diabetic skin induced an oxidative damage of fibroblasts and thus contributed to the thinner thickness of diabetic abdominal dermis. In vivo, less hydroxyproline, higher myeloperoxidase activity, and increased malondialdehyde (MDA) content were found in the diabetic skin. In vitro, the time- and dose-dependent inhibitory effects of AGE-bovine serum albumin (BSA) on fibroblast viability and the promotion of MDA production were shown [63].

5. Measurement of AGEs

Since the biochemistry of AGEs has been widely discussed, the effort to develop the measurement has been made as well. Blood is more accessible for repeated measurements of AGEs than tissue-requiring biopsies, but plasma AGEs assays have not yet been shown to be directly related to tissue AGEs content [64]. As tissue accumulation of AGEs proves a long-term course with low reversibility, the AGEs accumulated in long-lived tissue proteins like skin collagen may be a carrier of metabolic memory over a long period, even years [65]. Because certain AGEs have intrinsic fluorescence properties, tissue AGEs accumulation can be assessed as skin autofluorescence (SAF) by the AGE Reader™ (Diagn-Optics, Groningen, the Netherlands) easily and noninvasively [66], instead of other traditional invasive techniques (**Figure 3**). Several studies demonstrated that the SAF value obtained from the skin of the lower arm correlated with content of both fluorescent and nonfluorescent AGEs measured from skin biopsy specimens on the same site [67]. It is strongly related to AGEs accumulation in healthy subjects, and diabetic and hemodialysis patients over a broad age range [68]. There is no surprise that SAF values of the diabetic patients were significantly higher than the healthy population [69, 70], and SAF values of diabetes with complications were elevated compared with those without complications [71, 72]. So far, there have been SAF referential values and its influential factors for healthy Dutch, Slovakian, and Chinese people, and this offers the baseline values to further analyze diabetes and its chronic complications [73–75].

However, studies of SAF on predicting the diabetic vascular complications were of considerable clinical heterogeneity, and different experimental results were adjusted in different conditions [76, 77]. Recent publications have suggested that SAF serves as a marker of vascular damage [78], as well as a predictor of cardiac mortality in patients with type 1 and 2 diabetes. In Shuliang Lu's group, Liu Chuanbo et al. did a cross-sectional survey consisting of 118 consecutive hospitalized diabetic foot patients. The diabetic microvascular (retinopathy, nephropathy, and neuropathy) and macrovascular referring to coronary heart disease (CHD), cerebrovascular disease (CVD), or peripheral artery disease (PAD) complications were evaluated .The mean SAF value was 2.8 ± 0.2 AU. SAF was significantly associated with diabetes duration and blood urea nitrogen (R^2 = 62.8%; P < 0.01). Moreover, in logistic regression analysis, SAF was significantly associated with retinopathy (odds ratio [OR] = 40.11), nephropathy (OR = 8.44), CHD (OR = 44.31), CVD (OR = 80.73), and PAD (OR = 5.98 × 109). Therefore, SAF, reflecting tissue accumulation of AGEs is independently associated with the presence of micro-and macro-vascular complications in diabetic foot ulcer (DFU) patients [79]. Similarly, SAF values were significantly higher in type 1 diabetic patients with microvascular complications, like neuropathy, compared to those without complications [80]. Lisanne et al. reported that SAF was independently associated with all-cause mortality and fatal or non-fatal major adverse cardiovascular events in patients with peripheral artery disease after a 5-year follow-up [81].

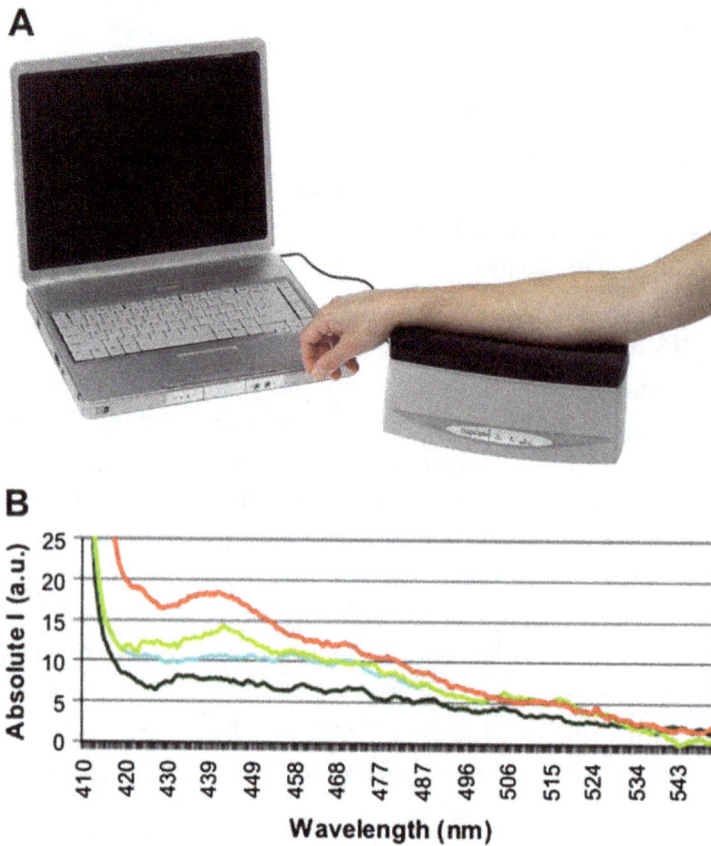

Figure 3. (A) The autofluorescence reader illuminates a skin surface with an excitation light source between 300–420 nm. Only light from the skin is measured with a spectrometer. (B) Various fluorescence spectrum results from different subjects: healthy subject (black line), diabetic patient without cardiovascular complications (blue line), diabetic patient with peripheral artery occlusive disease (green line), hemodialysis patient with recent myocardial infarction (red line). I = intensity (a.u.). (Illustrated from Meerwaldt R, van der Vaart MG, van Dam GM, et al. Clinical relevance of advanced glycation end products for vascular surgery. Eur J Vasc Endovasc Surg. 2008;36(2):125–31).

The use of SAF in the diabetic wound was also discussed. Meerwaldt et al. showed that SAF was increased and correlated with the Wagner score in DFU with neuropathy. SAF correlated inversely with nerve conduction velocity and amplitude [82]. Lapolla et al. found that AGEs were higher in type 2 diabetics with PAD compared to those without PAD; AGEs were correlated inversely to ABPI, even after correction for other cardiovascular risk factors [83]. SAF is independently associated with diabetic foot ulcerations. It might be a useful screening method for foot ulceration risk of diabetic patients [77].

Use of SAF measurement to assess foot vulnerability and to predict DFU events in high-risk patients seems to be promising. Yet, Vouillarmet et al.'s study in a subgroup of patients with an active DFU showed a nonsignificant correlation (P = 0.06) between SAF and the incidence of healing at 2 months, but the magnitude of effect is still high. Therefore, researchers deemed that the small number of patients may be the reason for the lack of statistical power. SAF method deserves attention because of its prognostic value for healing [84].

However, long-term studies validating both the specificity and sensitivity of this investigation, and its link to certain AGEs, remain to be confirmed. The importance of its use in the follow-up of DFU is not reported. Thus, AGEs might have some value as a screening tool for DFU, but there is no strong evidence for other clinical use in diabetic wound, and AGEs measurements should not be considered a replacement for HbA1c as a marker of glycemic control.

6. Anti-AGEs strategies

Since AGEs were considered as an important factor in diabetes, the development of strategies against AGEs has been of interest. Substances, which can prevent or inhibit the formation of AGEs, as well as agents that can break AGEs or antagonize their signaling have been identified.

6.1. Inhibit the formation of AGEs

The first approach is to reduce the formation of AGEs by intervention at one of the steps involved such as aminoguanidine [85]. Aminoguanidine was one of the first substances identified limiting the formation of AGEs [86]. It is a highly reactive nucleophilic reagent that prevents the formation of AGEs by reacting with the carbonyl groups as well as alpha- and beta-dicarbonyl compounds such as methylglyoxal, glyoxal, and 3-deoxyglucosone. Particularly, long-term aminoguanidine treatment improved the nerve conduction deficit and myelinated fiber pathology in diabetic rats in vivo [87]. A double-blinded, multiple-dose, placebo-controlled, randomized clinical trial of aminoguanidine in diabetic patients with overt diabetic nephropathy (ACTION) was completed in 1998; ACTION I involved 690 type 1 diabetic patients and ACTION II involved 599 type 2 diabetic patients. These studies were designed to evaluate the safety and efficacy of aminoguanidine in slowing the rate of renal disease progression in patients with overt diabetic nephropathy. However, ACTION II was terminated prematurely due to safety concerns and apparent lack of efficacy. Reported side effects included gastrointestinal disturbance, liver function abnormalities, flu-like symptoms, and a rare vasculitis [88]. Its use in clinical practice is limited due to adverse effects in clinical trials with diabetic patients. Despite the earlier promising results, aminoguanidine is unlikely to be used for therapeutic purpose due to safety concerns and lack of efficacy [89]. Studies on topical application of aminoguanidine on the skin are still lacking.

Metformin that is routinely used in the treatment of type 2 diabetic patients has some structural similarities to aminoguanidine and it was shown that in type 2 diabetes, treatment with metformin reduced levels of methylglyoxal [90]. Pyridoxamine is a natural intermediate of vitamin B6 metabolism and a potent inhibitor of the formation of AGEs [91]. Pyridoxamine traps reactive carbonyl intermediates and scavenges ROS. In addition, it inhibits post-Amadori stages of AGEs formation. Marked effects of pyridoxamine such as delayed development of nephropathy and retinopathy have been demonstrated in diabetic rats. Its oral intake could result in potent inhibition of skin collagen CML formation in diabetic rats as well [92].

6.2. Anti-RAGE

RAGE is the most studied receptor for advanced glycation end products. AGER1 has been shown to counteract AGEs-induced oxidative stress via inhibition of RAGE signaling [93]. sRAGE is a truncated splice variant of RAGE containing the ligand-binding domain but not the transmembrane domain and has been found in plasma. sRAGE is a soluble extracellular protein without signaling properties and it is considered as a natural decoy receptor of RAGE [30].

Blockage of RAGE by sRAGE may be a new target for therapeutic intervention in diabetic disorders. Potential protective effects of sRAGE have been shown in various diabetes and inflammatory models [94]. Interestingly, sRAGE could also attenuate impaired wound healing in diabetic mice. Other promising effects in various systems have been shown in vitro and in vivo with neutralizing anti-RAGE antibodies [31]. Possible approaches include gene knock-down of RAGE by siRNA or anti-sense and antagonism of RAGE with putative small molecular inhibitors against RAGE-induced signaling [95].

6.3. AGEs breakers

Chemical substances and enzymes that are able to recognize and break the Maillard reaction crosslinks have been identified. Such chemical AGEs breakers are dimethyl-3-phenayl-thiazolium chloride (ALT-711) [64], N-phenacylthiazolium and N-phenacyl-4,5-dimethylthia-zolium. Promising results against diabetic cardiovascular complications have been reported, though their actual ability to cleave existing protein crosslinks in tissues has been questioned [96]. However, treatment with ALT-711 for 2 weeks had no effects on motor nerve conduction deficit, C-fiber-mediated nociceptive dysfunction, or impaired pressure-induced vasodilation in diabetic mice [97].

Interference with intrinsic AGE-detoxifying enzymes like fructosyl-amine oxidases (FAOXs), fructosamine-3-kinase (FN3K), and the enzymatic system of glyoxalase I is another interesting strategy to remove AGEs, because enzymes could recognize specific substrates [60]. It is reported that overexpression of glyoxalase I significantly inhibits hyperglycemia-induced intracellular formation of AGEs in bovine aortic endothelial cells and in mouse mesangial cells by reduction of intracellular oxidative stress and apoptosis [98]. The pharmacological induction of such enzymes could represent a novel future strategy against AGEs.

Other anti-AGE agents, including the thiazolidine derivative named OPB-9195, have been investigated [99]. OPB-9195 has been shown to prevent the progression of diabetic nephropathy in rats. It has also been demonstrated to improve motor nerve conduction slowing without affecting body weight and blood glucose levels. The improvement was associated with reduced serum AGEs levels and peripheral nerve expression of AGEs and immunoreactive 8-hydroxy-2-deoxyguanosine, which is a marker for oxidative stress-related DNA damage as well as an increase in peripheral nerve (Na+, K+)-ATPase activity [100].

Diabetic rats were found to have increased mesenteric vascular AGEs accumulation and mesenteric vascular hypertrophy, both of which were prevented by treatment with N-phenacylthiazolium bromide (PTB) [101]. A more recent study has demonstrated that although AGE-breakers such as PTB and N-phenacyl-4,5-dimethylthiazolium cleave model crosslinks in vitro, they do not significantly cleave AGE crosslinks formed in vivo in skin collagen of diabetic rats [59].

Benfotiamine, a lipophilic analogue of thiamine, is a transketolase activator that inhibits three of the four major biochemical pathways implicated in the pathogenesis of hyperglycemia-induced vascular damage: the hexosamine pathway, PKC activation, and AGEs formation [102]. In diabetic rats, nearly normalized nerve conduction velocity and inhibition of neural imidazole-type AGEs and CML formation after 6 months of benfotiamine treatment were observed [103]. In both nondiabetic and diabetic rats, benfotiamine also reduced inflammatory and neuropathic nociception [104].

6.4. Nutrient substance

An increasing list of natural antioxidants and chelating agents such as ascorbic acid, α-tocopherol, niacinamide, pyridoxal, sodium selenite, selenium yeast, trolox, rivoflarin, zinc, and manganese has been shown to inhibit glycation of albumin in vitro [105]. Many spices and herbs could inhibit glycation of albumin in vitro as well, such as ginger, cinnamon, cloves, rosemary, and tarragon [106]. Besides, green tea, vitamins C and E, and a combination of N-acetylcystein with taurine and oxerutin could inhibit skin collagen glycation in mice [107]. In healthy human subjects, supplementation of vitamin C significantly decreased serum protein glycation [108].

Alpha-lipoic acid could reverse tail tendon collagen glycation in fructose-fed rats, an effect which was attributed to its endogenous antioxidant action, its ability to recycle ascorbic acid and GSH, as well as to its positive influence on glucose uptake and glycemia [109]. Blueberry extract, an AGE-inhibitor and C-xyloside, was tested for 12 weeks in female diabetic subjects. This treatment resulted in significant improvement of skin firmness, wrinkles, and hydration. However, it failed to show a significant decrease in the cutaneous content of AGEs [110].

6.5. Molecular chaperones

Molecular chaperones like carnosine have shown promise in improving skin appearance in part by reducing the amounts of skin AGEs [111]. Yet, more studies are needed to address the accumulation of AGEs in diabetic wound.

In conclusion, AGEs are a heterogeneous group of molecules that form from the non-enzymatic addition of sugar moieties onto arginine and lysine residues of proteins, free amino groups on lipids, or guanine nucleic acids. The AGE-RAGE interactions play an important role in the diabetic wound healing process. The measurement of AGEs on the skin, namely, skin autofluorescence might have some value as a screening tool for diabetic foot ulcer, but until now, there is no strong evidence for other clinical use in diabetic wound. In addition, substances which can prevent or inhibit the formation of AGEs, as well as agents that can break AGEs or antagonize AGE/RAGE signaling have been identified.

Author details

Junna Ye[1*], Ting Xie[2], Yiwen Niu[1], Liang Qiao[1], Ming Tian[1], Chun Qing[1] and Shuliang Lu[1*]

*Address all correspondence to: 13901738685@139.com

1 Institute of Burns, Ruijin Hospital, Shanghai Jiao Tong University, Shanghai, China

2 Department of Wound Healing, Shanghai Ninth Hospital, Shanghai Jiao Tong University, Shanghai, China

References

[1] Nolan CJ, Damm P, Prentki M. Type 2 diabetes across generations: from pathophysiology to prevention and management. Lancet. 2011;378:169e81.

[2] Jeffcoate WJ, Harding KG. Diabetic foot ulcers. Lancet. 2003;361:1545–51.

[3] Jiang Y, Huang S, Fu X, et al. Epidemiology of chronic cutaneous wounds in China. Wound Repair Regen. 2011;19(2):181–8.

[4] Yao H, Ting X, Minjie W, et al. The investigation of demographic characteristics and the health-related quality of life in patients with diabetic foot ulcers at first presentation. Int J Low Extrem Wounds. 2012;11(3):187–93.

[5] Brownlee M. The pathobiology of diabetic complications: a unifying mechanism. Diabetes. 2005;54:1615e25.

[6] Armstrong DG, Lavery LA, Wu S, et al. Evaluation of removable and irremovable cast walkers in the healing of diabetic foot wounds: a randomized controlled trial. Diabetes Care. 2005;28(3):551–4.

[7] Boulton AJ, Kirsner RS, Vileikyte L. Clinical practice. Neuropathic diabetic foot ulcers. N Engl J Med. 2004;351:48–7.

[8] Kislinger T, Fu C, Huber B, et al. N(epsilon)-(carboxymethyl)lysine adducts of proteins are ligands for receptor for advanced glycation end products that activate cell signaling pathways and modulate gene expression. J Biol Chem. 1999;274(44):31740–9.

[9] Haslbeck KM, Schleicher E, Bierhaus A, et al. The AGE/RAGE/NF-(kappa)B pathway may contribute to the pathogenesis of polyneuropathy in impaired glucose tolerance (IGT). Exp Clin Endocrinol Diabetes. 2005;113(5):288–91.

[10] Monnier VM, Stevens VJ, Cerami A. Maillard reactions involving proteins and carbohydrates in vivo: relevance to diabetes mellitus and aging. Prog Food Nutr Sci. 1981;5:315–27.

[11] Peppa M, Stavroulakis P, Raptis SA. Advanced glycoxidation products and impaired diabetic wound healing. Wound Repair Regen. 2009;17:461–72.

[12] Singh R, Barden A, Mori T, et al. Advanced glycation endproducts: a review. Diabetologia. 2001;44:129–146.

[13] Ulrich P, Cerami A. Protein glycation, diabetes, and aging. Recent Prog Horm Res. 2001;56:1–21.

[14] Ahmed N. Advanced glycation endproducts – role in pathology of diabetic complications. Diab Res Clin Pract. 2005;67:3–21.

[15] Huijberts MS, Schaper NC, Schalkwijk CG. Advanced glycation end products and diabetic foot disease. Diab Metab Res Rev. 2008;24 Suppl. 1:S19–24.

[16] Giardino I, Edelstein D, Brownlee M. BCL-2 expression or antioxidants prevent hyperglycemia-induced formation of intracellular advanced glycation endproducts in bovine endothelial cells. J Clin Invest. 1996;97:1422–1428.

[17] Ruderman NB, Williamson JR, Brownlee M. Glucose and diabetic vascular disease. FASEB J. 1992;6:2905–2914.

[18] Westwood ME, Thornalley PJ. Molecular characteristics of methylglyoxal-modified bovine and human serum albumins. Comparison with glucose-derived advanced glycation endproduct-modified serum albumins. J Protein Chem. 1995;14:359–372.

[19] Phillips SA, Thornalley PJ. Formation of methylglyoxal and Dlactate in human red blood cells in vitro. Biochem Soc Trans. 1993;21:163S.

[20] Shinohara M, Thornalley PJ, Giardino I, et al. Overexpression of glyoxalase-I in bovine endothelial cells inhibits intracellular advanced glycation endproduct formation and prevents hyperglycemia-induced increases in macromolecular endocytosis. J Clin Invest. 1998;101:1142–47.

[21] Peppa M, He C, Hattori M, et al. Fetal or neonatal low-glycotoxin environment prevents autoimmune diabetes in NOD mice. Diabetes. 2003;52(6):1441–8.

[22] Lin RY, Choudhury RP, Cai W, et al. Dietary glycotoxins promote diabetic atherosclerosis in apolipoprotein E-deficient mice. Atherosclerosis. 2003;168(2):213–20.

[23] American Diabetes Association. Peripheral arterial disease in people with diabetes. Diabetes Care. 2003;26:3333–41.

[24] Koschinsky T, He CJ, Mitsuhashi T, et al. Orally absorbed reactive glycation products (glycotoxins): an environmental risk factor in diabetic nephropathy. Proc Natl Acad Sci U S A. 1997;94:6474–6479.

[25] Kankova K. Diabetic threesome (hyperglycaemia, renal function and nutrition) and advanced glycation end products: evidence for the multiple-hit agent? Proc Nutr Soc. 2008;67:60e74.

[26] Peppa M, Uribarri J, Vlassara H. Aging and glycoxidant stress. Hormones 2008;7:123–32.

[27] Cai W, He JC, Zhu L, et al. AGE-receptor-1 counteracts cellular oxidant stress induced by AGEs via negative regulation of p66shc-dependent FKHRL1 phosphorylation. Am J Physiol Cell Physiol. 2008;294:C145–52.

[28] Vlassara H. The AGE-receptor in the pathogenesis of diabetic complications. Diabetes Metab Res Rev. 2001;17:436–43.

[29] Yamagishi S, Matsui T. Soluble form of a receptor for advanced glycation end products (sRAGE) as a biomarker. Front Biosci (Elite Ed). 2010;2:1184–95.

[30] Ramasamy R, Yan SF, Schmidt AM. RAGE: therapeutic target and biomarker of the inflammatory response-the evidence mounts. J Leukoc Biol. 2009;86:505–12.

[31] Bierhaus A, Humpert PM, Morcos M, et al. Understanding RAGE, the receptor for advanced glycation end products. J Mol Med. 2005;83:876–86.

[32] Ishihara K, Tsutsumi K, Kawane S, et al. The receptor for advanced glycation end-products (RAGE) directly binds to ERK by a D-domain-like docking site. FEBS Lett. 2003;550(1–3):107–13.

[33] Loughlin DT, Artlett CM. Precursor of advanced glycation end products mediates ER-stress-induced caspase-3 activation of human dermal fibroblasts through NAD(P)H oxidase 4. PLoS One. 2010;5:e11093.

[34] Lohwasser C, Neureiter D, Weigle B, et al. The receptor for advanced glycation end products is highly expressed in the skin and upregulated by advanced glycation end products and tumor necrosis factor-alpha. J Invest Dermatol. 2006;126(2):291–9.

[35] Fujimoto E, Kobayashi T, Fujimoto N, et al. AGE-modified collagens I and III induce keratinocyte terminal differentiation through AGE receptor CD36: epidermal-dermal interaction in acquired perforating dermatosis. J Invest Dermatol. 2010;130:405–14.

[36] Zhu P, Ren M, Yang C, et al. Involvement of RAGE, MAPK and NF-kB pathways in AGEs-induced MMP-9 activation in HaCaT keratinocytes. Exp Dermatol. 2012;21:123–9.

[37] Berg TJ, Snorgaard O, Faber J, et al. Serum levels of advanced glycation end products are associated with left ventricular diastolic function in patients with type 1 diabetes. Diab. Care. 1999;22(7):1186–90.

[38] Stern DM, Yan SD, Yan SF, et al. Receptor for advanced glycation endproducts (RAGE) and the complications of diabetes. Ageing Res Rev. 2002;1:1–15.

[39] Fisher GJ, Kang S, Varani J, et al. Mechanisms of photoaging and chronological skin aging. Arch Dermatol. 2002;138:1462–70.

[40] Tian M, Qing C, Niu Y, et al. The relationship between inflammation and impaired wound healing in a diabetic rat burn model. J Burn Care Res. 2016;37(2):e115–24.

[41] Bernhard D, Moser C, Backovic A, et al. Cigarette smoke – an aging accelerator? Exp Gerontol. 2007;42(3):160–5. Epub 2006 Nov 3.

[42] Niu YW, Miao MY, Dong W, et al. Effects of advanced glycation end products and its receptor on oxidative stress in diabetic wounds. Zhonghua Shao Shang Za Zhi. 2012;28(1):32–5.

[43] Zhu P, Yang C, Chen LH, et al. Impairment of human keratinocyte mobility and proliferation by advanced glycation end productsmodified BSA. Arch Dermatol Res. 2011;303:339–50.

[44] Giardino I, Edelstein D, Brownlee M. Nonenzymatic glycosylation in vitro and in bovine endothelial cells alters basic fibroblast growth factor activity. A model for intracellular glycosylation in diabetes. J Clin Invest. 1994;94:110–7.

[45] Wondrak GT. Let the sun shine in: mechanisms and potential for therapeutics in skin photodamage. Curr Opin Investig Drugs. 2007;8:390–400.

[46] Miao M, Niu Y, Xie T, et al. Diabetes-impaired wound healing and altered macrophage activation: a possible pathophysiologic correlation. Wound Repair Regen. 2012;20(2): 203–13.

[47] Tseng JY, Ghazaryan AA, Lo W, et al. Multiphoton spectral microscopy for imaging and quantification of tissue glycation. Biomed Opt Express. 2010;2:218–30.

[48] Lee C, Yim MB, Chock PB, et al. Oxidation-reduction properties of methylglyoxal-modified protein in relation to free radical generation. J Biol Chem. 1998;273:25272–8.

[49] Kazuhiro Y, Tomohide O, Tomonobu Y, et al. Inhibitory effect of peptide free forms of advanced glycation end products on the proliferation and extracellular matrix production of cultured cells. J Health Sci. 2001;47:296–301.

[50] Alikhani Z, Alikhani M, Boyd CM, et al. Advanced glycation end products enhance expression of pro-apoptotic genes and stimulate fibroblast apoptosis through cytoplasmic and mitochondrial pathways. J Biol Chem. 2005;280:12087–95.

[51] Berlanga J, Cibrian D, Guillén I, et al. Methylglyoxal administration induces diabetes like microvascular changes and pertubs the healing process of cutaneous wounds. Clin Sci (Lond). 2005;109:83–95.

[52] Duraisamy Y, Slevin M, Smith N, et al. Effect of glycation on basic fibroblast growth factor induced angiogenesis and activation of associated signal transduction pathways in vascular endothelial cells: possible relevance to wound healing in diabetes. Angiogenesis. 2001;4:277–88.

[53] Teixeira AS, Andrade SP. Glucose-induced inhibition of angiogenesis in the rat sponge granuloma is prevented by aminoguanidine. Life Sci. 1999;64:655–62.

[54] Gkogkolou P, Böhm M. Advanced glycation end products: key players in skin aging? Dermatoendocrinology 2012;4(3):259–70.

[55] Niu Y, Xie T, Ge K, et al. Effects of extracellular matrix glycosylation on proliferation and apoptosis of human dermal fibroblasts via the receptor for advanced glycosylated end products. Am J Dermatopathol. 2008;30(4):344–51.

[56] Bakris GL, Bank AJ, Kass DA, et al. Advanced glycation end-product cross-link breakers. A novel approach to cardiovascular pathologies related to the aging process. Am J Hypertens. 2004;17:23S–30S.

[57] Yang S, Litchfield JE, Baynes JW. AGE-breakers cleave model compounds, but do not break Maillard crosslinks in skin and tail collagen from diabetic rats. Arch Biochem Biophys. 2003;412:42–6.

[58] Monnier VM, Wu X. Enzymatic deglycation with amadoriase enzymes from *Aspergillus* sp. as a potential strategy against the complications of diabetes and aging. Biochem Soc Trans. 2003;31:1349–53.

[59] Voziyan PA, Hudson BG. Pyridoxamine: the many virtues of a Maillard reaction inhibitor. Ann N Y Acad Sci. 2005;1043:807–16.

[60] Vasan S, Foiles P, Founds H. Therapeutic potential of breakers of advanced glycation end product-protein crosslinks. Arch Biochem Biophys. 2003;419:89–96.

[61] Smit AJ, Gerrits EG. Skin autofluorescence as a measure of advanced glycation endproduct deposition: a novel risk marker in chronic kidney disease. Curr Opin Nephrol Hypertens. 2010;19:527–33.

[62] Genuth S, Sun W, Cleary P, et al. Glycation and carboxymethyllysine levels in skin collagen predict the risk of future 10-year progression of diabetic retinopathy and nephropathy in the diabetes control and complications trial and epidemiology of diabetes interventions and complications participants with type 1 diabetes. Diabetes. 2005;54:3103–11.

[63] Niu Y, Cao X, Song F, et al. Reduced dermis thickness and AGE accumulation in diabetic abdominal skin. Int J Low Extrem Wounds. 2012;11(3):224–30.

[64] Foell D, Wittkowski H, Roth J. Mechanisms of disease: a 'DAMP' view of inflammatory arthritis. Nat Clin Pract Rheumatol. 2007;3(7):382–90.

[65] Holman RR, Paul SK, Bethel MA, et al. 10-year follow-up of intensive glucose control in type 2 diabetes. N Engl J Med. 2008;359(15):1577–89.

[66] Meerwaldt R, Graaff R, Oomen PH, et al. Simple non-invasive assessment of advanced glycation endproduct accumulation. Diabetologia. 2004;47:1324–30.

[67] Mácsai E, Takáts Z, Derzbach L, et al. Verification of skin autofluorescence values by mass spectrometry in adolescents with type 1 diabetes: brief report. Diabetes Technol Ther. 2013;15(3):269–72.

[68] Meerwaldt R, Hartog JW, Graaff R, et al. Skin autofluorescence, a measure of cumulative metabolic stress and advanced glycation end products, predicts mortality in hemodialysis patients. J Am Soc Nephrol. 2005;16(12):3687e93.

[69] Samborski P, Naskręt D, Araszkiewicz A, et al. Assessment of skin autofluorescence as a marker of advanced glycation end product accumulation in type 1 diabetes. Pol Arch Med Wewn. 2011;121(3):67–72.

[70] Tanaka K, Tani Y, Asai J, et al. Skin autofluorescence is associated with severity of vascular complications in Japanese patients with type 2 diabetes. Diabet Med. 2012;29:492–500.

[71] Noordzij MJ, Mulder DJ, Oomen PH, et al. Skin autofluorescence and risk of micro- and macrovascular complications in patients with type 2 diabetes mellitus – a multi-centre study. Diabet Med. 2012;29:1556–1561.

[72] Hu H, Han CM, Hu XL, et al. Elevated skin autofluorescence is strongly associated with foot ulcers in patients with diabetes: a cross-sectional, observational study of Chinese subjects. J Zhejiang Univ Sci B. 2012;13(5):372–7.

[73] Koetsier M, Lutgers HL, de Jonge C, et al. Reference values of skin autofluorescence. Diabetes Technol Ther. 2010;12(5):399–403.

[74] Yue X, Hu H, Koetsier M, et al. Reference values for the Chinese population of skin autofluorescence as a marker of advanced glycation end products accumulated in tissue. Diabet Med. 2011;28(7):818–23.

[75] Simon Klenovics K, Kollárová R, Hodosy J, et al. Reference values of skin autofluorescence as an estimation of tissue accumulation of advanced glycation end products in a general Slovak population. Diabet Med. 2014;31(5):581–5.

[76] Meerwaldt R, Lutgers HL, Links TP, et al. Skin autofluorescence is a strong predictor of cardiac mortality in diabetes. Diabetes Care. 2007;30:107–12.

[77] Gerrits EG, Lutgers HL, Kleefstra N, et al. Skin autofluorescence: a tool to identify type 2 diabetic patients at risk for developing microvascular complications. Diabetes Care. 2008;31:517–521.

[78] Pietzsch J, Hoppmann S. Human S100A12: a novel key player in inflammation? Amino Acids. 2009;36(3):381–9.

[79] Liu C, Xu L, Gao H, et al. The association between skin autofluorescence and vascular complications in Chinese patients with diabetic foot ulcer: an observational study done in Shanghai. Int J Low Extrem Wounds. 2015;14(1):28–36.

[80] Araszkiewicz A, Naskret D, Niedzwiecki P, et al. Increased accumulation of skin advanced glycation end products is associated with microvascular complications in type 1 diabetes. Diab Technol Ther. 2011;13(8):837–42.

[81] de Vos LC, Mulder DJ, Smit AJ, et al. Skin autofluorescence is associated with 5-year mortality and cardiovascular events in patients with peripheral artery disease. Arterioscler Thromb Vasc Biol. 2014;34(4):933–8.

[82] Meerwaldt R, Links TP, Graaff R, et al. Increased accumulation of skin advanced glycation end-products precedes and correlates with clinical manifestation of diabetic neuropathy. Diabetologia. 2005;48(8):1637–44. Epub 2005 Jul 14.

[83] Lapolla A, Piarulli F, Sartore G, et al. Advanced glycation end products and antioxidant status in type 2 diabetic patients with and without peripheral artery disease. Diab Care. 2007;30(3):670–6.

[84] Vouillarmet J, Maucort-Boulch D, Michon P, et al. Advanced glycation end products assessed by skin autofluorescence: a new marker of diabetic foot ulceration. Diab Technol Ther. 2013;15(7):601–5.

[85] Thornalley PJ. Use of aminoguanidine (Pimagedine) to prevent the formation of advanced glycation endproducts. Arch Biochem Biophys. 2003;419:31–40.

[86] Edelstein D, Brownlee M. Mechanistic studies of advanced glycosylation end product inhibition by aminoguanidine. Diabetes. 1992;41:26–9.

[87] Yagihashi S, Kamijo M, Baba M, et al. Effect of aminoguanidine on functional and structural abnormalities in peripheral nerve of STZ-induced diabetic rats. Diabetes. 1992;41(1):47–52.

[88] Freedman BI, Wuerth JP, Cartwright K, et al. Design and baseline characteristics for the aminoguanidine clinical trial in overt type 2 diabetic nephropathy (ACTION II). Control Clin Trials. 1999;20(5):493–510.

[89] Bolton WK, Cattran DC, Williams ME, et al. Randomized trial of an inhibitor of formation of advanced glycation end products in diabetic nephropathy. Am J Nephrol. 2004;24:32–40.

[90] Beisswenger P, Ruggiero-Lopez D. Metformin inhibition of glycation processes. Diab Metab. 2003;29(4 Pt 2):6S95–103.

[91] Haus JM, Carrithers JA, Trappe SW, et al. Collagen, cross-linking, and advanced glycation end products in aging human skeletal muscle. J Appl Physiol (1985). 2007;103(6):2068–76. Epub 2007 Sep 27.

[92] Degenhardt TP, Alderson NL, Arrington DD, et al. Pyridoxamine inhibits early renal disease and dyslipidemia in the streptozotocin-diabetic rat. Kidney Int. 2002;61(3):939–50.

[93] Cai W, He JC, Zhu L, et al. Oral glycotoxins determine the effects of calorie restriction on oxidant stress, age-related diseases, and lifespan. Am J Pathol. 2008;173:327–36.

[94] Yan SF, Ramasamy R, Schmidt AM. Soluble RAGE: therapy and biomarker in unraveling the RAGE axis in chronic disease and aging. Biochem Pharmacol. 2010;79:1379–86.

[95] Chen Y, Akirav EM, Chen W, et al. RAGE ligation affects T cell activation and controls T cell differentiation. J Immunol. 2008;181:4272–8.

[96] Monnier VM, Sell DR. Prevention and repair of protein damage by the Maillard reaction in vivo. Rejuvenation Res. 2006;9:264–73.

[97] Demiot C, Tartas M, Fromy B, et al. Aldose reductase pathway inhibition improved vascular and C-fiber functions, allowing for pressure-induced vasodilation restoration during severe diabetic neuropathy. Diabetes. 2006;55:1478–83.

[98] Kim KM, Kim YS, Jung DH, et al. Increased glyoxalase I levels inhibit accumulation of oxidative stress and an advanced glycation end product in mouse mesangial cells cultured in high glucose. Exp Cell Res. 2012;318:152–9.

[99] Nakamura S, Makita Z, Ishikawa S, et al. Progression of nephropathy in spontaneous diabetic rats is prevented by OPB-9195, a novel inhibitor of advanced glycation. Diabetes. 1997;46:895–9.

[100] Wada R, Nishizawa Y, Yagihashi N, et al. Effects of OPB-9195, anti-glycation agent, on experimental diabetic neuropathy. Eur J Clin Invest. 2001;31:513–20.

[101] Vasan S, Zhang X, Kapurniotu A, et al. An agent cleaving glucose-derived protein crosslinks in vitro and in vivo. Nature. 1996;382:275–8.

[102] Hammes HP, Du X, Edelstein D, et al. Benfotiamine blocks three major pathways of hyperglycemic damage and prevents experimental diabetic retinopathy. Nat Med. 2003;9:294–9.

[103] Stracke H, Hammes HP, Werkmann D, et al. Efficacy of benfotiamine versus thiamine on function and glycation products of peripheral nerves in diabetic rats. Exp Clin Endocrinol Diabetes. 2001;109:330–6.

[104] Sanchez-Ramirez GM, Caram-Salas NL, Rocha-Gonzalez HI, et al. Benfotiamine relieves inflammatory and neuropathic pain in rats. Eur J Pharmacol. 2006;530:48–53.

[105] Tarwadi KV, Agte VV. Effect of micronutrients on methylglyoxal-mediated in vitro glycation of albumin. Biol Trace Elem Res. 2011;143:717–25.

[106] Dearlove RP, Greenspan P, Hartle DK, et al. Inhibition of protein glycation by extracts of culinary herbs and spices. J Med Food. 2008;11:275–81.

[107] Odetti P, Pesce C, Traverso N, et al. Comparative trial of N-acetylcysteine, taurine, and oxerutin on skin and kidney damage in long-term experimental diabetes. Diabetes. 2003;52:499–505.

[108] Vinson JA, Howard HB. Inhibition of protein glycation and advanced glycation end products by ascorbic acid and other vitamins and nutrients. J Nutr Biochem. 1996;7:659–63.

[109] Thirunavukkarasu V, Nandhini AT, Anuradha CV. Lipoic acid prevents collagen abnormalities in tail tendon of high-fructose-fed rats. Diab Obes Metab. 2005;7:294–7.

[110] Draelos ZD, Yatskayer M, Raab S, et al. An evaluation of the effect of a topical product containing C-xyloside and blueberry extract on the appearance of type II diabetic skin. J Cosmet Dermatol. 2009;8:147–51.

[111] Babizhayev MA, Nikolayev GM, Nikolayeva JG, et al. Biologic activities of molecular chaperones and pharmacologic chaperone imidazole-containing dipeptide-based compounds: natural skin care help and the ultimate challenge: implication for adaptive responses in the skin. Am J Ther. 2012;19(2):e69–89.

2

The Need for Increased Attention to Low-Level Laser Therapy as Treatment for Wounds and Ulcers

Mohammad Bayat

Abstract

Light amplification by stimulated emission of radiation (lasers) is a device that typically generates electromagnetic radiation of uniform wavelength, phase, and polarization. The term low-level laser therapy (LLLT) is broadly defined as the therapeutic benefit of lasers. This review aims to discuss the positive effects of LLLT on skin wounds, diabetic foot ulcers, and burn healing. Different LLLT protocols have been widely used as treatment for these conditions to accelerate tissue regenerative processes. We have classified eligible papers in the fields of skin wounds, ulcers, and burns into in vivo and in vitro experimental studies and clinical trials that evaluated the use of LLLT as treatments that promote healing. An electronic search of scientific peer reviewed papers was conducted in the PubMed database. Our search has shown that the use of LLLT in biology and medicine is growing rapidly, and advancements in LLLT research dramatically improved the clinicians' ability to safely and effectively treat wounds and ulcers. There is increased clinical use of laser for wound and ulcer treatment. Several recent studies have confirmed the potential beneficial effects of LLLT for wound healing.

Keywords: low-level laser therapy, skin wound, diabetic foot ulcer, burn

1. Introduction

The term low-level laser therapy (LLLT) is broadly defined as the therapeutic benefit of lasers. After Professor Mester from Hungary first revealed the therapeutic importance of lasers, different wavelengths of continuous wave (CW) LLLT have been shown to promote healing in skin from healthy humans and animals, as well as a number of experimental pathological cases. Different LLLT protocols have been widely used in numerous medical situations with the intent to accelerate the regenerative processes of tissues.

In this review, the author characterized eligible papers into in vivo and in vitro experimental studies and clinical trials that evaluated the use of LLLT on skin wounds for promotion of healing. The author conducted an electronic search of scientific peer reviewed papers in the PubMed database of English language studies published from 2004 to 2016 with the keyword "low-level laser therapy." As inclusion criteria, the author chose articles with availability of access to the full text. This review intended to show the positive effects of LLLT on healing of skin wounds, diabetic foot ulcers, and burns. Initially, the author introduced wounds, ulcers, and burns and showed their importance. Next, a number of important related papers in the field were reported.

2. Definition

Devices that provide light amplification by stimulated emission of radiation (LASERS) typically generate electromagnetic radiation of a uniform wavelength, phase, and polarization. In 1960, Theodore Maiman has originally described a ruby laser. A laser is described as a source of light or radiation energy [1].

3. History

The term "LLLT" is broadly applied to the therapeutic effects of lasers; other terms, such as low power laser therapy, laser biomodulation, laser bioactivation, laser biostimulation, laser irradiation, and laser photostimulation, may be substituted for LLLT. In this review, the author have chosen the term LLLT photostimulation because of the observed stimulatory effects of the laser beam and photochemical nature of its interaction with biological systems. LLLT is a special type of laser that influences biologic systems through nonthermal means [2]. The use of LLLT as a therapeutic modality has originated from Eastern Europe approximately 50 years ago [2]. In 1967, Professor Mester, an employee of Semmelweis University in Budapest, Hungary, observed that applying laser light to the shaven backs of mice could cause more rapid regrowth of hair compared to unshaven mice [3]. He reported that the helium-neon (He-Ne) laser had the capability to promote wound healing in mice [4]. Professor Mester applied these findings to humans when he used lasers to treat patients with nonhealing skin ulcers [5, 6]. The clinical applications of LLLT have become the leading edge of clinical research in several countries, such as the former USSR, Japan, Canada, Australia, United Kingdom, China, and several Scandinavian countries. The history, origin, and development of various lasers are well authorized [2]. The clinical application of laser photobiostimulation is growing rapidly. Several review articles that explain the clinical applications of LLLT have been published [2]. LLLT is currently considered not only as a therapeutic procedure primarily used for relief of inflammation, edema, and chronic joint disorders; escalate healing of the wounds, deeper tissues, and nerves; but also as a treatment for neurological disorders and pain [7].

4. Objective

LLLT exposes tissues and cells to low levels of red and near infrared (NIR) and IR light. This treatment is introduced to as "low level" because of usage of light at lower energy densities in comparison to other types of laser therapy such as cutting, ablation, and thermal coagulation of tissue. LLLT is also defined as "cold laser" therapy because of the lower power densities used compared to those needed to produce tissue heating [7]. LLLT is currently used to treat a wide variety of diseases in which a large number of laser parameters such as the energy density, wavelength, pulse structure, power density, and timing of the applied light must be chosen for each treatment. A less than optimal choice of parameters can lead to not only reduced effectiveness of the treatment but also result in negative therapeutic outcomes. Thus, numerous published results on LLLT include negative findings simply because of an inappropriate choice of light source and dosage. This choice is particularly important because of the optimal dose of light needed for any particular application; doses higher or lower than this optimal value may have no therapeutic effect. LLLT is defined by a biphasic dose response: lower doses of light are often more advantageous than high doses [7]. This review aims to discuss the positive effects of LLLT on healing diabetic wounds and burns. Low-level laser energy density (J/cm^2) calculation: power (W) × duration of laser radiation (s)/laser beam surface area (cm^2).

5. Wound healing

Wound healing, which is a normal physiological process, takes places in four particular phases: hemostasis, inflammation, proliferation, and remodeling. For a successful healing process, all four phases must follow in the appropriate sequence and time. Numerous factors can put adverse effects on different phases of this process, resulting in an inappropriate wound healing process. The most important factors that influence healing of the cutaneous wound and the potential cellular and/or molecular mechanisms involved consist of local and systemic factors. Local factors include oxygenation, infections, foreign bodies, and venous sufficiency, whereas systemic factors comprise age and gender, sex hormones, stress, diseases, such as diabetes mellitus (DM), keloids, fibrosis, hereditary healing disorders, jaundice, uremia, obesity, medications (glucocorticoid steroids, nonsteroidal anti-inflammatory drugs), chemotherapy, alcoholism, and smoking, as well as immunocompromised conditions (cancer, radiation therapy, AIDS, and nutrition). A better understanding of the effects of these factors on the wound healing process may lead to therapeutics that accelerate wound healing and resolve impaired wounds. However, the influences of these factors are not mutually exclusive. One or multiple factors may play a role in any of the individual phases by contributing to the overall outcome of the healing process [8].

6. Diabetic wound healing in animals and patients (diabetic foot ulcers (DFU))

DM is the general name for a heterogeneous group of metabolic disorder characterized by high blood glucose levels that result from defects in insulin secretion and/or action [9]. The percentage of the population diagnosed with DM continues to increase. A study projects that as many as one in three US adults may have DM by the year 2050 if current trends continue. The expense of DM in the United States, at more than $174 billion per year in 2007, is anticipated to become an increasingly large financial burden in the future [10].

DFUs are a common problem among individuals with DM. These ulcers are among the most serious complications of DM that may result in amputation and mortality [11]. The prevalence of DFU in people with DM vary from 4% to 10% with a lifetime incidence as high as 25% [12]. Treatment of diabetic foot is extremely hard because these wounds are delineated by delayed healing; often result in chronic wound [13]. It has been reported that the 5-year mortality leading to lower extremity amputations may be as high as 68% [14]. Therefore, successful treatment of diabetic ulcers is a field of huge importance [15].

Many elements considered to be sources for the lack of healing in diabetic wounds involve peripheral neuropathy, the presence of an impaired immune system, peripheral microvascular disease, glycation of hemoglobin that leads to inadequate oxygen delivery to tissues, alterations in the red blood cell membrane [13] due to glycation, interchange in the proportion of type III to type I collagen in the skin [16], impaired biomechanical properties of the diabetic skin [17], impaired proliferation of skin fibroblasts [18], and impaired L-lactate production [19]. The diabetic wound is a disorder of the wound healing process, especially in the inflammatory and proliferative phases [13], pathologic angiogenesis [20], and a significant diminishing of the tensile strength of wound repair, detected in studies on diabetic animal models [21].

According to a review of the literature, numerous in vitro and in vivo studies, as well as clinical trials have reported positive effects of LLLT on the wound healing process both in animals and human patients.

7. Literature review

Dahmardehei et al. have stated that significant numbers of patients in burn centers are diabetics. The healing process in these patients is more difficult due to complications attributed to diabetes. Despite the fact that the gold standard treatment for a grade 3 burn ulcer patient is split-thickness skin grafting (STSG), however in diabetic patients, the rate of graft rejection and organ amputation is high due to impaired tissue perfusion. Previous studies show that LLLT accelerates fibroblast proliferation, increases collagen synthesis and tissue perfusion, and accelerates wound healing. Dahmardehei et al. have recommended a new therapeutic method for improving the healing process with better prognosis for these patients. Their study enrolled type II diabetes patients with 13, grade 3 burn ulcers considered candidates for amputation.

In these patients, the grade 3 burn ulcers were treated by a 650 nm red laser light at 2 J/cm² for the bed of the ulcer and an 810 nm infrared laser light at 6 J/cm² for the margins, along with intravenous LLLT with a 660 nm red light, before and after STSG. The results showed complete healing for all patients considered candidates for amputation [22]. Góralczyk et al. reported that that chronic hyperglycemia was the source of endothelial activation. On the other hand, the inflammatory process in DM has been associated with the secretion of inflammatory cytokines by endothelial cells, such as tumor necrosis factor-alpha (TNF-α) and interleukin 6 (IL-6). Góralczyk et al. evaluated the effects of 635 and 830 nm wavelength LLL irradiation on the secretion of inflammatory factors (TNF-α and IL-6) in an endothelial cell culture-human umbilical vein endothelial cell (HUVEC) line under hyperglycemic conditions. Adverse effects of hyperglycemia on vascular endothelial cells might be recovered by the action of LLLT, especially at a wavelength of 830 nm. LLLT decreased TNF-α concentration in the supernatant and improved cell proliferation [23]. Lau et al. carried out a study to investigate the biophotonic effect of irradiance on collagen production in a rat model of a diabetic wound. The skin's tensile strength was a parameter to characterize the wound. The rat models received intravenous injections of streptozotocin (STZ) to induce diabetes. Skin-breaking strength was measured. The experimental animals were treated with an 808 nm diode laser at two power densities of 0.1 and 0.5 W/cm². The tensile strength was optimized after treatment with a high-power diode laser. The photostimulation effect was shown by the accelerated healing process and enhanced tensile strength of the wound. Lau et al. concluded that LLLT facilitated collagen production in diabetic wound healing [24]. Sharifian et al. assessed the influence of pulsed wave (PW) LLLT on healing of the diabetic wound in diabetic (STZ-D) rats. They divided rats into two groups: nondiabetic and diabetic. They induced type I DM in the diabetic rat group through injection of STZ. The rats were submitted to two full-thickness skin incisions on the dorsal region of each one. One month after the injection of STZ, wounds of the nondiabetic and diabetic rats were subjected to a pulsed, infrared 890 nm wavelength laser with an 80 Hz frequency and 0.2 J/cm² energy density for each wound point. PW LLLT significantly accelerated the numbers of macrophages, fibroblasts, and blood vessel sections in comparison with the corresponding control groups. Semiquantitative analysis of basic fibroblast growth factor (bFGF) gene expression indicated significant increase in gene expression in both nondiabetic and diabetic rats following LLLT [25]. Houreld reported that due to advancements in laser technology, irradiation of diabetic wounds with low-intensity laser irradiation (LILI) or phototherapy has vastly accelerated wound healing. At the correct laser parameters, LILI increased migration, viability, and proliferation of diabetic cells in vitro. A stimulatory effect on the mitochondria that resulted in increased adenosine triphosphate (ATP) was observed. In addition, LILI also showed anti-inflammatory and protective effects on these cells. In light of the continual threat of diabetic foot, infection, and amputation, new better therapies and the developing of wound healing research deserves better prioritization [26]. Esmaeelinejad and Bayat evaluated the effects of LLLT on human skin fibroblasts (HSFs) cultured in high glucose concentration and physiological glucose condition media. Release of IL-6 and bFGF was evaluated by enzyme-linked immunosorbent assay (ELISA). Statistical analysis demonstrated that certain previously mentioned laser doses (energy densities) promoted the release of IL-6 in HSFs which were cultured in high glucose concentration medium in comparison with nonirradiated HSFs cultured in the same medium. LLLT with 2 J/cm^2 energy density enhanced secretin of bFGF and IL-6 from fibroblast cultured in media mentioned above (hyperglycemic condition media). When HSFs were cultured in physiologic glucose concentration medium during laser irradiation, LLLT more effectively released IL-6 and bFGF [27]. In a single case study, Dixit et al. outlined the possible effect of LLLT on delayed wound healing and pain in a diabetic patient with chronic dehiscent sternotomy. After irradiation, they observed proliferation of healthy granulation tissue with decreased scores from the pressure ulcer scale of healing for sternal According to the results, LLLT could be a new potential treatment for chronic sternal dehiscence following coronary artery bypass graft, as it reinforced wound healing with an early closure of the wound deficit [28]. Fathabadie et al. conducted a study on the influence of PW LLLT on mast cells in wounds of nondiabetic and diabetic rats. The induction of type I DM and LLLT protocol was the same as Sharifian et al.'s study [25]. They assessed mast cell numbers and degranulation in all subgroups at 4, 7, and 15 days after infliction of the wounds. According to the paired t-test, there were significantly more total numbers of laser-treated mast cells compared to the placebos in the nondiabetic and diabetic groups. They observed significantly more granulated mast cells compared with degranulated mast cells for all laser-treated mast and placebo mast cells in the nondiabetic and diabetic groups [29]. Aparecida Da Silva et al. performed a study not only to determine if LLLT restored the balance between mRNA expression of matrix metalloproteinases (MMP)-2 and MMP-9 but also to determine the ratio between collagen types I and III during the diabetic wounds healing. The diabetes model was induced efficiently by STZ as demonstrated through increased levels of blood glucose. A diode laser (50 mW, 660 nm, 4 J/cm^2, 80 s) was administered once after scare induction. After LLLT, the rats were euthanized. The scarred areas were collected for MMP-2 and MMP-9 mRNA and histological analyses (inflammation and types I and III collagen). The results determined that scare significantly increased MMP-2 and MMP-9 expressions in untreated diabetic rats compared to nondiabetic rats. LLLT significantly reduced MMP-2 and MMP-9 expressions compared with untreated diabetic rats. Aparecida Da Silva et al. concluded that LLLT altered the expression of MMP-9, stimulated collagen production, and increased the total percentage of collagen type III in diabetic animals [30]. Esmaeelinejad et al. evaluated the effects of LLLT on HSFs cultured in high glucose concentration medium. HSFs were cultured either in physiologic glucose (5.5 mM/l) or high glucose (11.1 and 15 mM/l) media. LLLT was performed with a He-Ne laser unit at energy densities of 0.5, 1, and 2 J/cm^2. The viability and proliferation rate of these cells were determined by MTT assay. The results indicate that LLLT stimulate the viability and proliferation rate of HSFs, which were cultured in physiologic glucose medium compared to their control cultures. LLLT had stimulatory effects on the proliferation rate of HSFs cultured in high glucose concentrations compared with their control cultures. Esmaeelinejad et al. announced that HSFs originally cultured for 2 weeks in high glucose concentration attended to culture in physiologic glucose during laser irradiation increase cell viability and proliferation. Therefore, LLLT had a stimulatory effect on these HSFs [31]. Dadpay et al. studied the effect of LLLT in experimentally induced diabetic rats. They generated two full thickness skin incisions on the dorsal regions of each rat. The healthy (nondiabetic) groups received a pulsed-infrared 890 nm laser with an 80 Hz frequency and 0.03 J/cm^2 for each wound point in the first group and 0.2 J/cm^2

in the second group. Laser-treated diabetic wounds of the animals subjected to the same pulsed-infrared laser treatments as the second group for each wound point. Laser irradiation with 0.03 J/cm^2 significantly diminished the maximum load for wound repair in healthy rats. Laser irradiation with 0.2 J/cm^2 significantly escalated the maximum load in wounds from the healthy control and diabetic groups [32]. Peplow et al. have used a 660 nm laser diode in genetic diabetic mice to promote the healing process of wounds covered with a Tegaderm™ HP dressing that causes delayed contraction (splinted wounds). Possibly, the stimulation of healing could be due to the potential diabetes-modifying properties of laser light. Nonwounded diabetic mice and wounded diabetic mice was subjected to the 660 nm laser to at the same dose and location. They measured body weight and water intake of the mice. The left flank in the experimental group received 660 nm and 100 mW of irradiation 20 s/day for 7 days. There were no significant differences in body weight and water intake over 22 days between mice in the experimental and control groups. On day 14, the mean blood plasma glucose level did not significantly differ between the two groups. There was no glycated hemoglobin A1c detected in the samples. Peplow et al. concluded that irradiation of the left flank in diabetic mice with the 660 nm laser system did not have a significant hypoglycemic effect. The laser-stimulated healing of wounds in diabetic mice resulted from cellular and biochemical changes to the immediate wound environment [33]. Jahangiri et al. studied the effects of combined 670 and 810 nm diode lasers on diabetic wound healing parameters in rats. Two intervention (laser) groups underwent LLLT using 670 nm diode laser (500 mW, 10 J, 48 s) in the wound context and 810 nm diode laser (250 mW, 12 J, 50 s) to the wound margins. Never could they find statistically significant differences between the diabetic and nondiabetic groups in the wound area, percentage of open wound area, and wound healing rate by the repeated measurements. After 7 days of LLLT in the nondiabetic group, urine excretion significantly increased compared with the control group. Jahangiri et al. showed that no significant difference existed between the LLLT and control groups. The increased urine volume in nondiabetic rats after LLLT was an incidental observation that deserved future study [34]. Mirzaei et al. examined the impact of LLLT on cellular changes in organ culture and cell culture of skin from STZ-D rats. Type I DM was induced in rats by STZ. Fibroblasts extruded from the samples were proliferated in vitro and another set of samples were cultured as the organ culture. The researchers used an He-Ne laser. They administered 0.9–4 J/cm^2 energy densities four times to each organ and cell culture. The organ cultures were analyzed by light and transmission electron microscopy. Cell proliferation was evaluated by the MTT assay. Statistically, 4 J/cm^2 irradiation significantly increased the fibroblast numbers compared with the sham-exposed cultures [35].

8. Skin burn healing

Burn injuries are common traumatic injuries that cause considerable mortality and morbidity. Additionally, they are among the most expensive traumatic injuries due to the extended hospitalization and rehabilitation, as well as costly wound and scar treatments [36]. Annually in the United States, 1.25 million burn patients are treated. Of these, at least 50,000 require hospitalization [36]. Burn wounds generate special interest due to the large numbers of burn cases encountered. These wounds can generate a destructive effect functionally and cosmetically, which necessitates the search for a more efficient cure [37]. LLLT has beneficial effects on burn healing.

9. Literature review

Khoshvaghti et al. studied the effects of LLLT on mast cells in a third-degree burn rat model. Rats from all groups each received third-degree burns at three different locations. The first burn site on group I rats subjected to 890 nm pulsed laser, with 0.924 J/cm^2 energy density. 0.2% nitrofurazone cream was administrated for treatment of the second burn site on both groups of rats. They evaluated mast cell degranulation and numbers at each burn site on each group of rats. Analysis of variance on day 4 showed significantly lower total numbers of mast cells in the laser-treated burn sites compared with the other burn sites in both groups of rats. On day 8, the total numbers of mast cells were significantly lower at the laser-treated burn sites compared with the other burn sites. On day 13, there were significantly lower numbers of types I and II mast cells at the laser-treated burn sites compared with the other burn sites. Khoshvaghti et al. [38] concluded that LLLT significantly declined total numbers of mast cells through the proliferation and remodeling phases of healing in a rat model of third-degree burn. Ezzati et al. investigated the influence of PW LLLT on healing of a deep second-degree burn model in rats. In their study, two groups of laser-treated burns were treated by a 3000 Hz pulsed infrared diode laser that had 2.3 or 11.7 J/cm^2 energy densities, respectively. Treatment response was assessed both microbiologically and macroscopically. The incidence of *Staphylococcus aureus* diminished significantly in group 3 in comparison to group 1 on day 28. Analysis of variance showed that the 11.7 J/cm^2 LLLT significantly increased the wound closure rate at 2 and 3 weeks after infliction of the burn when compared with placebo burns. Independent sample t-tests demonstrated that LLLT with 11.7 J/cm^2 significantly enhance the wound closure rate though 4 weeks after infliction of the burn in comparison to the control burns. Ezzati et al. concluded that pulsed LLLT with 11.7 J/cm^2/890 nm of a deep second-degree burn model in rats significantly escalated the rate of wound closure compared with the control burns [39]. Ezzati et al. studied the influence of PW LLLT on the healing process of a third-degree burn in a rat model. They treated two groups of rats with a 3000 Hz-pulsed infrared diode laser that had 2.3 or 11.7 J/cm^2 energy densities and evaluated the response to treatment both microbiologically and macroscopically. They indicated that the incidence of *Staphylococcus epidermidis*, Lactobacillus, and Diphtheria diminished significantly in the laser-treated groups compared to the other groups by the chi-square test. The independent sample t-test illustrated that LLLT with 11.7 J/cm^2 energy density significantly escalated the wound-closure rate at 3 and 4 weeks after infliction of the burn compared with the control burns [40]. Vasheghani et al. evaluated 80 Hz pulsed infrared diode LLLT for third-degree burn healing in rats. The laser-treated burns were exposed to an 80 Hz pulsed 890 nm infrared diode laser at 0.396 J/cm^2, three times per week. Burn wounds were clinically examined. There were a significantly higher number of laser-treated burns that closed compared to the controls. The paired Student's *t*-test indicated that the wound closure rate of laser-treated burns was significantly longer than the control burns. Chi-square tests showed no significant difference between each microorganism (*Staphylococcus epidermis, S. aureus*, and *Pseudomonas aeruginosa*). Vasheghani et al. concluded that LLLT with an 80 Hz pulsed infrared diode laser accelerated third-degree burn healing in rats [41]. Bayat et al. studied the effects of LLLT on mast cell number during the inflammation, proliferation, and remodeling phases of the wound healing process of experimental burns. In the two laser-treated groups, burned areas were subjected to the LLLT with a He-Ne laser at energy densities of 38.2 or 76.4 J/cm^2. They observed that on day 7 in the first laser group, there were significantly more total numbers of mast cells compared with the other groups. On day 16 in the nitrofurazone-treated group, the total number of mast cells was significantly higher compared with the control, first laser, and normal groups [42]. In another study, Vashghani et al. investigated the effect of LLLT administered with a He-Ne laser on mast cell number and degranulation in rats with second-degree burns. All rats received deeply inflicted second-degree burns. In the two laser-treated groups, the burns received daily LLLT, with energy densities of 1.2 or 2.4 J/cm^2. In the fifth group, the burns were treated topically with daily administration of 0.2% nitrofurazone cream. Vashghani et al. concluded that administration of LLLT for deep second-degree cutaneous burns in rats not only significantly enhanced the number of intact mast cells during the inflammatory and proliferative phases of healing but also diminished the total number of mast cells during the remodeling phase [43]. In another study, Bayat et al. researched the effects of LL He-Ne LT on burn healing. The two laser treated groups, underwent daily treatment with LL He-Ne LT at energy densities of 1.2 or 2.4 J/cm^2. The response to treatment was assessed histologically and microbiologically. Analysis of variance demonstrated significantly greater mean blood vessel sections in the 1.2 J/cm^2 laser group compared with the other groups. Compared with the nitrofurazone-treated group, the mean depth of new epidermis in the 2.4 J/cm^2 laser group on day 16 was significantly lower. *P. aeruginosa* and *S. aureus* grew in more than 50% of samples obtained from control group, however these bacteria did not grow in the samples from the 2.4 J/cm^2 laser group. Bayat et al. concluded that LL He-Ne LT stimulated the destruction of *S. aureus* and *P. aeruginosa* in rats with third-degree burns. However, the histological evaluation demonstrated that LL He-Ne LT not only made a significant escalation in the mean blood vessel sections on day 7 after infliction of the third degree burns but also reduced the mean of the depth of new epidermis on day 16 after infliction of these burns in rats [44]. Bayat et al. studied the effects of two different doses of LLLT on healing deep second-degree burns. They inflicted a deep second-degree burn in each rat. The control group burns remained untreated. The two laser treated group burns were irradiated daily with LL He-Ne LT with energy densities of 1.2 or 2.4 J/cm^2. The response to treatments was assessed histologically and microbiologically. *S. epidermidis* was found in the 70% of the rats' wounds in the laser-treated groups in comparison to 100% of rats in the control group. Despite the fact that they found *S. aureus* in 40% of the rat wounds which were treated by nitrofurazone, they did not find this bacterium in the wounds of the laser treated and control groups. Bayat et al. determined that LLLT of deep second-degree burns made significant reduction in the number of macrophages and depth of the new epidermis.

Moreover, this treatment diminished the incidence of *S. epidermidis* and *S. aureus* [45]. It seems that special LLLT protocols have potential antimicrobial activity.

10. Cellular and tissue mechanisms of LLLT

It appears that LLLT not only has a great range of effects at the molecular, cellular, and tissue levels and also its specific modes of action may vary among different applications. Within the cell, there is strong evidence to suggest that LLLT causes the mitochondria [46] to enhance ATP production [27, 31], modification of reactive oxygen species (ROS), and induce transcription factors [47].

LLLT also enhances the proliferation, maturation, and motility of fibroblasts, and increases the production of bFGF [48]. When a chromophore absorbs a photon of light (laser) in the treated cells, an electron in the chromophore has the potential to become excited and move from low-energy orbit to a higher energy orbit [49]. The system can then use this stored energy to achieve various cellular tasks. There are several pieces of data that suggest that a mitochondria chromophore is as the initial LLLT target. Radiation of tissue with light makes mitochondrial products such as ATP, nicotinamide adenine dinucleotide (NADH), proteins, and RNA, as well as a reciprocal augmentation in oxygen consumption to increase. Various in vitro experiments have showed that cellular respiration is upregulated when mitochondria are subjected to a He-Ne laser or other forms of illumination [50]. The relevant chromophore can be detected by matching the action spectra for the biological response to light in the NIR range to the absorption spectra of the four membrane-bound complexes identified in mitochondria. This procedure demonstrates that complex IV or cytochrome *c* oxidase (CCO) is the essential chromophore in the cellular response to LLLT. CCO that consists of two copper and two heme-iron centers (components of the respiratory electron transport chain) is a large transmembrane protein complex [51]. The high-energy electrons are passed from electron carriers through a series of transmembrane complexes (such as CCO) to the final electron acceptor which makes a proton gradient used to produce ATP. Therefore, the administration of light directly affects ATP production by influencing one of the transmembrane complexes in the chain. Especially, LLLT increases ATP production and electron transport [52].

11. Contraindications and precautions

11.1. Contraindications

Direct irradiation of the eyes, within 4–6 months after radiotherapy, hemorrhaging region, locally to the endocrine glands [53].

11.2. Precautions

Epilepsy, fever, malignancy, to the low back or abdomen during pregnancy or menstruation, embryo or fetus, over the gonads, epiphyseal lines in children confused or disoriented patient, area of decreased sensation, infected tissue, sympathetic ganglia, vagus nerves, or cardiac region in patients with heart disease [53].

12. Conclusion

The effects of LLLT depend on the physiological state of the target cells, type of laser, radiation wavelength, energy density, and number of laser sessions. The biostimulation efficiency of LLLT is also dependent on the delivered energy density, which appears to be restricted to a very narrow therapeutic window. Compared with CW LLLT devices, PW LLLT devices provide more laser parameters. By investigating different values of these parameters, research models can be more effectively studied in these devices (PWLLLT) in comparison with CW LLLT devices, with the purpose of achieving better outcomes [54]. There were different LLLT protocols for different tissues. Clinical applications of LLLT have significantly impacted medicine and attracted the interest of clinicians, the public, and the media. The use of LLLT in biological applications and medicine is growing rapidly; advances in LLLT research have dramatically improved the clinician's ability to safely and effectively treat various medical conditions. According to several studies if the general condition of patients (such as blood glucose level, hydration, Na level, etc.) is controlled, LLLT can be useful for the treatment of diabetic foot ulcer. Nevertheless, additional research is required to elucidate the exact mechanism of laser photostimulations action at the cellular and molecular levels. Standardized treatment parameters of LLLT should be followed. Efforts should be made to evaluate precise dosimetry for skin wounds, DFUs, and burns.

Author details

Mohammad Bayat

Address all correspondence to: bayat_m@yahoo.com

Cellular and Molecular Biology Research Center, and Department of Biology and Anatomical Sciences, School of Medicine, Shahid Beheshti University of Medical Sciences, Tehran, Iran

References

[1] Farivar S, Malekshahabi T, Shiari R. Biological effects of low level laser therapy. J Lasers Med Sci. 2014;5:58–62.

[2] Reddy GK. Photobiological basis and clinical role of low-intensity lasers in biology and medicine. J Clin Laser Med Surg. 2004;22:141–50. doi: 10.1089/104454704774076208.

[3]   Mester E, Szende B, Gartner P. The effect of laser beams on the growth of hair in mice. Radiobiol Radiother. 1968;9:621–6.

[4]   Mester E, Spiry T, Szende B, Tota JG. Effect of laser rays on wound healing. Am J Surg. 1971;122:532–5. doi: 10.1016/0002-9610(71)90482-X.

[5]   Mester E, Nagylucskay S, Doklen A, Tisza S. Laser stimulation of wound healing. Acta Chir Acad Sci Hung. 1976;17(1):49–55.

[6]   Mester E, Szende B, Spiry T, Scher A. Stimulation of wound healing by laser rays. Acta Chir Acad Sci Hung. 1972;13:315–24.

[7]   Chung H, Dai T, Sharma SK, Huang YY, Carroll JD, Hamblin MR. The nuts and bolts of low-level laser (light) therapy. Ann Biomed Eng. 2012;40:516–33. doi: 10.1007/s10439-011-0454-7.

[8]   Guo S, Dipietro LA. Factors affecting wound healing. J Dent Res. 2010;89(3):219–29.

[9]   Couch R, Jetha M, Dryden DM, Hooton N, Liang Y, Durec T, et al. Diabetes education for children with type 1 diabetes mellitus and their families. Evid Rep/Technol Assess. 2008;(166):1–144.

[10] Boyle JP, Thompson TJ, Gregg EW, Barker LE, Williamson DF. Projection of the year 2050 burden of diabetes in the US adult population: dynamic modeling of incidence, mortality, and prediabetes prevalence. Popul Health Metrics. 2010;8:1. doi: 10.1186/1478-7954-8-29.

[11] Noble-Bell G, Forbes A. A systematic review of the effectiveness of negative pressure wound therapy in the management of diabetes foot ulcers. Int Wound J. 2008;5:233–42. doi: 10.1111/j.1742-481X.2008.00430.x.

[12] Singh N, Armstrong DG, Lipsky BA. Preventing foot ulcers in patients with diabetes. JAMA. 2005;293(2):217–28. doi: 10.1001/jama.293.2.217.

[13] Breitbart AS, Laser J, Parrett B, Porti D, Grant RT, Grande DA, et al. Accelerated diabetic wound healing using cultured dermal fibroblasts retrovirally transduced with the platelet-derived growth factor B gene. Ann Plastic Surg. 2003;51:409–14. doi: 10.1097/01.SAP.0000084461.83554.71.

[14] Reiber GE, Boyko EJ, Smith DG. Lower extremity foot ulcers and amputations in diabetes. In Aubert R, editor. Diabetes in America. Diane Publishing Co. National Institutes of Health, USA; 1995. p. 409–27.

[15] Kawalec J, Pfennigwerth T, Hetherington V, Logan J, Penfield V, Flauto J, et al. A review of lasers in healing diabetic ulcers. Foot. 2004;14:68–71. doi: 10.1016/j.foot.2003.11.001.

[16] Kern P, Moczar M, Robert L. Biosynthesis of skin collagens in normal and diabetic mice. Biochem J. 1979;182:337–45. doi: 10.1042/bj1820337.

[17] Bermudez DM, Herdrich BJ, Xu J, Lind R, Beason DP, Mitchell ME, et al. Impaired biomechanical properties of diabetic skin: implications in pathogenesis of diabetic wound complications. Am J Pathol. 2011;178:2215–23. doi: 10.1016/j.ajpath.2011.01.015.

[18] Loots MA, Lamme EN, Mekkes JR, Bos JD, Middelkoop E. Cultured fibroblasts from chronic diabetic wounds on the lower extremity (non-insulin-dependent diabetes mellitus) show disturbed proliferation. Arch Dermatol Res. 1999;291(2–3):93–9.

[19] Hehenberger K, Hansson A, Heilborn JD, Abdel-Halim SM, Östensson CG, Brismar K. Impaired proliferation and increased l-lactate production of dermal fibroblasts in the GK-rat, a spontaneous model of non-insulin dependent diabetes mellitus. Wound Repair Regener. 1999;7:65–71. doi: 10.1007/s004030050389.

[20] Francis-Goforth KN, Harken AH, Saba JD. Normalization of diabetic wound healing. Surgery. 2010;147:446–9. doi: 10.1016/j.surg.2009.04.038.

[21] Kwon DS, Gao X, Liu YB, Dulchavsky DS, Danyluk AL, Bansal M, et al. Treatment with bone marrow-derived stromal cells accelerates wound healing in diabetic rats. Int Wound J. 2008;5:453–63. doi: 10.1111/j.1742-481X.2007.00408.x.

[22] Dahmardehei M, Kazemikhoo N, Vaghardoost R, Mokmeli S, Momeni M, Nilforoush-zadeh MA, et al. Effects of low level laser therapy on the prognosis of split-thickness skin graft in type 3 burn of diabetic patients: a case series. Lasers Med Sci. 2016 31:497–502. doi: 10.1007/s10103-016-1896-9.

[23] Góralczyk K, Szymańska J, Szot K, Fisz J, Rość D. Low-level laser irradiation effect on endothelial cells under conditions of hyperglycemia. Lasers Med Sci. 2016:1–7.

[24] Lau PS, Bidin N, Krishnan G, Nassir Z, Bahktiar H. Biophotonic effect of diode laser irradiance on tensile strength of diabetic rats. J Cosmet Laser Ther. 2015;17:86–9.

[25] Sharifian Z, Bayat M, Alidoust M, Farahani RM, Bayat M, Rezaie F, et al. Histological and gene expression analysis of the effects of pulsed low-level laser therapy on wound healing of streptozotocin-induced diabetic rats. Lasers Med Sci. 2014;29:1227–35. doi: 10.1007/s10103-013-1500-5.

[26] Houreld NN. Shedding light on a new treatment for diabetic wound healing: a review on phototherapy. Scientific World J. 2014;2014. doi: 10.1155/2014/398412.

[27] Esmaeelinejad M, Bayat M. Effect of low-level laser therapy on the release of interleu-kin-6 and basic fibroblast growth factor from cultured human skin fibroblasts in normal and high glucose mediums. J Cosmet Laser Ther. 2013;15:310–7. doi: 10.3109/14764172.2013.803366.

[28] Dixit S, Maiya A, Umakanth S, Borkar S. Photobiomodulation of surgical wound dehiscence in a diabetic individual by low-level laser therapy following median sternotomy. Indian J Palliat Care. 2013;19:71. doi: 10.4103/0973-1075.110242.

[29] Fathabadie FF, Bayat M, Amini A, Bayat M, Rezaie F. Effects of pulsed infra-red low level-laser irradiation on mast cells number and degranulation in open skin wound

healing of healthy and streptozotocin-induced diabetic rats. J Cosmet Laser Ther. 2013;15:294–304. doi: 10.3109/14764172.2013.764435.

[30] Aparecida Da Silva A, Leal-Junior ECP, Alves ACA, Rambo CS, Dos Santos SA, Vieira RP, et al. Wound-healing effects of low-level laser therapy in diabetic rats involve the modulation of MMP-2 and MMP-9 and the redistribution of collagen types I and III. J Cosmet Laser Ther. 2013;15:210–6. doi: 10.3109/14764172.2012.761345.

[31] Esmaeelinejad M, Bayat M, Darbandi H, Bayat M, Mosaffa N. The effects of low-level laser irradiation on cellular viability and proliferation of human skin fibroblasts cultured in high glucose mediums. Lasers Med Sci. 2014;29:121–9. doi: 10.1007/s10103-013-1289-2.

[32] Dadpay M, Sharifian Z, Bayat M, Bayat M, Dabbagh A. Effects of pulsed infra-red low level-laser irradiation on open skin wound healing of healthy and streptozotocin-induced diabetic rats by biomechanical evaluation. J Photochem Photobiol B: Biol. 2012;111:1–8. doi: 10.1007/s10103-013-1289-2.

[33] Peplow PV, Chung TY, Baxter GD. Laser photostimulation (660 nm) of wound healing in diabetic mice is not brought about by ameliorating diabetes. Lasers Surg Med. 2012;44:26–9. doi: 10.1002/lsm.21133. Epub 2011 Nov 22.

[34] Jahangiri Noudeh Y, Shabani M, Vatankhah N, Hashemian SJ, Akbari K. A combination of 670 nm and 810 nm diode lasers for wound healing acceleration in diabetic rats. Photomed Laser Surg. 2010;28(5):621–7.

[35] Mirzaei M, Bayat M, Mosafa N, Mohsenifar Z, Piryaei A, Farokhi B, et al. Effect of low-level laser therapy on skin fibroblasts of streptozotocin-diabetic rats. Photomed Laser Surg. 2007;25:519–25. doi: 10.1089/pho.2009.2634.

[36] Gamelli RL. Cost-utility analysis applied to the treatment of burn patients in a specialized center—invited critique. Arch Surg. 2007;142:57. doi: 10.1001/archsurg. 142.1.50.

[37] Ghieh F, Jurjus R, Ibrahim A, Geagea AG, Daouk H, El Baba B, et al. The use of stem cells in burn wound healing: a review. Biomed Res Int. 2015;684084:7. doi: 10.1155/2015/684084.

[38] Khoshvaghti A, Zibamanzarmofrad M, Bayat M. Effect of low-level treatment with an 80-Hz pulsed infrared diode laser on mast-cell numbers and degranulation in a rat model of third-degree burn. Photomed Laser Surg. 2011;29:597–604. doi: 10.1089/pho. 2010.2783.

[39] Ezzati A, Bayat M, Khoshvaghti A. Low-level laser therapy with a pulsed infrared laser accelerates second-degree burn healing in rat: a clinical and microbiologic study. Photomed Laser Surg. 2010;28:603–11. doi: 10.1089/pho.2009.2544.

[40] Ezzati A, Bayat M, Taheri S, Mohsenifar Z. Low-level laser therapy with pulsed infrared laser accelerates third-degree burn healing process in rats. J Rehabil Res Dev. 2009;46:543. doi: 10.1089/pho.2009.2544.

[41] Vasheghani MM, Bayat M, Dadpay M, Habibie M, Rezaei F. Low-level laser therapy using 80-Hz pulsed infrared diode laser accelerates third-degree burn healing in rat. Photomed Laser Surg. 2009;27:959–64. doi: 10.1089/pho.2008.2366.

[42] Bayat M, Vasheghani MM, Razavie N, Jalili MR. Effects of low-level laser therapy on mast cell number and degranulation in third-degree burns of rats. J Rehabil Res Dev. 2008;45:931.

[43] Vasheghani MM, Bayat M, Rezaei F, Bayat A, Karimipour M. Effect of low-level laser therapy on mast cells in second-degree burns in rats. Photomed Laser Surg. 2008;26:1–5. doi: 10.1089/pho.2007.2103.

[44] Bayat M, Vasheghani MM, Razavi N. Effect of low-level helium–neon laser therapy on the healing of third-degree burns in rats. J Photochem Photobiol B: Biol. 2006;83:87–93. doi: 10.1016/j.jphotobiol.2005.12.009.

[45] Bayat M, Vasheghani MM, Razavi N, Taheri S, Rakhshan M. Effect of low-level laser therapy on the healing of second-degree burns in rats: a histological and microbiological study. J Photochem Photobiol B: Biol. 2005;78:171–7. doi: 10.1016/j.jphotobiol. 2004.08.012.

[46] Greco M, Guida G, Perlino E, Marra E, Quagliariello E. Increase in RNA and protein synthesis by mitochondria irradiated with helium-neon laser. Biochem Biophys Res Commun. 1989;163:1428–34. doi: 10.1016/0006-291X(89)91138-8.

[47] Karu T. Primary and secondary mechanisms of action of visible to near-IR radiation on cells. J Photochem Photobiol B: Biol. 1999;49:1–17. doi: 10.1016/S1011-1344(98)00219-X.

[48] Chen AC, Arany PR, Huang Y-Y, Tomkinson EM, Sharma SK, Kharkwal GB, et al. Low-level laser therapy activates NF-kB via generation of reactive oxygen species in mouse embryonic fibroblasts. PLoS One. 2011;6:e22453. doi: 10.1371/journal.pone.0022453.

[49] Karu TI. Photobiological fundamentals of low-power laser therapy. Quant Electron. IEEE J. 1987;23:1703–17. doi: 10.1109/JQE.1987.1073236.

[50] Karu T, Afanas' eva N. Cytochrome c oxidase as the primary photoacceptor upon laser exposure of cultured cells to visible and near IR-range light. Dokl Akad Nauk/[Rossiiskaia akademii nauk]. 1995;342:693–5.

[51] Fuller S, Capaldi R, Henderson R. Structure of cytochrome c oxidase in deoxycholate-derived two-dimensional crystals. J Mol Biol. 1979;134(2):305–27.

[52] Karu T, Pyatibrat L, Kalendo G. Irradiation with He-Ne laser increases ATP level in cells cultivated in vitro. J Photochem Photobiol B: Biol. 1995;27(3):219–23. doi:10.1016/1011-1344:07078-3.

[53] Cameron MH. Physical agents in rehabilitation: from research to practice. Elsevier Health Sciences; St Louis, Missouri, USA; 2012.

[54] Bayat M. The necessity for increased attention to pulsed low-level laser therapy. Photomed Laser Surg. 2014;32:427–8. doi: 10.1089/pho.2014.9858.

3

Pressure Ulcers

Jill M. Monfre

Abstract

Pressure ulcers or pressure injuries occur in all health care settings and are considered a quality care indicator. Individuals in every health care setting must routinely be assessed for factors that place them at risk for development of pressure ulcers and have routine skin assessments to assess for the presence of pressure ulcers. If risks for pressure ulcer development or actual pressure ulcers are identified, it is crucial that a prevention and treatment plan be developed and implemented to address the risks and treat the wounds. For a prevention and treatment plan to be comprehensive and effective, it must be evidence based and multidisciplinary. The plan needs to address the risk factors or wound concerns specific to the individual and include education for the providers, caregivers and individuals at risk for pressure ulcer development and/or with pressure ulcers. Expert consensus panels concur that despite evidence-based multidisciplinary comprehensive pressure ulcer prevention plans, there are clinical situations in which pressure ulcers are deemed unavoidable.

Keywords: Pressure, Ulcer, pressure injury, decubitus, bed sore, prevention, treatment

1. Introduction

Pressure ulcers, also referred to as decubitus ulcers, pressure sores or bed sores and recently referred to as pressure injures by the National Pressure Ulcer Advisory Panel (NPUAP) [1], are a common occurrence in all health care settings, including acute care hospitals, long-term care facilities, rehabilitation centers and subacute care centers [2]. Pressure ulcers have a significant impact on patients, families and health care facilities. These wounds can cause pain and suffering to individuals, produce emotional distress for families and significant others, increase the length of a hospital stay and increase the costs to facilities. The incidence of a pressure ulcer can also lead health care providers to feel as though they have failed to deliver quality care to those who have been entrusted to their care [3]. It is important to identify individuals who are at risk for pressure ulcer development or those who have developed a pressure ulcer, in order to implement preventative or treatment measures; these individuals also require close monitoring.

2. Definition

The National Pressure Ulcer Advisory Panel (NPUAP), an organization comprised of leading experts in health care dedicated to the prevention and management of pressure ulcers, during a consensus conference held in the spring of 2016 replaced the term pressure ulcer with pressure injury to more accurately reflect injuries related to pressure in both intact and ulcerated skin [1]. The NPUAP also revised their definition of a pressure injury as *localized damaged to the skin and/or underlying soft tissue usually over a bony prominence or related to a medical or other device. The injury can present as intact skin or an open ulcer and may be painful. The injury occurs as a result of intense and/or prolonged pressure or pressure in combination with shear. The tolerance of soft tissue for pressure and shear may also be affected by microclimate, nutrition, perfusion, comorbidities and condition of the soft tissue* [1]. The European Pressure Ulcer Advisory Panel (EPUAP), also a leading organization of wound care experts, continues to use the term pressure ulcer as well as the definition originally developed in conjunction with the NPUAP, which states a pressure ulcer is a *localized injury to the skin and/or underlying tissue usually over a bony prominence, as a result of pressure, or pressure in combination with shear* [4].

3. Etiology

Pressure ulcers, the term that will be used throughout this chapter, occur across all health care settings with the most common setting for the occurrence of pressure ulcers being acute care hospitals followed by long-term care facilities then equally in occurrence in an individual's home and nursing facilities [5]. Pressure ulcers usually occur on the lower half of the body with two-thirds occurring in the pelvic region such as the sacrum, coccyx or hip areas and one-third occurring on the lower extremities. The occurrence of pressure ulcers on the heels is increasing. **Table 1** indicates bony prominences of the body, the location where pressure ulcers occur most often [6].

Approximately 10% of pressure ulcers are device related [7]. Multiple medical devices or pieces of medical equipment can lead to pressure ulcer development. Items such as endotracheal tubes, feeding tubes, cervical collars, tracheostomy tubes and positive pressure airway masks all have the potential for creating pressure ulcers due to pressure points created by the device. Transfer boards or slide boards place an individual at risk for shear injuries due to sliding over the firm surface.

The most common age group for the incidence of pressure ulcers is the elderly, especially those 70 and older. The occurrence of a pressure ulcer in an elderly individual increases their mortality rate fivefold. In hospital, when a patient has developed a pressure ulcer, mortality increases by 25% in the over 70 age group [5].

Prone position (lying on stomach)

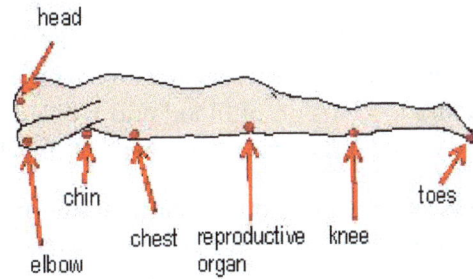

Supine position (lying on back)

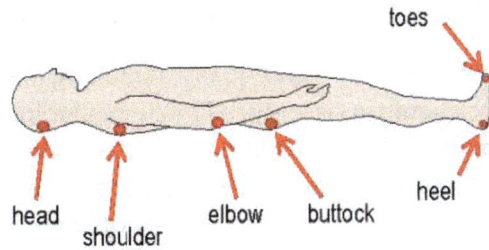

Lateral position (lying on side)

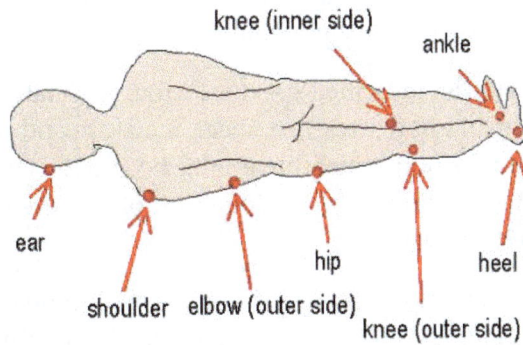

Sitting position

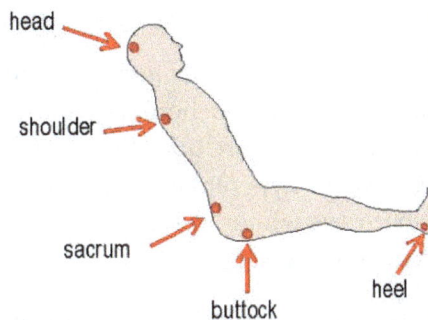

Table 1. Pressure ulcer pressure points.

4. Pathogenesis

The development of a pressure ulcer is not solely dependent upon pressure [8]. Multiple factors that modify the effect of pressure on tissues play a role in the development of pressure ulcers. The tolerance tissues have to external load depends on the duration of the exerted load. High loads can be tolerated for short periods of time, while relatively low loads can be tolerated for longer periods of time. The internal load in the tissues, as a result of the external load, causes cell deformation, occlusion of blood and lymphatic vessels and ischemia. If the internal load could be measured a risk for pressure ulcer, development could potentially be quantified [8].

A pressure ulcer results from sustained compression of soft tissues [5]. This compression occurs most often between a bony prominence and an external surface. Blood flow supplies oxygen and nutrients to the tissues. If pressure is sustained, the blood supply to the tissues is interrupted. When the blood flow is interrupted, oxygen and nutrients are not delivered to the tissues. Without oxygen and nutrients, the tissue will be damaged and eventually die [5].

Not all types of pressure are equally damaging to tissues [9]. Hydrostatic pressure, the pressure exerted by a liquid, as is endured by divers for long periods of time does not result in pressure ulcer formation. Yet localized pressure, as is exerted on the sacrum of a bedbound patient in the supine position for an extended period of time, often causes tissue distortion and blockage of the blood vessels resulting in much more damage. Studies related to localized pressure have found that pressure applied over a bony prominence resulted in more damage to the muscle than to the skin causing the study team to conclude that the muscle is more sensitive to pressure than is the skin or subcutaneous tissue [9].

Further studies identified specific factors associated with the development of a pressure ulcer including; interface pressure, shear, moisture and friction [4]. The NPUAP, after investigating shear and friction which have long been associated with pressure ulcer development, has eliminated friction from its definition of a pressure ulcer the explanation of which will be discussed below [10].

Interface pressure contributes to pressure ulcer development, as it is the pressure that develops between the skin and a surface upon which an individual is sitting or lying. Interface pressure is a measure commonly used to evaluate the effectiveness of a support surface [11]. Pressure mapping measures interface pressures and helps to determine appropriate positioning [8].

Not all localized pressure results in a pressure ulcer. When the pressure of short duration is relieved, blood flow returns to the area. This occurrence is known as reactive hyperemia, blood vessels in the area of pressure dilate in an attempt to overcome the ischemia that occurs with the pressure. Reactive hyperemia is transient and is also described as blanchable erythema — an area that becomes white when pressed with a finger and returns to erythema when the compression is removed [11].

Pressure that is not relieved and is of longer duration leads to further decreased capillary blood flow, occlusion of lymphatic vessels and tissue ischemia. Over a bony prominence, pressure of 20 mmHg can increase to as much as 300 mmHg. If this pressure is sustained, destruction of deep tissues can occur including destruction of muscle, subcutaneous tissue, dermis and epidermis [11].

When capillaries are occluded metabolic waste begins to accumulate in the surrounding tissues due to the lack of oxygen and nutrients. Capillaries that are damaged become more permeable and leak fluid into the interstitial space-causing edema. Perfusion is slowed through the edematous tissue; therefore, hypoxia worsens. Hypoxia increases cell death that results in an increased metabolic waste released into the surrounding tissues [11]. The ensuing edema further compresses small vessels causing increased edema and ischemia. Local tissue death occurs, which results in a pressure ulcer [7].

Shear is an applied force that causes an opposite yet parallel sliding motion such as when an individual slides in a bed or chair. The individual's skeletal structure slides in one direction yet the skin layer is restrained in the original position secondary to friction forces. In these situations, when shear is involved, multiple studies have found the pressure needed to occlude the blood vessels is much less than in an area where shear force is not involved [5, 8]. Elderly individuals are at higher risk for the effects of shear due to the decreased amount of elastin in their skin which is a normal consequence of aging [5].

Moisture, another factor associated with the development of pressure ulcers, alters the resiliency of the epidermis to external forces [11]. The effects of friction and shear are increased in the presence of moisture. Increased moisture is often associated with incontinence, perspiration or wound exudate [5].

Friction was originally determined to be a causative factor in the development of pressure ulcers after a study by Sidney Dinsdale was published in 1974 [10]. The results of this study showed that significantly less pressure was needed to stimulate the development of a full or partial thickness wound when the pressure was applied in conjunction with friction.

There are several forms of friction as they relate to the development of pressure ulcers. Friction, as a general term, is the rubbing of two body parts together. It is also a force that resists the motion of two bodies and/or material elements sliding against each other. In relation to skin breakdown, the type of friction, that is of concern is dry friction, of which there are two types, namely static and kinetic. Static friction is the force that resists the motion between two bodies when there is no sliding. There are multiple aspects that impact the amount of static friction at the skin surface including an individual's hydration level and what the individual is in contact with, for example bed linen. Moisture is an important factor relative to static friction as humidity and liquid moisture increases the friction and may cause an individual to adhere to a surface. Dynamic friction, also known as kinetic friction, is the force between two bodies relative to one another as they are sliding. Dynamic friction occurs when an individual slides downward in bed or rubs a foot in a shoe causing a blister. Such a blister may be misdiagnosed as a pressure ulcer.

In relation to the Dinsdale study, the type of friction applied during the study was not noted. The results of this study showed that the blood flow to the epidermis in a given area was not significantly different when pressure and friction were applied together and when pressure was applied alone. Investigators concluded that increased susceptibility of lesions with friction was not due to ischemia in the epidermis. Three decades later, it has been hypothesized that the friction used in Dinsdale's study was creating shear strain or deformation in deeper layers of tissue. Current hypothesis is that friction causes mechanically damaging shear strain of superficial tissue cells and tissue damage results directly from excessive deformation not ischemia as previously thought.

Friction is an important factor as it leads to shear stress and strain yet does not alone lead to the development of a pressure ulcer. Friction contributes to the development of a pressure ulcer due to the shear forces it can create. In other words, friction causes the shear forces in the tissue, which can increase the risk of tissue breakdown and lead to the development of a pressure ulcer. Therefore, shear remains in the current NPUAP definition of a pressure ulcer yet friction is eliminated. Including friction would be redundant as friction is now thought to be a cause of shear. Also, eliminating friction may decrease the number of wounds that are misdiagnosed as pressure ulcers when they are caused solely by friction [10].

5. Pressure ulcer stages

Pressure ulcers are classified by the amount of visible tissue loss [4]. Depth of tissue loss is important, as it determines a treatment plan of care and can impact payment. Once a wound is determined to be a pressure ulcer, it is assigned a pressure ulcer-specific stage or category. No other wound utilizes this same staging/categorizing system. A stage or category is assigned after careful and thorough assessment of the pressure ulcer to determine the extent of tissue destruction. To complete this assessment, one must have a competent understanding of the anatomy of the tissue layers involved and of the physiology of pressure ulcer development.

The NPUAP has defined the stages or categories of pressure ulcers as follows (**Table 2**):

EPUAP staging guideline	
Stage I	Nonblanchable erythema—Intact skin with nonblanchable redness of a localized area usually over a bony prominence. Darkly pigmented skin may not have visible blanching; its color may differ from the surrounding area. The area may be painful, firm, soft, warmer or cooler as compared to adjacent tissue. Category I may be difficult to detect in individuals with dark skin tones. May indicate "at-risk" persons.
Stage II	Partial thickness skin loss—partial thickness loss of dermis presenting as a shallow open ulcer with a red pink wound bed, without slough. May also present as an intact or open/ruptured serum-filled or sero-sanguinous-filled blister. Presents as a shiny or dry shallow ulcer without slough or bruising. This category should not be used to describe skin tears, tape burns, incontinence-associated dermatitis, maceration or excoriation
Stage III	Full-thickness skin loss—Full-thickness tissue loss. Subcutaneous fat may be visible but bone, tendon or muscles are not exposed. Slough may be present but does not obscure the depth of tissue loss. May

	include undermining and tunneling. The depth of a category/stage III pressure ulcer varies by anatomical location. The bridge of the nose, ear, occiput and malleolus do not have (adipose) subcutaneous tissue and category/stage III ulcer can be shallow. In contrast, areas of significant adiposity can develop extremely deep category/stage III pressure ulcers. Bone/tendon is not visible or directly palpable.
Stage IV	Full-thickness tissue loss—Full-thickness tissue loss with exposed bone, tendon or muscle. Slough or eschar may be present. Often includes undermining and tunneling. The depth of a category/stage IV pressure ulcer varies by anatomical location. The bridge of the nose, ear, occiput and malleolus do not have (adipose) subcutaneous tissue and these ulcers can be shallow. Category/stage IV ulcers can extend into muscle and/or supporting structures (e.g., fascia, tendon or joint capsule) making osteomyelitis or osteitis likely to occur. Exposed bone/muscle is visible or directly palpable.
Unstageable	Full-thickness skin or tissue loss—depth unknown—Full-thickness tissue loss in which actual depth of the ulcer is completely obscured by slough (yellow, tan, gray, green or brown) and/or eschar (tan, brown or black) in the wound bed. Until enough slough and/or eschar are removed to expose the base of the wound, the true depth cannot be determined, but it will be either a category/stage III or IV. Stable (dry, adherent, intact without erythema or fluctuance) eschar on the heels service as "the body's natural (biological) cover" and should not be removed
Suspected deep tissue injury (sDTI)	SDTI depth unknown—Purple- or maroon-localized area of discolored intact skin or blood-filled blister due to damage of underlying soft tissue from pressure and/or shear. The area may be preceded by tissue that is painful, firm, mushy, boggy, warmer or cooler as compared to adjacent tissue. Deep tissue injury may be difficult to detect in individuals with dark skin tomes. Evolution may include a thin blister over a dark wound bed. The may further evolve and become covered with thin eschar. Evolution may be rapid exposing additional layers of tissue even with optimal treatment.

Table 2. Pressure ulcer staging [4].

An illustration of the pressure ulcer stages/categories is seen in **Table 3** [1].

As pressure ulcers heal, the lost muscle, subcutaneous fat or dermis are not replaced with like tissue before they re-epithelialize [12]. A pressure ulcer fills in with scar tissue, which is composed primarily of endothelial cells, fibroblasts, collagen and extracellular matrix. Therefore, a stage-III pressure ulcer, for example, cannot, as the wound heals, become a stage-II pressure ulcer and progress on to a stage-I pressure ulcer because the term stage I would not accurately reflect the structures that are now present under the newly re-epithelialized tissue. Referring to a healing stage-III pressure ulcer as a stage II, then a stage-I pressure ulcer is known as reverse staging or down staging and is not acceptable. The stage needs to reflect the scar tissue that has developed. Therefore, the stage for this healing pressure ulcer is "healing stage-III pressure ulcer" and when the pressure ulcer has healed, the stage is a "healed stage-III pressure ulcer," indicating the pressure ulcer is now filled with granulation or scar tissue and resurfaced with epithelium [12].

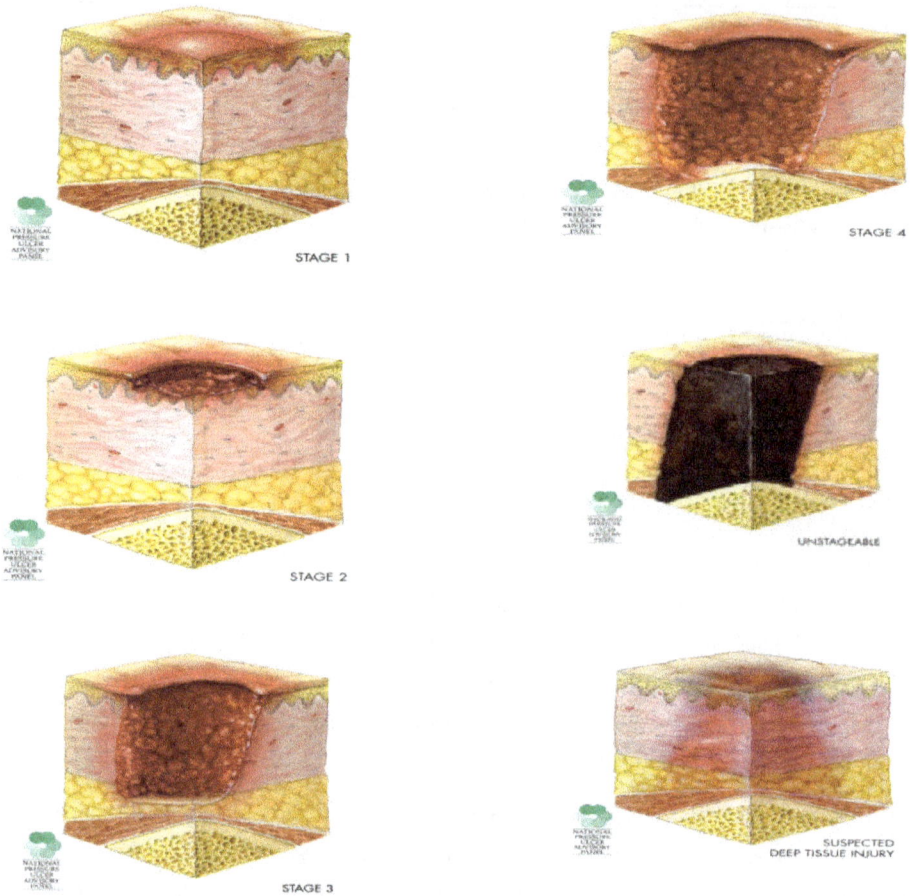

Table 3. Pressure ulcer injury/ulcer stages/categories.

Mucosal pressure injuries are *pressure injuries found on mucous membranes with a history of a medical device in use at the location of the ulcer* [1]. A mucous membrane is the moist lining of a body cavity, such as the gastrointestinal tract, nasal passages, urinary tract and vaginal canal, that communicates with the exterior. When pressure is applied to a mucous membrane, ischemia can result that can lead to a pressure ulcer. Mucous membranes are vulnerable to pressure especially related to medical devices such as oxygen tubing, feeding tubes, urinary catheters and fecal containment devices [13].

The anatomy of mucous membranes impacts the staging or categorizing of a mucous membrane pressure injury [13]. There are two types of mucous membrane tissue; nonkeratinized stratified squamous epithelium and an underlying connective tissue layer, the lamina propria. These layers are similar to the epidermis and dermis and are connected via rete pegs. At the interface of the two layers is a basal laminal layer. The epithelial layer is continuously renewed through migration of lower layers of epithelium to the surface. The epithelium of the mucosa, although is not keratinized like the epithelium of the skin. The lamina propria generally contains blood vessels, elastin and collagen fibers [13].

Injured mucosa heals similarly as skin with the exception of scar formation [13]. There is an increasing evidence that the fibroblasts in mucosa resembles fetal fibroblasts. Most mucosal injuries heal without scar formation [13].

The staging or categorizing of pressure ulcers that is used for the skin cannot be used to stage mucosal pressure injuries [13]. Nonblanchable erythema cannot be seen in mucous membranes, as superficial tissue losses of the nonkeratinized epithelium are so shallow they cannot be differentiated from deeper, full thickness injuries. The coagulum seen on a mucous membrane pressure injury resembles slough yet it is actually soft blood clot. Muscle is seldom seen in a mucous membrane pressure injury and bone is not present in these tissues. Therefore, pressure injuries located on a mucous membrane are referred to as mucous membrane pressure injuries [13].

6. Pressure ulcer prevention

There are several factors that have been associated with the development of pressure ulcers. Many of these factors affect an individual's ability to withstand episodes of pressure and shear as well as decrease the length of time or amount of pressure necessary to cause tissue damage. Risk factors that can lead to pressure ulcer development include age, immobility, nutritional deficiencies, skin moisture and incontinence, vasopressor use, chronic diseases such as diabetes or stroke, smoking, behavioral issues leading to noncompliance, poor general health and sensory loss [14, 15]. No single factor can explain all pressure ulcers rather it is a complex interaction among factors which increases the probability of pressure ulcer development

Braden scale	Norton scale	Waterlow scale	Jackson Cubbin scale
Sensory perception	Physical condition	Sex	Age
Moisture	Mental status	Age	Weight
Activity	Activity	Appetite	Skin condition
Mobility	Mobility	Nurses' visual assessment of skin	Mental status
Nutrition status	Continence	condition	Mobility
Friction/shear		Mobility	Nutrition
		Continence	Respiration
		Factors contributing to tissue Malnutrition	Continence
		Neurologic deficits	Hygiene
		Major surgery or trauma	Hemodynamic status
		Medication	

Table 4. Pressure ulcer risk assessment tools.

Prevention begins with identifying those individuals at risk for pressure ulcer development. A pressure ulcer risk assessment instrument that has been validated for use in the specific age group should be utilized. In the Unites States, the most common adult risk assessment instruments are The Braden and Norton scales that have been tested for validity in predicting pressure ulcer development risk [7, 16]. In Britain, the most common scales are the Braden and the Waterlow. The Jackson Cubbin Scale is specific to European critical care (**Table 4**).

These scales will identify specific factors related to assessment categories that place an individual at risk for pressure ulcer development. Once specific factors are identified, a prevention plan to address those factors can be implemented to reduce or eliminate the risk of pressure ulcer development [3, 16]. With the implementation of an evidence-based pressure ulcer prevention plan, pressure reduction can occur which will preserve the microcirculation and prevent the development of pressure ulcers [17]. A pressure ulcer prevention plan is multifaceted. Factors related to prevention and discussed further in treatment, as these factors are also included in a treatment plan, include; mobility, moisture and continence care, nutrition and hydration, support surfaces, documentation and education. No single intervention has been found that will consistently, reliably and completely reduce pressure ulcer development. Pressure ulcer prevention involves multiple interventions and a multidisciplinary team to affect the identified factors and reduce the risk of pressure ulcer development.

7. Pressure ulcer treatment

The treatment of pressure ulcers is based on the physiology of wound healing. Wound healing is a complex process that changes with the health status of the individual [17]. A health care provider needs to have a basic knowledge of the phases of wound healing including; hemostasis, inflammation, proliferation and maturation. Once a provider understands wound healing, one has a significant piece of the knowledge necessary to develop a pressure ulcer treatment plan [18].

7.1. Phases of wound healing

The first phase of wound healing is hemostasis. Briefly, in this phase, damaged blood vessels are sealed when platelets form a stable clot to seal the blood vessel. The platelets also stimulate the clotting cascade through the production of thrombin that initiates the production of fibrin. The fibrin mesh ultimately strengthens the platelet aggregate into a hemostatic plug. Hemostasis occurs within minutes of injury unless the injured individual has underlying clotting disorders [18].

In the second phase of wound healing, the inflammation phase, the erythema, swelling and warmth that occur are often associated with pain. This phase of wound healing usually lasts up to 4 days after injury. During this phase, neutrophils or PMN's (polymorphonucleocytes) and plasma are leaked from the blood vessels into the surrounding tissue. These factors clean debris from the surrounding tissue and provide the first line of defence against infection. Macrophages are also active in the second phase of wound healing acting to destroy bacteria and secreting growth factors which direct the third phase of wound healing.

Chronic wounds, wounds that take longer than 12 weeks to heal, often remain in the inflammatory stage longer than occurs with acute wounds. Cellular and molecular abnormalities within a wound bed prevent progression through the stages of healing [19]. Chronic wounds contain elevated inflammatory cytokines and proteases. Chronic wounds do not respond to growth factors in the same manner in which acute wounds do. Specifically related to pressure ulcers, the volume of exudate is often times increased in chronic wounds. Secondary to infection, the exudate may be more purulent. If protein levels are low, the exudate may appear thinner [19]. Chronic wounds often have inadequate blood supply that also contributes to delayed healing and the formation of unhealthy granulation tissue.

The third phase of wound healing, the proliferation phase, begins approximately 4 days after injury and usually lasts until day 21 postinjury. The activity during this phase is replacement of dermal tissue and possibly subdermal tissue and contraction of the wound. Fibroblasts secrete collagen, which is the framework upon which new dermal regeneration, can occur. Angiogenesis, development of new capillaries, also occurs during this phase of wound healing. Keratinocytes differentiate to form the protective outer layer.

In the final phase of wound healing, maturation, remodeling of the dermal layer occurs to produce greater tensile strength. The cells that are involved in this process are fibroblasts. This process can take up to 2 years to complete [18].

7.2. Principles of wound healing

In addition to knowledge of wound healing, a provider must also be aware of the principles of wound treatment and intervention. For a wound to progress to healing, the wound bed must be well vascularized, free of devitalized tissue, free of infection and moist. Continual evaluation of a wound is necessary as the wound progresses through the stages of wound healing.

7.3. Dressings

No one dressing is appropriate for all wounds. There are multiple factors that will affect the dressing selected for a particular wound **Table 5**.

Knowledge of the properties of available wound dressings and an understanding that a treatment plan may need to change as the wound progresses through the stages of healing is vital. Wounds that do not advance through the process of healing in a reasonable or expected time frame must be assessed for issues that have not been previously identified or wound changes that have occurred and the treatment plan re-evaluated **Table 6**.

The principles in selecting dressings for pressure ulcer treatment include eliminate dead space, control exudate, prevent bacterial overgrowth, ensure proper moisture balance, cost-efficiency, and manageability for the individual, caregiver and providers.

Several adjuvant therapies/advanced dressings have been used to treat pressure ulcers. These therapies include (a) platelet-derived growth factor (PDGF) applied to the wound bed, which will stimulate the growth of cells involved in wound healing and granulation tissue formation; (b) negative pressure wound therapy (NPWT), which utilizes subatmospheric pressure applied to a wound via a sealed dressing to promote wound healing, the applied suction removes drainage and increases blood flow to the wound; and (c) hyperbaric oxygen therapy, delivered in multiple modes—total body, body part or mask—exposes the body to 100% oxygen at a higher pressure than normally experienced, this therapy provides oxygen necessary to stimulate wound healing and combats infection by enhancing leukocyte and macrophage activity [20]. PDGR and hyperbaric oxygen, although supported for use, have less support than does NPWT in studies conducted on individuals with pressure ulcers [20].

Wound depth	Partial thickness
	Full thickness
Wound description	Necrotic
	Slough
	Granulating
	Epithelializing
Wound characteristics	Dry
	Moist
	Heavily exudating
	Malodorous
	Excessively painful
	Difficult to dress
Bacterial description	Colonized
	Infected

Table 5. Wound description.

Alginate	Highly absorbent, useful for wounds with copious exudate. Alginate rope is particularly useful to pack exudate cavities or tracts
Hydrofiber	Absorbent dressing used for exudative wounds
Debriding agents	Useful for necrotic wounds, often used as an adjunct to surgical debridement
Foam	Useful for clean granulating wounds with minimal exudate
Hydrocolloid	Useful for dry necrotic wounds, wounds with minimal exudate or clean granulating wounds
Hydrogel	Useful for dry, sloughy, necrotic wounds
Transparent film	Useful for clean, dry wounds with minimal exudate, protect high friction areas
Negative pressure wound therapy	Conforms to the wound bed by suction and stimulates wound contraction while removing exudate

Table 6. Dressings [17].

There is limited evidence, although moderate strength, indicating support for the use of radiant heat dressings to improve pressure ulcer healing. Radiant heat dressings are noncontact dressings attached to a heating element. These dressings provide warmth to the wound and have been found to increase capillary blood flow to the area and thus increase wound healing. Also with limited yet moderate strength of evidence is the use of electrical stimulation, which provides a direct electrical current through the wound bed using electrodes on the surface of the wound. One hour daily session has been shown to be most effective. Caution has been noted not to use electrical stimulation on individuals with cancer as the treatment could stimulate the cancerous cells. The American College of Physicians specifically notes electrical stimulation in its guidelines [15].

7.4. Treatment plan

Prior to the development of a comprehensive pressure ulcer treatment plan, consideration should be given to an individual's psychological, behavioral and cognitive status. The individual's goals and prognosis need to be determined as well as the resources an individual has available, both financially and as caregivers.

A multidisciplinary team is needed to develop a comprehensive pressure ulcer prevention and treatment plan, as numerous factors are addressed. The team may include the individual's primary care provider, a wound care specialist, nurses or medical assistants who will provide wound care or education, social workers who will assist the individual and family members with resources and emotional concerns, a physical therapist who will provide assistance with mobility therapy and any other necessary consultants.

Within the plan, the following needs may need to be addressed.

Debridement of necrotic tissue within an acute wound may be necessary to be able to completely assess the wound. Necrotic tissue may obscure underlying fluid collections that need to be identified. Necrotic tissue also promotes bacterial growth that impairs wound healing and therefore should be debrided [17]. However, debridement is not recommended for stable dry eschar on heel wounds with no edema, erythema or fluctuance. Debridement can be achieved by multiple methods including sharp debridement, mechanical, enzymatic or autolytic debridement. Most sharp debridement can be completed at bedside, yet if more extensive sharp debridement is needed it may need to be performed in an operating room [17].

Mobilization of an individual is an important component to a pressure ulcer treatment plan. Since, by definition, a pressure ulcer is caused, in part, by pressure, if an individual begins to mobilize pressure will be relieved individuals who cannot ambulate redistributing pressure on a support surface needs to be investigated.

Moisture management, controlling incontinence and excess perspiration by wicking moisture away from the skin, will impact the effect of moisture. Managing moisture will increase the ability of the epidermis to return to its original state after being exposed to pressure. Shear and friction also will not be as detrimental to the skin when moisture is not allowed to be in contact with the skin for prolonged periods of time.

Nutrition studies indicated weak evidence that nutritional interventions provide benefits in the prevention or treatment of pressure ulcers [15]. A guideline presented by the American College of Physicians in 2015 cited moderate quality evidence supporting protein supplements in treating pressure ulcers. A Cochrane review in 2014 concluded that there is no evidence to support nutritional interventions, including protein, provide any benefits in preventing or treating pressure ulcers. A study regarding vitamin C supplements concluded that there was no change in wound healing. No results were noted related to zinc due to insufficient evidence. Although, evidence supports that providing adequate nutrition is important. Oral nutrition is preferred, yet if not possible; provide nutrition by the most appropriate route.

Oxygenation and perfusion must be ensured. A primary reason for inadequate tissue oxygenation is vasoconstriction as a result of sympathetic over activity. Blood volume deficit, pain and hypothermia are common causes of sympathetic overactivity for which the end result could be increased risk for pressure ulcer development.

Infection is usually determined clinically [15]. All open wounds contain some degree of bacteria. Healing is most often not impaired until bacteria reach a high colony count. If a wound culture needed, evidence indicates the Levine technique should be used. This technique involves rotating a swab over a 1 cm^2 patch of wound with enough pressure to express fluid from the wound for 5 s. A tissue or bone biopsy is the preferred method of identification of osteomyelitis, although biopsies of this nature are not always feasible. Magnetic resonance imaging (MRI) and nuclear medicine tests are more sensitive and specific than conventional plain radiography in identifying osteomyelitis. When bone is exposed in a pressure ulcer, osteomyelitis is often presumed.

An individual with increasing pain may be exhibiting a sign of a wound infection. Other signs of an acute wound infection include erythema around the ulcer's edges, induration, warmth and purulent drainage, no progression toward healing for 2 weeks, friable granulation tissue, foul odor, new necrotic tissue or lack of even spread of granulation tissue across the base of the wound. An individual may also exhibit systemic symptoms of a wound infection including fever, delirium and confusion [15].

Repositioning is replacing the term turning. The aim of repositioning individuals at risk for pressure ulcer development is to relieve pressure and/or redistribute pressure. It has been found that a slight change in position can be adequate to aid in relieving pressure. A turn of 30°, as previously encouraged for an individual in bed, for pressure relief, is not always needed to relieve pressure from bony prominences.

There is no research to support repositioning individuals every 2 h will aid in preventing the development of pressure ulcers; this recommendation is based on expert opinion [15]. The frequency of repositioning will, in part, be determined by an individual's tissue tolerance or the ability of both the individual's skin and its underlying structures to withstand pressure without an adverse effect.

As a provider or caregiver, when an individual at risk for pressure ulcer development is in bed, avoid positions with the head of the bed elevated to the point in which excess pressure and shear are applied to the sacrum and coccyx. This is most often any point beyond 30°.

In the seated position, the greatest exposure to pressure is to the ischial tuberosities. The area of the ischial tuberosities is relatively small; therefore, the pressure will be high. Without pressure relief, a pressure ulcer will develop quickly.

If a patient has a reddened area as a result of a previous episode of pressure loading, it is not advisable to position the individual on the same body surface. The reddened area indicates the body has not recovered from the previous position on the body surface and continues to require relief from the pressure load.

If heels are left in contact with a surface for a prolonged period of time, it is not unusual for heel pressure ulcers to develop due to the significant volume of bony structure in relation to the soft tissue in the heel. For the protection of the heels or treatment of heel, pressure ulcers assure that heels are elevated off any surface. Heels should be elevated so as to distribute the weight of the leg along the calf without putting pressure on the Achilles tendon. To avoid obstruction of the popliteal vein, which begins behind the knee, which may lead to a deep vein thrombosis, care must be taken to not hyperextend the knee.

Physical conditions of certain populations require additional care in positioning. These populations include those with spinal cord injuries, those that are insensate, older adults, individuals that have sustained hip fractures or those that do not maintain a healthy lifestyle.

Support surface use has been validated in studies for the prevention of pressure ulcers in high-risk individuals and for the treatment of individuals with pressure ulcers. A support surface reduces pressure by spreading the tissue load over a larger area, thus decreasing the load over bony prominences. A support surface also manages the microclimate including moisture and temperature.

Support surface selection is based on mobility, comfort and circumstances of care. In a home setting, consideration is given to the structure of the home including width of doors, power supply and available ventilation for heat from the motor as these factors relate to the support surface to be utilized. If a spouse or significant, other will share the bed consideration should be given to his or her comfort also.

Regular foam does not distribute patient weight uniformly and may worsen or cause pressure ulcers. A higher specification foam mattress is more effective in preventing pressure ulcers

When an individual is placed on a low-air loss, surface consideration must be given to the linens and pads used on the surface. Linens and pads should not be of materials that will block the air flow.

An issue that can negatively impact an individual at risk for pressure ulcer development or with a pressure ulcer that is related to any support surface is bottoming out. Bottoming out occurs when an individual's pelvic region or buttocks sink down and the support surface no longer provides adequate redistribution of pressure. An assessment for bottoming out can be performed with a hand check. Place a hand, palm side up under the support surface directly below the individual's buttocks region. If the individual can feel your hand or if less than an inch of support material is evident, the individual has bottomed out and the surface should be replaced [16].

Physician consults are generally part of a comprehensive treatment plan for individuals with pressure ulcers. Specialists may be consulted to debride wounds or with more complex wounds to perform flap procedures. Infectious disease physicians may be consulted to provide input or to monitor infected wounds especially if osteomyelitis is suspected or confirmed.

Education of providers, caregivers and individuals with pressure ulcers is a vital component to any prevention or treatment plan. Without adequate education, failure of a plan is probable. Education of providers should include how to complete a comprehensive skin and wound assessment as well as documentation of the assessments. Providers also require education on the facilities process for wound care treatment, including the principles of wound care and the products available on the wound care formulary.

Caregivers or the individual with a pressure ulcer need to be educated on the cause of the pressure ulcer, the contributing factors, prevention measures, proper nutrition, appropriate wound treatment and appropriate times to contact a provider. Education should include materials in a format understandable for the caregivers and individuals. For individuals with chronic conditions, such as spinal cord injuries, there are often times formal education programs in rehabilitation centers. It is also common to request a caregiver to receive education in the hospital prior to a patient being discharged. Education is crucial to an effective prevention and treatment plan.

8. Unavoidable pressure ulcers

In 2014, the NPUAP hosted a multidisciplinary international conference to explore the issue of unavoidable pressure ulcers. This conference brought experts together to explore, within the context of organ systems, the issue of unavoidable pressure ulcers [14]. At a previous conference in 2010, also hosted by the NPUAP, an unavoidable PU was defined *as one that may occur even though providers have evaluated the individual's clinical condition and PU risk factors have been evaluated and defined and interventions have been implemented that are consistent with individual needs, goals and recognized standards of practice.*

It was agreed upon by those in attendance at the 2014 conference that unavoidable pressure ulcers do occur. This conference also established consensus on risk factors that have in some situations been shown to increase the likelihood of the development of unavoidable pressure ulcers. In summary, the organ systems which were identified that may in some situations contribute to the development of unavoidable pressure ulcers included; (a) impaired tissue oxygenation/cardiopulmonary dysfunction—an individual cannot be repositioned due to the potential for a fatal event related to hemodynamic status, (b) hypovolemia—an individual is hemodynamically unstable which often leads to an inability to reposition an individual, (c) body edema/anasarca–leads to decrease pressure-loading tolerance and increased risk of pressure ulcer development, (d) peripheral vascular disease, lower extremity arterial and venous disease—compromised circulation that contributes to ischemia which leaves tissues more vulnerable to pressure ulcer development. Within this category, other subcategories were identified including chronic kidney disease, whereas the change in tissue tolerance may increase the likelihood of pressure ulcer development, hepatic injury which results in hypo-albuminemia that leads to edema and anasarca, sensory impairment, skin issues related to extremes in age, multiorgan dysfunction syndrome, critical status and burns all which leave patients prone to pressure ulcer development, (e) body habitus—obesity compromises an individual's ability to prevent shear injury during movement, pressure ulcer development related to moisture due to increased diaphoresis and inability to redistribute pressure over bony prominences and (f) immobility—associated with vascular congestion, dependent edema, compromised lung aeration, decreased red blood cell mass, dyspnea and activity tolerance leading to increased risk for unavoidable pressure ulcer development. The consensus panel also agreed that further research is necessary to examine the issue of unavoidable pressure ulcers [21].

9. Summary

A pressure ulcer rate is considered a quality care indicator in most health care settings and being an international health care concern. Most pressure ulcers are preventable. With a thorough assessment, including an assessment of an individual's skin and an assessment of pressure ulcer development risk, a comprehensive prevention and treatment plan can be developed and implemented to enhance positive outcomes.

Author details

Jill M. Monfre

Address all correspondence to: jmonfre@uwhealth.org

University Hospital, University of Wisconsin, Madison, Wisconsin, USA

References

[1] National Pressure Ulcer Advisory Panel. NPUAP Pressure Injury Stages [Internet]. April 13, 2016. Available from: http://www.npuap.org/resources/educational-and-clinical-resources/npuap-pressure-injury [Accessed: April 27, 2016]

[2] Lyder C. H. Pressure ulcer prevention and management. JAMA. 2003;289(2):223–226.

[3] Satekova L., Ziakova K. Validity of pressure ulcer risk assessment scales: review. Central European Journal of Nursing and Midwifery. 2014;5(2):85–92.

[4] National Pressure Ulcer Advisory Panel. NPUAP Pressure Ulcer Stages/Categories [Internet]. 2014. Available from: http://www.npuap.org/resources/educational-and-clinical-resources [Accessed: February 18, 2016]

[5] Grey J. E., Enoch S., Harding K. G. ABC of wound healing: pressure ulcers. BMJ. 2006;332(25):472–475.

[6] Images of Imgarcade. [Internet]. April 2015, Available from: http://www.Imgarcade.com [accessed February 13, 2016]

[7] Cooper K. L. Evidence-based prevention of pressure ulcers in the intensive care unit. Critical Care Nurse. 2013;33(6):57–66.

[8] Reenalda J., Jannink M., Nederhand M., Ijzerman M. Clinical use of interface pressure to predict pressure ulcer development: a systematic review. Assistive Technology. 2009;21:76–85.

[9] Loerakker, S. Aetiology of pressure ulcers [thesis]. Eindhoven, Netherlands: Eindhoven University of Technology; 2007. 24 p.

[10] National Pressure Ulcer Advisory Panel. Friction Induced Skin Injuries-Are They Pressure Ulcers? A National Pressure Ulcer Advisory Panel White Paper [Internet]. November 20, 2012. Available from: http://NPUAP.org [Accessed: February 14, 2016]

[11] Pieper B. Mechanical forces: pressure, shear and friction. In: Ruth A. Bryant, editor. Acute & Chronic Wound Nursing Management. 2nd ed. St. Louis: Mosby; 2000. pp. 221–264.

[12] National Pressure Ulcer Advisory Panel. The Facts about Reverse Staging in 2000. The NPUAP Position Statement [Internet]. 2000. Available from: http://www.NPUAP.org [Accessed: February 26, 2016]

[13] National Pressure Ulcer Advisory Panel. Mucosal Pressure Ulcers [Internet]. August 2008. Available from: http://www.NPUAP.org [Accessed: February 23, 2016]

[14] Edsberg L. E., Langemo D., Baharestani M. M., Posthauer M. E., Goldberg M. Unavoidable pressure injury. J Wound Ostomy Continence Nurs. 2014;41(4):313–334.

[15] Raetz J., Wick K. Common questions about pressure ulcers. American Family Physician. 2015;92(10):888–894.

[16] Ratliff C. R. Pressure ulcer prevention. Advance for NP's and PA's. 2016;18(6):24–29.

[17] Bluestein D., Javaheri A. Pressure ulcers: prevention, evaluation, and management. American Family Physician. 2008;78(10):1186–1194.

[18] The Canadian Association of Wound Care. The Basic Principles of Wound Healing [Internet]. Available from: http://cawc.nwt [Accessed: February 24, 2016]

[19] Ousey, K. Chronic wounds-an overview. Journal of Community Nursing 2009;23(7):20–24.

[20] National Pressure Ulcer Advisory Panel, European Pressure Ulcer Advisory Panel, PAN Pacific Pressure Ulcer Injury Alliance, editors, London England. Prevention and Treatment of Pressure Ulcers: Clinical Practice Guideline. 2nd ed. Australia: Cambridge Media; 2014. 308 p.

[21] Black J. M., Edsberg L., Baharestani M. M., Langemo D., Goldberg M., McNichol L., Cuddigan J. Pressure ulcers: avoidable or unavoidable? results of the national pressure ulcer advisory panel consensus conference. Ostomy Wound Management. 2011;57(2): 24–36.

4

Ischemic Ulcer Healing: Does Appropriate Flow Reconstruction Stand for All That We Need?

Vlad-Adrian Alexandrescu and François Triffaux

Abstract

During the recent decades, soaring progresses in vascular disease knowledge, particularly in critical limb ischemia (CLI) treatment, enhanced novel diagnostic and interventional strategies with high serviceableness in patient's selection, arterial recanalization, and dedicated ischemic ulcer follow-up. However, despite undeniable advances in medical technology and clinical judgment, limb salvage, the ambulation recovery, and patient's survival seem only scarcely affected in this heterogeneous CLI group, particularly concerning the diabetic and renal patients. Innovative strategies such as *"end artery occlusive disease"* treatment or *"wound-targeted revascularization"* were equally proposed by following the angiosomal anatomical distribution associating individual foot collateral assessment in a unified *macro*- and *micro*-circulatory judgment. However, despite encouraging clinical results, prospective evidence still lacks on this concern. It also appears that specific wounds could not always stand for the lowest perfusion areas according to current CLI criteria, since severe neuropathy, inflammatory swelling, local infection, and skin trauma may add complementary hindrances to tissue viability.

The present chapter endeavor to summarize main available treatment principles for ischemic ulcer recovery that every modern practitioner eventually disposes in an updated contemporary view."

Keywords: wound healing, critical limb ischemia, diabetic foot, angiosome, limb revascularization

Motto: *'Each ulcer is unique in complexity and deserves flexible understanding and control of whole individual tissue recovery challenges'* (Current clinical observation)

1. Introduction

During centuries, wound healing was believed to be part of a mysterious process that addresses only inspirational approaches of secret practitioner's experience. Outstanding scientific advances over the last 50 years revealed real complexity of this staged process, astonishing as life's unfolding itself. This natural course seems to bear thousands of overlapping and indissoluble processes [1]. Today's knowledge, beyond new high-performance techniques for revascularization and tissue engineering [1], affords additional key data about intimate mechanisms of ischemic threat, ulcer formation, and steps to wound recovery [1, 2]. In the recent decades, this proper knowledge enhanced complementary diagnostic and interventional strategies with high serviceableness in patient's selection, arterial recanalization, and dedicated ulcer follow-up [1, 3]. However, despite soaring progress in medical technology and clinical judgment for critical limb ischemia (CLI) wound treatment, limb salvage, and patient's survival seem only scarcely affected [1–3]. This assertion dwells particularly true in diabetic and renal patients who exhibit ischemic foot wounds [1, 2]. Outstanding advances in basic research and clinical management toward better tissue regeneration, unfortunately, seem to confront with parallel increasing of CLI subjects each year [1]. It becomes obvious nowadays that ischemic ulcer healing implies a convergent treatment for multifaceted presentations in patients with multiple arterial and systemic affectations [1–3].

The present chapter endeavor to summarize main treatment principles for CLI ulcer recovery that every modern practitioner eventually disposes in an updated contemporary view.

2. Historical perspectives and advancements in ischemic wounds treatment

Wound healing approaches are probably old as the history of medicine. During centuries, several significant breakthroughs, however, marked significant progress in wound repair, following thorough scientific understanding. Starting with the Ancient World, according to the oldest medical record found on a Sumerian clay tablet (2100 BC) [4], cleansing and bandaging the wound was noted to represent the central "healing gestures" to be practiced in the healing course [4]. The Ancient Egyptians (1600 BC–1550 BC) also mention the use of mixtures (honey, grease, and lint) for wound regeneration, however, without apparent etiologic segregation [5, 6]. They also displayed an impressive science of bandaging, including herbal extracts and resins (probably the first coordinated bandages ever mentioned) [5]. Hippocrates in the ancient Greece originally devised approach methods for acute and chronic wounds [6]. Later on, Cornelius A. Celsius marked a momentous step in wound care history by his original description of the "four cardinal signs of inflammation," including first "gangrenous foot" delineation in his eight-volume *Compendium of Medicine* (41 BC) [6]. A substantial contribution to ulcer's classification and healing understanding is appointed by outstanding surgical work of Ambroise Parré in the Renaissance era about the treatment of gunshot wounds including "the gangrenous battlefield limb" [7]. During the next centuries, many new ideas in wound management were unfortunately rejected by lack of validation and time-related historical tendencies. Wound healing understanding was subsequently developed by Joseph Lister's [8] and by Louis Pasteur's remarkable clinical research [8, 9] adding relevant knowledge for bacterial colonization and sepsis development, particularly in the ischemic ground [9]. More recently, notable breakthroughs in comprehending the complexity of wound healing cascade were added by Virchow [10], owning establishment of histopathology as an autonomous discipline [6, 10], and by first isolation of "epidermal growth factor" as a mitotic stimulant in 1962 [11].

Probably one of the most ponderous discoveries in the same period was the defining structure of DNA and RNA by Franklin, Watson, and Crick [6]. Parallel advances were noted in surgical and interventional revascularization techniques for *tissue healing* perceived in a hemodynamic ischemic perspective. Leading milestones in arterial flow imaging were marked by first arteriographic diagnostic reported by Brooks in 1924 [12], followed by first translumbar aortography described by Dos Santos in 1929 [13], both with considerable influence in more accurate inferior limb arterial disease diagnostic. First Doppler ultrasound assessment of atherosclerotic occlusive disease by noninvasive method was reported by Strandness [14] in 1966. All these diagnostic methods have borne huge influence first in distinguishing arterial from nonischemic wounds, and further for separating arterial from venous limb ulceration. The current ischemic injury diagnostic era yet institutes since the computed tomography (CT) scanning and magnetic resonance imaging (MRI) have become an integrated part of ongoing peripheral arterial flow evaluation [15]. For that arterial surgery enables high limb salvage nowadays, the achievement of several important steps was mandatory. The first lumbar sympathectomy in 1924 by Labat [16], the heparin use since 1937 [17], the Kunlin's first saphenous vein graft in 1951 [18] and the first Dacron [19], and polytetrafluoroethylene (PTFE) [20] prothesis utilization, all had tremendous influences in modern surgical revascularization for wound healing [1–3, 20].

Traditionally during years, open surgical bypass represented the main effective treatment strategy for tissue recovery and limb salvage [1, 21]. In addition to outstanding surgical revascularization advances, new transcatheter endovascular techniques emerged and rapidly evolved in CLI treatment arena during the last three decades [21]. They seem to improve the perioperative morbidity-mortality and the length of hospital stay, affording comparable limb preservation rates [1 3, 21]. Owning remarkable low invasiveness and reproducibility, the percutaneous transluminal angioplasty (PTA) and stenting (first promoted by Gruntzig in 1974 and by Dotter [20] in 1964) rapidly gained a wide utilization in the coronary, but also in the peripheral arterial disease (PAD) current treatment [21]. Although the "stent" term derives from Charles Stent (1807–1885), an English dentist who used this term for creating customed dental molds [21], the idea to modulate vascular lumen by diligent metallic implants had great issues in vascular practice. During the next decades, new "bare" or "covered stents" were imagined, together with new "stent grafts" originally pioneered by Volodos and Parodi in the treatment of aortic aneurysmal disease around 1985–1990s [22]. Novel "drug eluted" devices including balloons and stents have been successfully launched during the last decade with promising clinical results [1, 21].

Following parallel scientific emancipation, new strategies as to improve ischemic tissue healing were cast in parallel medical disciplines. Thus, in 1987, Taylor and Palmer initially described the "angiosome" model of human body vascularization [23] and auspiciously implemented the concept among particular plastic reconstructive surgery applications. This significant breakthrough in tissue perfusion understanding was succeeded by its first use in CLI limb salvage by Attinger and colleagues 20 years later [24], using "topographical" or angiosome-guided bypasses to the foot ischemic wounds [24]. Not surprisingly, starting with 2008–2010s, and up to the contemporary period, new endovascular "wound-directed" revascularization applications were described with promising wound healing and limb preservation results [25, 26]. All these progresses have added and undoubtedly will add complementary understanding in ischemic ulcer treatment, owning more precise revascularization selection since specific "wound-targeted" revascularization is performed [24–26].

3. Demographics, etiologic factors, and social implications of PAD with its most severe presentation represented by critical limb ischemia

Recent demographic data suggest that more than 200 million individuals worldwide suffer from varied forms of the PAD that represent a 24% increase over the last decade and concern all socioeconomic strata [27, 28]. The economic weight of PAD was proven to be ponderous [28]. It has meant that the total costs of vascular-related hospitalizations climbed to 21 billion dollars in the USA in 2004, and this threshold seems to rise each year continually [28]. Critical limb ischemia as a consequence of severe infra-inguinal atherosclerosis embodies extreme forms of PAD and currently associates rest pain and ischemic ulcers (corresponding to Fontaine stages III/IV and Rutherford categories 4-5 ischemic limb presentations) [1–3].

The term of CLI is commonly used for patients who exhibit symptoms of severe arterial hypoperfusion for more than 2 weeks [3, 27]. Elementary CLI diagnosis is made by clinical exam, anatomical stratification, and hemodynamic evaluation of flow disturbances over accessible arterial paths [1, 3, 27]. Defining and analyzing large CLI groups of patients, however, prove to be difficult [2–4].

These hindrances are mainly determined by (1) the vast heterogeneity of underlying arterial diseases [1, 27], (b) the various appended risk factors [1–3, 27], (c) the multilevel spread of arterial lesions [1, 27] (d) by concurrent systemic pathologies [27], (e) the scarce follow-up data [3, 27], and (f) the lack of synchronous macro- and microvascular apprehension for gradual hypoxic limb changes [1, 27–31]. It is known that without precocious recognition and aggressive treatment, CLI invariably inflicts significant morbidity and high rates of major amputation and mortality [1–3, 27–30].

To date, the likelihood of death within the first 6 months of CLI diagnosis has been estimated to reach 20% (all etiologies confounded) and exceeds 50% at 5 years following prime documented onset [27–32]. Contemporary studies reveal that patients with PAD (and particularly those with CLI) are more likely to experience simultaneous coronary or cerebral vascular disease, bearing a higher risk of early death [1–3, 27]. The risk for developing PAD seems considerably increased in diabetic and renal patients, prone to more frequently experience systemic ischemic events compared to general population [1–3, 27–31].

Several risk factors that lead to lower limb major amputation in patients having ischemic wounds were described, including increasing age, being male, being African American, having peripheral neuropathy, and developing infected ulcers [1, 2, 27–29]. The Trans-Atlantic Inter-Society initial Consensus (TASC) II document showed that more than 15% of diabetic subjects will unfold a foot ulcer during their lifetime while 14–24% of them, unfortunately, will require amputation [3]. It is also valued that more than 170 million people suffer nowadays from diabetes mellitus, and their worldwide number is anticipated to attain 366 million by 2030 [1]. In this particular cohort of diabetic patients during the first year of CLI diagnosis, 40–50% among them may experience foot amputation while 20–25% among them will die [1, 2, 27].

Nevertheless, by applying optimal revascularization and local wound treatment as early as possible, up to 85% of amputations can be prevented [3].

The social burden of the metabolic syndrome and particularly the diabetic systemic athero-sclerotic disease is tremendous for the patient, the medical care organization, and public communities [1, 2, 28, 31].

Particularly concerning *arterial* inferior limb *ulcers* (all arterial pathologies confounded), current reports document 18–29% prevalence among 60 years or older patients who interest-ingly bear equal rates as much younger (50-year-old) individuals associating diabetes or tobacco use [33].

4. Critical limb ischemia ulcers: do we meet the current clinical needs?

Postischemic tissue recovery implies simultaneous alignment of several distinct physiological processes [33]. Inasmuch their entire clinical signification remains only partially controlled [27, 30, 33], their unaltered unfolding dwells prerequisite. Among numerous molecular and cellular events that clearly overpass the purposes of this chapter, some practical aspects may be however useful to be highlighted and are briefly summarized in the sections below.

4.1. Leading physiological mechanisms in wound recovery and appended phases of revascularization

It is accepted that mechanisms concerning tissue regeneration are strongly influenced by the type and thickness of tissue layer affectation, also by their capacity for healing [1, 33]. The retrieval of CLI threat resets in motion the regular "cascade" of reconstructive tissue events leading in normal circumstances (absence of systemic risk factors for healing) to long-lasting tissue repair [33, 34]. Full-thickness wound regeneration following most CLI revasculariza-tions concerns the skin, the underlying subcutaneous and the deep muscular compartments. Currently, this process is depicted in three schematic phases: the inflammatory stage (the "lag" phase), the "tissue formation" (or the "proliferative") phase, and the "tissue remodeling" phase [34]. It is important to note that this "allotment" is somewhat conventional since all three stages are commonly overlapping to some degree [33, 34]. Activating cells that participate in one phase usually produce biological triggers indispensable to interlock tissue molding into the next phase [34]. These stages are routinely *conditioned* by initial hemostasis and by intentional *arterial revascularization*, both representing fundamental activating processes [33–35]. Most details concerning these enthralling multimodal events are largely depicted in available histopathology literature and will not be further characterized in this section.

During the same sequential process, the ischemic burden relief sets in motion three parallel *hemodynamic* regenerative phases [35]. These stages are conceptualized as (1) *the initiatory* flow redistribution phase (concerning "large" remnant collaterals surrounding the ischemic wound zone), (2) *the early* or "mid-term" flow dispensation (regarding the "rescue" or "small" collaterals and arterioles), and (3) *the retarded* postischemic phase, essentially characterized by the arteriogenesis, the angiogenesis processes [33–35]. Alike most biological chain-processes, these three flow-redistribution phases exhibit specific time overlapping in their activation, according to concomitant vascular risk factors and individual patterns of arterial occlusive disease [35]. This particular knowledge may enable the clinician to choose better appropriate diagnostic and treatment methods in a timely approach for every ischemic wound follow-up [33, 35].

4.2. Main pathophysiological aspects in ischemic wound healing and related clinical presentations

To date, the exact mechanisms and time periods conducting to chronic ischemic ulceration are not completely understood [30, 31, 33, 34, 36]. Most arterial ulcers are encountered over the age of 65 as people live longer nowadays [3, 33]. Arterial ulcers are ranked to constitute about 12–19% among all leg ulcers [33, 37] while mixed venous-arterial or combined neuro-ischemic tissue defects may concern 15% [37] up to 24% [29–31] of these patients, respectively. There were described either as "spontaneous" ulcerations (typically involving the forefoot and toes as progressive collateral occlusion occurs) or as "post-minor trauma" wounds since inadequate arterial flow proves ineffective to increased oxygen demands for cicatrization [34, 38]. Bed-ridden patients with PAD represent another high-risk category to develop pressure heel ischemic ulcers on preexisting vascular impairment [37, 38]. For this particular cohort exhibiting ischemic hind foot ulcers, current guidelines emphasize that prevention by scrupulous heel elevation or soft tissue contact interposition is mandatory [3, 28, 38].

The TASC II fundamental CLI criteria [3] as absolute ankle pressure (AP) inferior to 50–70 mm Hg, or diminished toe pressure (TP) below 30–50 mm Hg are unanimously accepted [3]. A series of parallel predisposing factors for ischemic tissue damage were evinced in the last decade. They either concern the arterial perfusion (tobacco use, dyslipidemia, hypertension, weight excess, hyperglycemia, hyperhomocysteinemia, etc.), or specific foot conditions (peripheral neuropathy, inflammation, edema, infection, bedridden status, hypoalbuminemia, hyperglycemia, uremia, cortisone therapy, etc.), all with huge influence on peripheral tissue regeneration [1–3, 27, 33–35, 37, 38]. Although arterial ulcers theoretically may appear anywhere on the ischemic limb [3, 33], the presence of multilevel CLI arterial disease inflicts more distal localizations, particularly in subjects with deprived foot collateral reserve [1, 25, 29, 30].

Beyond common atherosclerotic arterial ulcers, other *arterial*-related ulcers were described such as superficial hypertensive wounds, peripheral embolic tissue defects (owning 0.01–0.2 mm. cholesterol particles), those associated with connective tissue arteritis, those affecting hypercoagulable states, or following microangiopathic lesions, within parallel to mixed nutritional, hemolytic, or neurologic disorders [33, 34, 36].

4.3. What determines ischemic tissue defects to slide toward chronicity and necrosis? Is there a conjuring threshold to consider?

It has been showed that in healthy individuals, peripheral wounds promptly tend to recover owning adapted cell's metabolism, appropriate oxygen supply, essential growth factors, cytokines, and matrix proteins inflow (Section 5.1.2.) that all endeavor to orient local tissue damage on "steady" sequential healing process [27, 33, 36].

Since initial ischemic changes last beyond local individual compensatory reserves [30, 35], the readapting mechanisms are gradually exhausted and local tissue homeostasis finally drifts toward biological extinction [36, 39, 40]. Inasmuch CLI wound onset may be commonly displayed over days or weeks [3], local infection and collateral depletion by septic thrombosis can urge irrecoverable tissue loss appearance and make it devastating [30, 32, 35]. Probably the real "tipping point" between viable or perished, for every inch of ischemic tissue around the wound relies on local collateral adaptation vigor [39]. Alike other ischemic models described in human tissues (stroke, myocardial infarction), the extent of necrosis core depends on rescue capacity inside the "penumbra" or intermediary neighboring zone [35]. For this transitional layer of undecided viability, a few factors strongly influence its fate. The timing and intensity of main ischemic threat, the type of arterial pathology, the remnant upstream arterial trunks and collaterals, and the elapsed interval to prompt debridement and revascularization, play a pivotal role in any arterial ulcer progress [30, 33, 36, 40].

Daily vascular practice proves that interventionists are more likely confronted with patients exhibiting more than one *long acting* adverse factors for tissue healing [39, 40]. These conditions can be summarized as malnutrition and hypoalbuminemia, lack of compensatory arterial collateral network, diminished arterio- and angiogenesis, peripheral edemas enhancing local compartmental syndromes, low cardiac output, and prolonged bony prominences pressure that collectively contribute as notable interferences in physiological cicatrization [34, 35, 37, 40].

4.4. Current CLI diagnostic: can we effectively assess the real ischemic burden?

A series of high-performance technologies conceived to assess tissue-related arterial disease were introduced in the last two decades. These methods afford high or low invasiveness and focus on different targets in evaluating CLI hemodynamic and tissue changes [29, 30]. With each passing year, novel or modernized diagnostic techniques strive for accurately scoring the degree of perfusion tissue impairment in mixed series of patients and arterial pathologies [1, 2, 27–32].

It has been showed that first *detailed clinical assessment* of each tissue defect is mandatory in all presentations [36, 38, 39, 40]. Basic characteristics of each ulcer (surface and depth), its precise location(s), and the appended inflammatory extensions before and after revascularization should be carefully analyzed and scored by trained clinical teams [38, 39].

The majority of available diagnostic techniques can be roughly divided into *macro-* and *microcirculatory* investigation tools. Some "routine" *noninvasive macro-vascular exams* such as the ankle-brachial index (ABI < 0.5, severe ischemia), the toe-brachial index (TBI < 0.7, presence of PAD), the ankle and toe pressure (<40 mm Hg, threat of the limb), the exercise stress testing, and the Doppler and Duplex assessments are well-documented and own undeniable benefits, and drawbacks [33–35, 37, 39]. Meticulous Doppler evaluation avails real usefulness for knowledgeable clinicians in determining antegrade versus retrograde tibial, pedal, or collateral flow toward the wound zone [24, 39]. It may also yield helpful information over the remnant "large caliber" collaterals in the targeted foot ischemic area [24, 35, 39]. A precise mapping of lower limb arteries specifying eventual stenosis, occlusions, and secondary collateral flow represents a valuable *preoperative* or *follow-up* guide for any interventionist in planning wound-directed revascularization [39].

Other low-invasiveness techniques for detecting "large" arteries and collaterals include last-generation multislice computed tomographic angiography (CTA with "Dual energy") and the magnetic resonance angiography (MRA adding "BOLD sequences") [33, 39]. The "Dual energy" CTA imaging represents a current evaluation method in our team experience for patients with normal renal function. This technology allows accurate calcific plaques removal in tibial and foot vessels and provides a true BTK "lumenograms" in these patients [39].

Despite notable progress in both techniques, these two methods host similar iodine or gadolinium-based contrast disadvantages, being contraindicated in allergic patients or for those suffering from chronic renal insufficiency [33, 39].

Unfortunately, in the daily clinical practice, most of diabetic or renal CLI patients with threatening foot ulcers often associate advanced nephropathy that challenges the use of Iodine or Gadolinium contrast agents.

Probably the most accustomed *macro-circulatory* yet *invasive* available test is represented by the digital subtraction arteriography (DSA) of the inferior limb arteries [1, 3, 28, 38].

DSA is currently recognized as a "key exam" in accurate ischemic flow assessment and classification [1–3, 38, 39]. It is cited to afford best available spatial resolution required to establish main arterial trunks and collaterals (>500 μm diameter) morphological details toward the wound zone [1, 3, 27, 35, 38]. DSA also enables appropriate diagnostic for eventual anatomical variables and their collateral network in each specific arterial pattern [1, 27, 35]. This *quantitative* information becomes essential in understanding individual vascular anatomy for performing eventual *direct* (wound targeted) or *indirect* (collateral supported) arterial revascularization to the wound zone [24–26, 39]. Peripheral angiography consequently helps in determining the most appropriate and "feasible" target vessel to be treated [23–26, 35].

It is shown that DSA affords the interventionist valuable *qualitative* information about *the severity* of distal leg ischemia (the "desert" foot presentation). It also provides accurate characteristics of run-off vessels, the integrity of foot arches, and clues about potential technical difficulties in long chronic total occlusions (CTO) recanalization (the presence of concave/convex atherosclerotic caps) [1, 21, 29, 39]. This technology provides corresponding information about extensive calcifications, tortuosities, and available arterial-arterial communicants or "blush" irrigation around the ulcer's zone [25, 26, 31, 35, 39]. Inasmuch DSA bears evoked drawbacks due to iodine contrast (allergic or renal failure reactions), it also carries the eventual access-related risk for hemorrhagic complications (0.8–3% of cases) [27, 33, 39].

Modern wound practitioners equally avail latest *micro-vascular noninvasive* diagnostic technology, with soaring applications in the last two decades. Among these methods, some showed promising results such as the consecrated transcutaneous oxygen pressure [1–3, 33, 39]; the novel vascular optical tomographic imaging (VOTI) [41]; the "real-time" Laser-Doppler skin perfusion pressure [33, 35, 39]; the continuous tissue oxygen saturation foot-mapping (StO$_2$); and the recent ^{99m}Tc Scintigraphic, the PET, and the single-photon emission computed tomography (SPECT) scans (owning specific CLI 3-D detection at molecular level) [35, 39]. Parallel *microcirculatory* yet, more *invasive* exploration was recently documented gathering intraoperative "Indocyanine green" angiography (ICGA) [42, 43], the "Indigo Carmine" angiography [44], and the foot "micro-oxygen sensors" (MOXYs) technology, all with encouraging applications during wound-targeted revascularization [45].

4.5. The CLI multimodal approach: a novel contemporary concern

Bell et al. first proposed the notion of critical limb ischemia in 1982 for defining severe arterial flow deprivation that currently inflicts major limb amputation threat [46]. In their original publication, the authors characterize CLI essentially on *macro-vascular hemodynamic criteria*, such as the measured AP <40 mm Hg in the presence of rest pain and <60 mm Hg when tissue necrosis is noted [46]. It should be mentioned that in the original form of this concept, the diabetic group of CLI patients was deliberately excluded since neuropathy and infection are often associated and make more complex real ischemic stratification [46]. During the next 30 years, the term of CLI was broadly, yet most of the times inappropriately, used [29–32, 47] as to characterize a much larger hierarchy of severe arterial presentations, including diabetic and renal subjects [27, 30, 46–49]. Although the particular threshold from "reversible" to "irrecoverable" limb ischemia still dwells imprecise [27, 29, 31, 34], it is accepted that CLI often implies a poor limb outcome without prompt revascularization [1–3, 27, 30, 46, 47]. An eloquent 1527 CLI subjects review analysis recently performed by Abu Dabrh et al. on the natural history of untreated "severe" or "critical" ischemic limbs revealed 22% all-cause mortality, 22% major amputation, and 35% worsening in wound evolution rates at 1 year [48]. The almost similar observation was reported in 2016 by Vallabhaneni et al. in a 443 CLI cohort assembling more than 60% diabetics and 20% dialyzed patients [49]. They found 32 and 56% mortality rate at 1 and 3 years, respectively, and 24 and 31% major amputation rates at the same time intervals [49]. The authors conclude that not all patients were encompassing current ABI- and TBI-accepted CLI *macro-vascular* criteria, obviously are at high risk for major amputation [49].

We know nowadays that CLI associates a modest quality of life to the high rate of major amputations and that about 60% of mortality is documented between 3 and 5 years following the initial diagnostic [1–3, 32, 46, 47–49].

Parallel papers focusing on equivalent *macro-vascular* hemodynamic standards (ABI, TBI, AP, TP, etc.), equally fail to explain this huge heterogeneity encountered in CLI "limb salvage" and dedicated treatments [47–49]. Struggling to provide more accurate CLI categorization, several conspicuous classifications systems were proposed in the last two decades [1, 3, 30, 47].

Owning the Bollinger angiographic scale [50], the Trans-Atlantic Inter-Society initial Consensus (TASC I and II) [3, 51], the Rutherford staging of PAD [52], and the European recommendations for CLI management [53], complementary definitions yet adding only TcPO$_2$ *microcirculatory* references were settled [27, 47, 53].

In the recent years, novel PAD classification systems were developed alike the Graziani morphologic arteriographic indexation in diabetics [54], the Toursarkissian angiographic scoring for distal limb salvage bypass [55], and the "Jenali" tibial run-off classification system, with appended below-the-knee intervention protocol [56]. This latest is based on three grades for main infragenicular arterial trunks fluency associating three levels of time-related collaterally filling (at 3–6–9 s) [56].

Undoubtedly, all abovementioned iconographic scoring systems excel in meticulous angiographic anatomy analysis, yet only partially address concomitant wound index or baseline *microcirculatory* perfusion status [30, 39].

Despite real efforts in stratifying CLI intimate mechanisms, to date, all evoked classifications add a little emphasis on coupled *macro-* and *microcirculatory* evaluation, including individual wound characteristics [30, 39].

They also fail to quantify eventual threshold [47] below which inferior limb perfusion becomes nonviable without opportune revascularization [27–30, 47]. The risk of developing CLI and ischemic wounds seems considerably increased in diabetic patients, although prone to more frequently endure systemic ischemic events compared to general population [3, 27, 31].

Contemporary clinical expertise allows better knowledge over the multifaceted "Diabetic Foot Syndrome" (DFS) presentation that gathers arteriopathy, neuropathy, sepsis, pressure injuries, and cellular and molecular metabolic disturbances, in myriads of different clinical archetypes [31, 57]. A vehement need for more specific CLI delineation in these patients was increasingly recollected in modern vascular literature.

4.6. Does healing process in diabetics follow same predictable "standards" alike other CLI patients?

Soaring progress in arterial ulcers treatment is however confronted with an exponentially increasing number of diabetic CLI subjects each year [1, 31]. To date, the prevalence of purely neuropathic, ischemic, and combined neuro-ischemic foot ulcers in patients with diabetes was estimated at 35, 15, and 50% rates, respectively [57–59].

Reported DFS singularities include (1) the regular tibial trunks *calcifications* [2, 30, 31, 57] that match the extent of local neuropathy [25, 31], (2) the "end-artery occlusive disease" (EAOD) concept [59], (3) an impaired *arterio-* and *angiogenesis* [60], (4) a specific *collateral deprivation* following chronic inflammation and septic thrombosis of small vessels [31, 35, 57–59], (5) intrinsic vascular or *matrix impaired regeneration* [61], and (6) characteristic neuro-ischemic *compartmental hyper pressure* foot syndromes [62].

The EAOD theory emphasizes that in the collateral-depleted diabetic limb, "each millimeter of skin" up to the "entire foot" may rely upon one particular artery with *terminal* distribution [59], while this valuable vessel may be auspiciously targeted by "wound directed" revascularization, according to the angiosome concept [24–26].

Modern diabetic ulcer understanding builds a complete design of multifaceted and potentially devastating CLI effects in these patients [2, 31, 57–62].

Enthralling scientific works in the last decade evoke a possible central mechanism playing a pivotal role in different DFS pathological changes [59, 63]. Thus, chronic hyperglycemia may enhance at the mitochondrial-level expanded free radicals production, altering normal metabolic and cellular activity [63]. This malfunction affects more particularly normal regeneration at the *microcirculatory* level (vasa-vasorum and vasa-nervorum) also the tissue binding matrix [58, 59–61].

Arteriopathy and neuropathy, albeit regular DFS features (in different proportions) [58, 59], may probably share the same pathological emergence in the vast diabetic complications puzzle [57–59, 63].

Trying to stratify main DFS characteristics, a few classification systems were proposed. It should be mentioned the "Wagner" stratification [64], the PEDIS (perfusion, extent/size, depth/tissue loss, infection, sensation/neuropathy) [65], the University of Texas (UT) [66], the sepsis, arteriopathy, denervation (SAD) scale [67], the diabetic ulcer severity score (DUSS) [68], the multiple ulceration, wound area, pedal pulse, and ulcer duration (MAID) classification [69], and the "St. Elian wound score system" [70], rejoicing unanimously recognized popularity and documented clinical benefits [57–59].

However, most of these classifications fail to provide concomitant *perfusion* information [35, 47]; individual *ulcer features* [47]; *infection, denervation,* or *gangrene* specifications [47]; systemic factors report [2, 30] (Section 4.5); and healing prognosis [2, 10, 47]. All these clinical entities seem to bear a huge interest in healing evaluation [2, 31, 37, 39].

In same effort to fully perceive each DFS presentation, the remarkable WIfI classification [47] recently brought together Wound grades, Ischemia levels, and foot Infection ranked in a unitary view, as important variables for appended wound prognosis [47]. However, diabetic neuropathy [36, 58, 71] and concurrent systemic variables influencing tissue recovery [57, 61, 72] are not included in this model of examination. In a parallel analysis, owing a consecutive 249 CLI wounds series, Azuma et al. [72] found that beyond diabetes (including neuropathy and infection), equally end-stage renal disease (ESRD), Rutherford category 6 (including or not the heel), and low albumin levels, represented significant factors in the complex tissue recovery cascade beyond prompt revascularization [72].

5. Contemporary landmarks in ischemic wounds revascularization

Expanding clinical evidence in the last three decades supports both bypass and the endovascular techniques as useful strategies in CLI revascularization [1–3, 29–31]. Providing low invasiveness, high reproducibility, and comparable limb salvage rate to open surgery [21–73], transcatheter strategies continue to evolve with new low-profile and high-performance devices in arterial reconstruction [21, 29, 74]. For most "high-risk" CLI patients [1, 2, 31, 34], new endovascular approaches and techniques were designed. In succinct overview, the "drilling," the "subintimal," or the "parallel wire" techniques via the ante- or retrograde accesses, the pedal-plantar "loop," and the femoral-femoral or transtibial collaterals angioplasties were recently described [29, 74, 75].

Not with standing with these spectacular transcatheter performances, the "classical" bypass for distal leg reperfusion is still imposed as a fundamental technique for CLI diabetic foot revascularization, tissue healing, and limb preservation [1, 3, 72, 76]. High-skill distal vein bypasses to the tibial [72], to the pedal [77], and up to the plantar or tarsal foot arteries [78] equally by targeting remote branches of pedal arteries in some particular cases [1, 76] were successfully documented. We now know that both surgical and endovascular techniques are more likely complementary than competitive techniques since each of them holds major advantages and inherent drawbacks [1, 29, 30, 79]. Endovascular techniques essentially provide minimal invasiveness, great accessibility, and reproducibility for one or multiple below-the-knee CTO recanalizations [1, 29, 73–75]. Alternatively, bypass offers a higher pressure on targeted arteries and more physiological and pulsatile flow inside collaterals around the wound zone [35, 53, 77–79]. This particularity heightens arterial-arterial collateral shear stress and enhances rising arteriogenesis [58–60] toward further tissue cicatrization [1, 29, 35, 60, 72].

Although still heterogeneously structured [1, 73, 79], increasing contemporary clinical observation documents equivalent limb salvage, clinical success, and survival outcomes for bypass versus endoluminal interventions in selected groups of CLI patients [1–3, 27, 29–31, 79, 80]. Notwithstanding with initial historical considerations [79], these two strategies appear nowadays more intricate than ever inside the conceptualized "team approach" as CLI treatment [29, 35].

Parallel advances concerning the DFS revascularization and ischemic wound healing were equally testified in the last two decades [1, 2, 75]. Beyond striking surgical arterial reconstructions [76–79], new tapered nitinol [81], drug-eluting stents (DES) [82], and original drug-eluting balloon, (DEB) [83] were imagined. Novel or redesigned directional or rotational atherectomy devices [84], together with latest "bioresorbable scaffolds" technologies [85], represent few additional of numerous achievements that challenge today ancient technical barriers [1, 29, 75, 81–86].

6. New strategies for "wound targeted revascularization"

The complex cascade of tissue regeneration needs precise circumstances to unfold [85]. Beyond high-performance techniques in reconstructing arterial flow [72–86], new strategies about "when" and "where" to perform appropriate revascularization emerge today [1, 27, 30, 35]. Contemporary practitioners equally avail key data on the molecular mechanisms generating ischemic threat and tissue regeneration [59–61]. This knowledge, part of a larger "integrated multidisciplinary medicine" [87, 88], supports new strategies in limb salvage [1, 29, 48] based on precise arterial flow mapping [23–26] and deliberate tissue healing reengineering [29–31]. A new conceptualization of ischemic wound treatment rises at present [1, 2, 33], with promising serviceableness in patient's stratification [47, 53, 57, 59], revascularization selection [35, 38], and dedicated postoperative follow-up [31].

According to this modern emphasis, novel "hybrid" surgical and endovascular techniques [89], synchronous ante- and retrograde arterial accesses [74, 90], and novel topographic "wound-directed" revascularization (WDR) [24, 35, 91–93] proved useful to save more limbs for major amputation. Alternatively, extreme venous limb arterialization [94, 95] and cell stem treatment [1, 29] parallel to rising "multidisciplinary team" practice [57, 87, 88] have also been developed and seem to revolutionize previous CLI paradigms of care [1, 29, 92–94].

6.1. The "angiosome concept" in ischemic wound healing: a succinct overview

Among all innovative strategies in CLI wound treatment, a remarkable leap was undoubtedly marked by *topographic*, or intentional, *wound directed* arterial reconstruction [23–26, 35, 72, 91–93]. This theory represents a unique clinical application of the *angiosome concept* initially pioneered in 1987 by Taylor et al. in the plastic reconstructive surgery field [23].

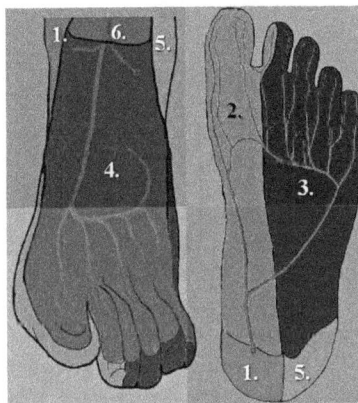

Figure 1. A schematic anatomic representation of the six angiosomes of the lower leg in a forefoot/hindfoot topographic view. (**1**) The *medial calcaneal* angiosome (from the posterior tibial artery). (**2**) The *medial plantar* angiosome (posterior tibial artery). (**3**) The *lateral plantar* angiosome (posterior tibial artery). (**4**) The *dorsalis pedis* angiosome (from the anterior tibial artery). (**5**) The *lateral calcaneal* angiosome (from the peroneal artery). (**6**) The *antero-lateral malleolar* angiosome (currently from the anterior tibial, also from the perforator branch of the peroneal artery).

The angiosome conceptualization describes more than 44 specific 3-D *tissue sectors* of the human body nourished by individual arterio-venous bundles called "the angiosomes" [23]. This anatomical representation was further referred to CLI treatment two decades later by Attinger et al. [24], owning encouraging clinical results.

The lower leg angiosome territories. The following skin and underlying tissue zones were earlier described as to nearly encompass six main *angiosomes* (**Figure 1**) of the foot and ankle [23–26, 91–93]:

- The *medial calcaneal* and appended *medial* and *lateral plantar* arteries angiosomes arising all from the *posterior tibial artery*. They supply the entire plantar heel and the medial and lateral plantar surface to the toes.

- The *dorsalis pedis* angiosome, downstream to the *anterior tibial artery* that nourishes the dorsal foot and toes areas, also ensures the upper and anterior peri-malleolar vascularization.

- The *lateral calcaneal artery* angiosome branching from the *peroneal artery* and that supplies the lateral, plantar heel.

- At a higher level of the superior ankle, other angiosomes were described, such as *the antero-lateral malleolar* owning its correspondent *antero-medial malleolar* angiosomes (both from the *anterior tibial artery*), and the *pstero-medial malleolar* angiosome following correspondent branch from the *posterior tibial artery*, respectively [23–26, 91–93].

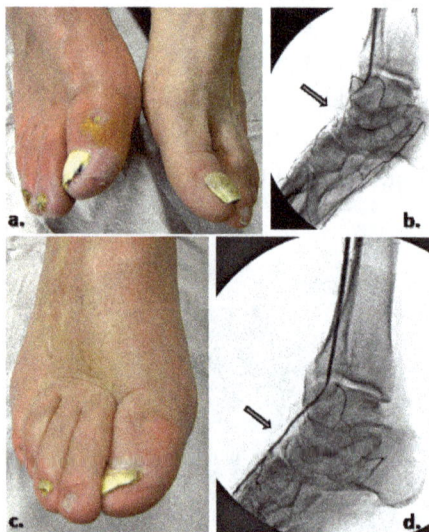

Figure 2. A diabetic neuro-ischemic ulcer associating cutaneous sepsis on the antero-medial aspect of the foot. (**a**) The initial clinical aspect (CLI, Rutherford 5). (**b**) The appended angiographic aspect showing complete occlusions of the dorsalis pedis and distal posterior tibial artery. (**c**) Healing aspect at three months, following (**d**) angiosome-targeted revascularization by deliberately opening the dorsalis pedis artery territory (arrow).

These vascular territories are closely interconnected by numerous *arterial-arterial* communicants [23, 24], whose caliber and density are strongly influenced by the age of patients, by each region's anatomy and by the manifest arterial disease triggering CLI [24, 35, 72, 96–98]. Every individual collateral system essentially assists blood supply between neighboring angiosomes. These compensatory branches the so-called "choke vessels" include *large-*, *middle-*, and *small-*sized arterial-arterial communicants, beyond the arterioles and capillary vessels in a vast "compensatory arterial foot network" [24, 29, 35]. All collateral interconnections between adjacent angiosomes are submitted to specific hemodynamic influences related to local *arterio*genesis and *angio*genesis processes [35, 59, 60].

The angiosome clinical model implies a conspicuous vascular anatomical order, although subject to specific pathophysiological changes in every CLI individual pattern. Optimal *wound-targeted revascularization* probably means correct angiosome-related anatomical evaluation associated with individual collateral-related pathophysiological judgment for each CLI presentation [30].

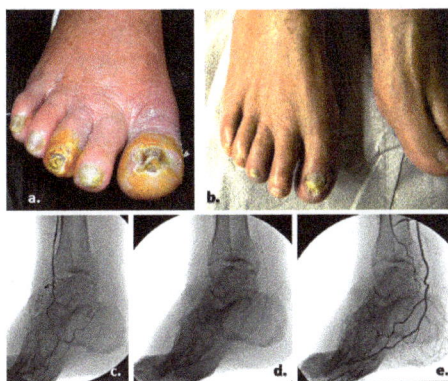

Figure 3. Wound-targeted revascularization for severe forefoot sepsis and tissue necrosis, extending to the plantar side of the hallux and toes. (**a**) The initial clinical aspect (CLI, Rutherford 5). (**b**) Healing after topographic revascularization and multidisciplinary team care at five months. (**c**) The starting angiographic image showing complete posterior tibial artery occlusion (the dominant wound territory), and the dorsalis pedis thrombosis. We can remark only a few remnant collaterals (the characteristic diabetic foot collateral deprivation) represented by two lasting diagonal arteries. (**d**) Endovascular plantar angiosomes-targeted revascularization by posterior tibial artery intentional reopening. (**e**) The end-procedural result showing the posterior tibial, the plantar arteries, and the plantar arch reperfusion in an intentional wound-directed revascularization.

In young subjects with unaltered collateral network possible post-traumatic or ischemic injuries activate unmitigated "choke vessels" that warrant (at some point) effective compensatory blood pressure between adjacent angiosomes [24, 39, 96, 97]. Atherosclerotic, inflammatory, or local thrombotic conditions may alter this unique natural compensatory system. As previously described [23, 24], the foot angiosomes are 3-D dynamic and continuously interacting structures [30]. Although their primary anatomical distribution seems accurately reproduced in more than 90% of subjects (owing 6–9% eventual anatomival variants) [23, 24, 26, 91], their interconnections ("choke vessels") are yet submitted to continuous changes, according to each type of CLI pathology [72, 95–98].

Assessing and treating ischemic wounds in the light of the angiosome theory imposes a flexible reflection upon *how* utilizing the remnant arterial-arterial connections (**Figures 2** and **3**) at best flow benefit for the patient [88, 97].

6.2. What group of ischemic ulcers may need WDR?

Inasmuch genetic collateral network warrants a remarkable "rescue system" in non-athero-sclerotic patients, it can be dramatically hindered in specific diabetic or uremic ischemic wounds [24, 35, 72, 96–98]. The interventionist should be aware of treating peculiar diabetic and ESRD *ischemic ulcers*, for that these patients may hide huge collateral decay and poor arterial-arterial connections among adjacent foot angiosomes [72, 97]. Eventual *indirect* [26] or *nonspecific* revascularization [25, 93] in these subjects may fail to afford correct arterial flow to the wound by a lack of collateral resources [25, 59, 72, 96].

Alternatively, the use of WDR principle in these cases seems to provide improved healing results [24, 39, 72, 96–98] owning scrupulous *macro-* and *microcirculatory* evaluation, planning for intervention and follow-up [39, 96, 97].

Despite encouraging tissue healing and limb salvage results for both, bypass and endovascular treatment [24–26, 91–93], uncertainty still dwells concerning the utility of angiosome-oriented revascularization in specific CLI groups of patients dysplaying different etiologies of arterial disease [35, 72, 96, 97]. Growing clinical expertise, however, seems to support WDR in "low-collateral" CLI patients such as those presenting DFS (**Figures 2** and **3**), or ESRD ischemic wounds [72, 91–93, 96–98].

6.3. Does topographic WDR allow unrestricted anatomical applications?

The angiosome-oriented revascularization theoretically offers superior chances for healing in selected ischemic wounds, yet this theory still awaits for further prospective validation in larger groups of equivalent CLI patients [92, 97].

Lower limb topographic anatomy addressed to date unnumbered ex vivo or clinical works [99–102] (most of them in the last 50 years) and their analysis largely overpasses the purposes of this chapter. However, some compelling points should be probably mentioned for better picturing this impressive graduation in the distribution of the arterial tree toward the target tissue [35, 101, 102]. The whole body vasculature can be delineated from a "fractal" point of view, as harmonious repetitive patterns of peripheral tissue irrigation [35, 101]. Particularly concerning the inferior limb vascularization, this archetype evinces some specific *levels of irrigation* [35]. A primary *level I* of perfusion contains the main arterial and venous bundles (i.e. iliac and common femoral), the *level II* gathers first rank arterial branches in the thigh and calf (i.e. the superficial and profonda femoris and the three tibial trunks), and the next *level III* features distinct ramifications for *specific skin and underlying tissue zones* in the foot [35]. This level also encompasses the *large* collaterals (around 1 mm diameter), including *the angiosomes branches*, the appended *foot arches*, and the *metatarsal perforators* [24, 35, 101], yielding specific interest in topographic revascularization [23–26, 35, 93, 100]. The next *level IV* holds the *medium-* and *small*-size (<0.5 mm) collaterals, while next microcirculatory ranks assemble *level V* that gathers *the arterioles* and the *level VI* connecting the *capillary* tier (around 8-μm diameter) [39, 101, 103]. This latest convenes several millions of small micrometric conduits in the whole human body, approximating 60,000 miles of estimated length [102].

Another parallel and more common anatomical partition used in CLI literature roughly distinguishes the *macrocirculatory* rank (that embodies previous *levels I–IV*) from the *microcirculatory* level (equivalent to other *levels V* and *VI*) of limb perfusion [1, 27, 29, 30, 103–106]. By bridging these two levels, the *medium* and *small* muscular arteries and adjacent *arterioles* contribute to a continuous *pacing system* of local tissular perfusion [103–105]. Since CLI threat appears, this function seems to be notably distorted until focused revascularization is applied [25, 60, 106].

According to the above considerations, several anatomical variants were equally described, mainly concerning level III of limb flow distribution [104, 105]. Following two recent meta-analysis gathering 7671 [107] or 5790 inferior limbs [108], and two "in vivo" analogous angiographic observations [109, 110], *native atypical leg arteries* were described in utmost 7.9–10% individuals out of general population [107–110]. Among these variants, hypoplastic or aplastic posterior tibial artery was encountered in 3.3% cases, whereas the anterior tibial trunk was absent in about 1.5% of instances [108]. The presence of highly emergent anterior tibial artery or irregular tibial trifurcation was described in 5.6–6% cases [109–110], while anomalous origins of the dorsalis pedis artery were encountered in 4.3–6% presentations [109, 111]. Aberrant first dorsal metatarsal artery and appended first toe dominant irrigation was described in 8.1% cases [112], parallel variants of the arcuate artery in 5% [113], and modified courses of the plantar arch and plantar arteries in 5% of presentations [114]. The intimate knowledge of these variants seems significant for the advised interventionist since *wound-directed revascularization* is planned [30, 100]. The presence of one anatomical popliteal variation (i.e. high origin of the anterior tibial trunk) on one side may indicate possible ipsilateral foot vessel abnormalities in about 21% of cases [107, 109], and similar contralateral leg variants in 48% of instances [109, 110]. Concomitant *acquired arterial flow disturbances* were also cited in lower leg ischemic presentations, most of them accompanying the diabetic neuro-ischemic foot syndrome [34, 53, 59]. The majority of these anomalies were represented by occlusions of at least two or all tibial arteries in more than 70% of CLI diabetic subjects [110, 115]. A higher prevalence of long (>15 cm) obstructions in the posterior tibial and plantar arteries [25, 116, 117] and extensive (type II) calcifications [25, 91] in most diabetic calf and foot arterial segments were also demonstrated [91]. Our group experience over 232 diabetic CLI limbs [91] with Wagner grade 2–4 foot wounds [64] availing *angiosome-targeted* revascularization [24, 96–98], also confirmed more frequent posterior tibial atherosclerotic occlusive disease (68% of cases versus 25% anterior tibial and 7% peroneal presentations) [91]. Moreover, the posterior tibial hypoperfusion showed significant (>90%) concordance with distinct plantar, heel and forefoot (on the plantar side) skin, and adjacent tissue trophic lesions [25–91].

Although precise below-the-knee arterial *anatomical knowledge* is of paramount importance in planning "angiosome-directed" revascularization [91–93], the skilled interventionist should also corroborate additional *hemodynamic information* enabled by each collateral pattern [24, 93, 96–98, 118].

Even in the presence of unusual anatomical variants to supply the foot, topographic revascularization still appears feasible [39] by taking advantage either on visible or on unmasked arterial branches (the "dormant" collaterals) that gradually reveal during CTO recanalization [24, 35, 56].

It becomes clearer that since all tibial trunks become occluded, the tipping point between hypoxic tissue regeneration versus chronic ulceration and necrosis hinges upon *the remnant individual collateral reserve* and ways to deliberately use it in addressing the ischemic threat [24, 30, 34, 59].

Despite encouraging results to date [91–93, 96], the angiosome concept may provide better, yet not complete, ischemic tissue control [35, 61, 72, 118].

Topographic WDR for ulcer healing remains an enthralling subject of discussion. Certainly, alike similar new openings of flourishing interest in tissue regeneration, the scarcer the available evidence, the acrider the current debate, mostly based on heterogeneous retrospective deliberations [35, 72, 92, 96–98, 118].

7. The state of foot collaterals: a key principle in modern CLI wound treatment

The TASC II recommendation [3] for prompt revascularization in CLI is generally accepted [1, 27], however, do all these interventions address similar extent of ischemic threat? Do all these interventions bear then, equivalent expectations for tissue recovery? [49] More concretely, does the modern vascular interventionist truly control all hemodynamic *macro-* and *microvascular* changes at the wound level while performing CLI revascularization? [49, 61, 97] Up-to-date research reveals that not all proven lower limb ischemic ulcers share the same TASC II/CLI criteria [3] and, consequently, harbor the corresponding amount of ischemic burden! [2, 31, 49, 61, 118, 119] Owning steady improvement in diagnostic and treatment, modern practitioners start to adapt current CLI standards to each type of arterial pathology [1, 35, 73, 107], and to resize ischemic ulcer appraisal in deeper *macro-* and *microcirculatory* perception [39, 59–61, 97, 106]. The contemporary medical community is now facing *a novel* challenge wherein specific strategies for revascularization in CLI patients *with* and *without* a convenient foot *collateral network* [92, 96–100, 119]. Thorough research in diabetic CLI treatment had already evinced good tissue cicatrization since topographic revascularization is performed in subjects having a poor collateral reserve [26, 92, 96–100, 119]. It is known that DFS currently alter common foot cutaneous, the underlying tissue and bony presentation, by iterative inflammation, scars, ischemic necrosis, sensorimotor neuropathy, and local pressure aggressions [57–60]. Even though that CLI/DFS severely distorts the "classically pictured" angiosomal foot vasculature [23–25, 96–98], *wound-targeted revascularization* using the *surviving collateral system* represents a valuable solution for better tissue regeneration [92, 96–100, 119].

Today's evidence suggests that both *macro-* and *microcirculation* evaluation should be routinely considered in each ischemic ulcer presentation toward deeper CLI understanding, as a whole limb circulatory pattern [39, 105].

7.1. Compensatory *collateral systems* relying the foot angiosomes and derived wound healing implications

An impressive compensatory collateral network interconnecting neighboring foot and ankle angiosomes was thoroughly documented by previous publications [23, 24, 101, 102], available as to counterbalance any possible ischemic threat [23, 24, 98].

The central *arterial-arterial* communicants relying upon different leg angiosomes encompass numerous *small* to *large* collaterals (the above-described *levels III and IV*), beyond the arterioles (*level V*) in a sequential model of perfusion [35, 101]. Numerous "large" foot collaterals hold particular importance in supplying adjacent angiosomes [24, 39, 118]. They also seem to play a pivotal role in intentional "wound-directed" revascularization and appropriate tissue regeneration [35, 96–98, 118]. These vessels assemble the *foot arches*, (acknowledging eventual 5–9% anatomical variations, Section 6.3) [108–114], the *metatarsal perforators*, the anterior *communicants*, and other sizable *arterial-arterial* branches such as the dorsal foot-to-plantar, or the peroneal-to-posterior tibial *rescue* heel collaterals (*level III* of perfusion) [35, 101].

In the same design, yet with narrow compensatory significance (Section 6.3), the *medium-* and *small*-sized muscular collateral arteries (*level IV*) [35] and *the arterioles (level V)*, also contribute in vital tissue flow preservation [103, 105, 106]. These "rescue" connections were also implicated in the "initiatory" phase of revascularization (Section 4.1) [35, 105] and actively partake throughout the vast "choke vessels" salvage system [23, 24], before or during the angio- and arteriogenesis processes [104–106]. Regardless individual variations, the following groups of arterial-arterial collateral connections were appointed in CLI flow compensation [24, 35, 39, 102, 118]:

- The communications between the posterior tibial and peroneal arteries (via the *medial* and *lateral calcaneal branches*, also via the *posterior peroneal branch*) play an important role in *ischemic heel ulcers* supply, equally for targeted hind foot or heel intentional revascularization [24, 72, 96–98].

- The connections between the *anterior* (dorsalis pedis) and the *posterior tibial* (plantar) arteries. These branches ensure either directly via diagonal arteries or following the first *metatarsal perforators* or through the metatarsal *paired anterior* and *posterior inter-digital collaterals*, a significant compensation in *forefoot* and *toes ischemic tissue* flow preservation and eventual tarsal/metatarsal reperfusion [24, 35].

- The arterial compensation around the *peri-malleolar wounds* is reinforced by the *lateral peri-malleolar anastomoses* linking the peroneal artery (via the *anterior perforating branch*) with the anterior tibial trunk (via the *antero-lateral malleolar branch*). Following similar, but more medial connections, *the medial peri-malleolar network* (sharing similar *medial malleolar branches* from the anterior and posterior tibial arteries) represent complementarily, yet distinct, pathways for blood compensation in the ankle [24, 35].

- The communicants between *both plantar arteries* (medial and lateral, from the posterior tibial artery) and the *lateral and medial tarsal arteries* (via the anterior tibial artery) seem to enable influential compensatory flow to eventual *plantar ischemic wounds* [24, 35, 39].

All these briefly schematized *arterial-arterial* communications constitute but a small part of the whole natural foot compensatory system against ischemic aggression [23, 24, 35]. Although severely compromised in distinct CLI categories of patients (diabetes, ESRD, and inflammatory arteritis) [59–61, 104], all these "rescue branches" [35, 59, 101, 102] or "choke-vessels" [23, 24] provide noticeable flow assistance during miscellaneous ischemic injuries. Their appropriate evaluation affords valuable diagnostic and therapeutic knowledge for better tissue preservation and limb salvage [39, 56–59].

In this exhaustive "regional view" of ischemic tissue perfusion, albeit more precise than blunt angiographic assessment (Section 4.5), it appears that *not all foot areas may express similar ischemic affliction* [59–61, 104]. Even more surprisingly, the ulcer's area could not always stand for the lowest perfusion point in the ischemic limb, since severe neuropathy, inflammatory swelling, sepsis, and local skin trauma may add complementary hindrance to main CLI threat [26, 27, 31, 33].

Future diagnostic tools focusing on *superficial* and *deep* tissue "wound-oriented" arterial flow may eventually complete this unique holistic view of the neuro-ischemic diabetic foot [33, 39, 53, 59].

We know today that diabetic and renal CLI patients express serious tissue regeneration handicap, inflicted by specific infragenicular arterial collateral depletion [29–31]. This significant decay in tissue regeneration also appears proportionate with the *type* and *time* of ischemic suffering [1, 2, 27, 30, 59]. In this perspective, recent researchers advise reasonable adaptation of current revascularization indications upon individual *macro* [3, 41] and *microvascular* CLI characteristics [29–31, 39], weighted in patients *with* and *without* available collateral reserve [29, 39, 59].

8. The essential role of multidisciplinary approach in ischemic ulcer healing

Increasing clinical evidence suggests that despite "well-suited" revascularization efforts, at least 25% of DFS ulcers will eventually not heal, and around 28% may end however with some form of amputation [58, 120].

It appears unmistakable that no current *single* therapy can enhance *alone* profitable healing results in a majority of CLI ulcers [1, 27, 58] without concomitant management of all risk factors, including ischemic, metabolic, septic, local pressure, neuropathic, and adequate off-loading appointed treatment [1–3, 120–123]. Wound healing embodies a complex cascade of molecular and clinical events in continuous dynamic interaction [34, 48]. It was stated that because CLI wound etiology is always multidimensional [1, 27, 58], specific therapy in turns requires a parallel multidisciplinary application [1–3, 120, 121].

Every individual risk factor requires accurate identification and management and represents a fundamental task for any multidisciplinary wound center to encourage [124]. Investing *healing* as the primary endpoint in care acts as a real benchmark for all collective therapeutic efforts [57, 87, 124].

The recent guidelines document of the Society for Vascular Surgery connecting with the American Podiatric Medical Association and the Society for Vascular Medicine acts as a great reference to current evidence of ischemic wound treatment [120]. This noteworthy analysis addresses best available proofs and guidelines to date on the following main indicators: (1) prevention of diabetic foot ulceration, (2) off-loading, (3) diagnosis of sepsis and foot osteomyelitis, (4) specific wound care, and (5) peripheral arterial disease in DFS [120].

Prevention following evidence-based program includes the patient and the referral General Practitioners (GP) as active members of the multidisciplinary group [120–123]. Knowing that peripheral neuropathy can generate about 45–65% of DFS ulcers, patients with neuropathy hold >3.5-fold complementary risk for iterative neuro-ischemic ulceration [26, 71, 87, 120]. Adequate *laboratory tests* surveillance also represents a critical method as to minimize detrimental obstacles in tissue regeneration [120–123]. It has been recorded that for every additional 1% increase in HbA_1C, there is a 0.028 cm/day healing decay in DFS wounds [120–125]. The major importance of *off-loading* devices in the global healing process is acknowledged [57, 58, 120–122]. Pressure reduction is reputed to allow superior healing effects to any revascularization strategy [2, 57, 58, 120–124]. Early diagnostic and treatment of *foot infection* also have paramount consequences in correct tissue regeneration [2, 57–59, 120–122]. Expeditious *local wound debridement* following timely reevaluation schedule bears huge implications for maintaining tissue viability, parallel to revascularization [57–59]. Since aggressively applied, early debridement can save millimeters of "time-dependent" irreversible damage [2, 57, 58, 61, 87, 120–124].

Appropriate *wound dressing* should help by maintaining a moist wound bed, providing exudate drainage, and urging granulation of tissue defect [53, 57, 120, 126].

The adapted dressing should match each specific CLI pathology, wound features and location, and individual amount of exudates, inflammation, and pain [87, 88, 120, 126].

New *complementary therapies* including negative pressure therapy, living cellular therapy, extracellular matrix products, and hyperbaric oxygen therapy were equally developed in the last years [57, 127]. Their application should follow multidisciplinary team advises [88, 120, 127] in ulcers that fail to demonstrate >50% area reduction per month, using standard therapy [120, 127].

Although revascularization still holds specific postoperative indicators [33, 39], the global efficacy of multidisciplinary approach can be timely rated by percentage reduction in wound extent as an early predictor of clinical success [120, 126]. Wound surface diminution of 10–15% per week, or >50% in 4 weeks strongly suggests increased likelihood of healing and diminished probability for amputation [120, 121, 126].

8.1. Ischemic wound healing as an integrated medicine concept

The contemporary practitioner becomes aware that every ischemic ulcer presentation should be carefully weighted and treated alike *distinct pathological prototype*. It appears reasonable that for every single ulcer puzzling (in various amounts) possible neuropathic, ischemic, hyperglycemic, uremic, venous hypoxic, septic, hypoproteic, or pressure threats, only a multimodal team approach may afford better healing expectations [121–126, 128, 129]. Every chronic ulceration case can be theoretically approached alike a 3-D graphical mold assembling in different proportions of some or the whole of the determinants mentioned above. The vital role of any multidisciplinary team is to decode each clinical presentation into basic pathological influences and treat them upon best available knowledge granted by all participant specialties [121, 123, 126].

9. Conclusions

In treating arterial ulcers it should be remembered that not all foot sectors share same ischemic affectation and that not all patients with comparable *macro*-vascular images bear same collateral reserve and related *micro*-vascular tissue recovery resources.

Contemporary research reveals astonishing multilevel anatomical and physiological intricacy of lower limb blood supply, viewed in a dynamic and time unfolding perspective. This apparent complexity represents but plausible challenges for the experienced interventionist availing high-performance macro and microcirculatory diagnostic and treatment methods for revascularization and tissue healing.

Author details

Vlad-Adrian Alexandrescu[1,2*] and François Triffaux[1]

*Address all correspondence to: v.alex@skynet.be

1 Department of General, Thoracic and Vascular Surgery, Princess Paola Hospital, IFAC/ Vivalia, Marche-en-Famenne, Belgium

2 Department of Cardio-Vascular and Thoracic Surgery, CHU Sart-Tilmant, University of Liège, Liège, Belgium

References

[1] Gulati A, Botnaru I, Garcia LA. Critical limb ischemia and its treatments: a review. *J Cardiovasc Surg (Torino)*. 2015; 56(5): 775–785.

[2] Hinchliffe RJ, Andros G, Apelqvist J, Bakker SF, Friederichs S, et al. A systematic review of the effectiveness of revascularization of the ulcerated foot in patients with diabetes and peripheral disease. *Diabetes Metab Res Rev.* 2012; 28(Suppl. 1): 179–217.

[3] Norgreen L, Hiatt WR, Dormandy JA, Nehler MR, Harris KA, et al. Inter-society consensus for the management of peripheral arterial disease (TASC II). *Eur J Vasc Endovasc Surg.* 2007; 33(Suppl 1): S1–S75.

[4] The Asu (Mesopotamia). In: Majno G: *The Healing Hand. Man and Wound in the Ancient World*, 2nd ed. 1975. Cambridge, MA: Harvard University Press: 30–67.

[5] The Swnw (Egypt). In: Majno G: *The Healing Hand. Man and Wound in the Ancient World*, 2nd ed. 1975. Cambridge, MA: Harvard University Press: 66–138.

[6] Cohen IK. The evolution of wound healing. In: Veves A: *The Diabetic Foot*, 2nd ed. 2006. New Jersey: Humana Press Inc.: 51–57.

[7] Buck AH. The development of surgery in France: Ambroise Parré. In: Buck AH: *The Growth of Medicine: From the Earliest Times to about 1800*. New Haven: Yale University Press; 1917: 499–515.

[8] Lister J. An address on the antiseptic management of wounds. *Br Med J.* 1893; 1(1): 161–162, 277–278.

[9] Wells TS. Some causes of excessive mortality after surgical operation. *Medical Times and Gazette.* 1864; 349–364.

[10] Virchow R. *Cellular Pathology.* 1860. London: John Churchill Ed.: 283–315.

[11] Cohen S. Isolation of a mouse submaxillary gland protein accelerating incisor eruption and eyelid opening in the new-born animal. *J Biol Chem.* 1962; 237: 1555–1562.

[12] Brooks B. Intraarterial injection of sodium iodine. *J Am Med Assoc.* 1024; 84: 1016.

[13] Dos Santos R, Lamas AC, Pereira-Caldas J. Arteriography of abdominal aorta, its branches and inferior limb arteries. *Bull Soc Nat Chir.* 1929; 55: 587.

[14] Strandness DE Jr, McCutcheon EP, Rushmer RF. Application of a transcutaneous Doppler flowmeter in evaluation of occlusive arterial disease. *Surg Gynecol Obstet.* 1966; 122: 1039.

[15] Jens S, Koelemay MJ, Reekers J, Bipat S. Diagnostic performance of computed tomography angiography and contrast-enhanced magnetic resonance angiography in patients with critical limb ischaemia and intermittent claudication: systematic review and meta-analysis. *Eur Radiol.* 2013; 3(11): 3104–3114.

[16] White JC, Smethwick RH. *The autonomic nervous system.* 1944. London: Macmillan Ed.

[17] Dos Santos JC. From embolectomy to endarterectomy or the fall of a myth. *J Cardiovasc Surg.* 1976; 17: 409–411.

[18] Kunlin J. Treatment of arteriopathic ischemia using long venous grafts. *Rev Chir (Paris)*. 1951; 70: 206–235.

[19] Crawford ES, De Bakey ME, Cooley DA, et al. Use of crimped knitted Dacron grafts in patients with occlusive disease of the aorta and of the iliac, femoral and popliteal arteries. In: Wesolowska SA, Denis C. *Fundamentals of Vascular Grafting*. 1963. New York: McGraw Hill: 864–872.

[20] Soyer T, Lempinen M, Cooper P, et al. A new venous prosthesis. *Surgery*. 1972; 72: 864–872.

[21] El-Sayed HF. Endovascular techniques in limb salvage: stents. *Methodist Debakey Cardiovasc J*. 2013; 9(2): 79–83.

[22] Volodos NL. The 30th anniversary of the first clinical application of endovascular stent-grafting. *Eur J Vasc Endovasc Surg*. 2015; 49(5): 495–497.

[23] Taylor GI, Palmer JH. The vascular territories (angiosomes) of the body: experimental studies and clinical applications. *Br J Plast Surg*. 1987; 40: 113–141.

[24] Attinger CE, Evans KK, Bulan E, et al. Angiosomes of the foot and ankle and clinical implications for limb salvage: reconstruction, incisions and revascularization. *Plast Reconstr Surg*. 2006; 117(7 Suppl): 261S–293S.

[25] Alexandrescu V, Hubermont G, Philips Y, et al. Selective angioplasty following an angiosome model of reperfusion in the treatment of Wagner 1-4 diabetic foot lesions: practice in a multidisciplinary diabetic limb service. *J Endovasc Ther*. 2008; 15: 580–593.

[26] Iida O, Nanto S, Uematsu M, et al. Importance of the angiosome concept for endovas-cular therapy in patients with critical limb ischemia. *Catheter Cardiovasc Interv*. 2010; 75: 830–836.

[27] Elsayed S, Clavijo LC. Critical limb ischemia. *Cardiol Clin*. 2015; 33(1): 37–47.

[28] Conte MS, Pomposelli FB, Clair DG, et al. Society for Vascular Surgery practice guidelines for atherosclerotic occlusive disease of the lower extremities: management of asymptomatic disease and claudication. *J Vasc Surg*. 2015; 61(Suppl): 3S–40S.

[29] Chin JA, Sumpio BE. New advances in limb salvage. *Surg Technol Int*. 2014; 25: 212–216.

[30] Alexandrescu V, Letawe A. Critical limb ischemia strategies in diabetics: present deeds and future challenges. *Curr Res Diabetes Obes J*. 2015; 1(1): 553–555.

[31] Marso SP, Hiatt WR. Peripheral arterial disease in patients with diabetes. *J Am Coll Cardiol*. 2006; 47(5): 921–929.

[32] Howell MA, Colgan MP, Seeger RW, et al. Relationship of severity of lower limb peripheral vascular disease to mortality and morbidity: a six-year follow-up study. *J Vasc Surg*. 1989; 9: 691–696.

[33] Doughty DB. Arterial ulcers. In: Bryant RA. *Acute and chronic wounds, current management concepts*. 2012. St. Louis: Elsevier Mosby: 178–194.

[34] Shai A, Maibach H. Natural course of wound repair versus impaired healing in chronic skin ulcers. In: *Wound Healing and Ulcers of the Skin, Diagnosis and Therapy*. 2005. San Francisco: Springer: 7–17.

[35] Alexandrescu VA. The angiosome concept: anatomical background and physiopathological landmarks in CLI. In: *Angiosomes Applications in Critical Limb Ischemia: In Search for Relevance*. 2012. Torino: Ed. Minerva Medica: 1–30, 71–88.

[36] Shai A, Maibach H. Etiology and mechanisms of cutaneous ulcer formation. In: *Wound Healing and Ulcers of the Skin, Diagnosis and Therapy*. 2005. San Francisco: Springer: 30–52.

[37] Hafner J. Management of arterial leg ulcers and combined (mixed) venous-arterial leg ulcers. *Curr Probl Dermatol*. 1999; 27: 211–219.

[38] Hirsch A, et al. ACC/AHA 2005 practice guidelines for management of patients with peripheral arterial disease (lower extremity, renal, mesenteric, and abdominal aortic): a collaborative report from the American Association for Vascular Surgery/raphy and Interventions, Society for Vascular Medicine and Biology, Society for Interventional Radiology, and the ACC/AHA Task Force on Practice Guidelines. *Circulation*. 2006; 113(11): 1474–1547.

[39] Alexandrescu VA, London V. Angiosomes: the cutaneous and arterial evaluation in CLI patients. Chapter 5. In: Mustapha JA: *Critical Limb Ischemia: CLI Diagnosis and Interventions*. 2015. Chicago: Ed. HMP: 71–88.

[40] Doughty DB, Sparks-DeFriese B. Wound-healing physiology. In: Bryant RA: *Acute and Chronic Wounds, Current Management Concepts*. 2012. St. Louis: Elsevier Mosby: 63–82.

[41] Khalil MA, Kim HK, Hoi JW, et al. Detection of peripheral arterial disease within the foot using vascular optical tomographic imaging: a clinical pilot study. *Eur J Vasc Endovasc Surg*. 2015; 49: 83–89.

[42] Igari K, Kudo T, Toyofuku T, et al. Quantitative evaluation of the outcomes of revascularization procedures for peripheral arterial disease using indocyanine green angiography. *Eur J Vasc Endovasc Surg*. 2013; 46(4): 460–465.

[43] Yamamoto M, Orihashi K, Nishimori H, et al. Indocyanine green angiography for intra-operative assessment in vascular surgery. *Eur J Vasc Endovasc Surg*. 2012; 43: 426–432.

[44] Higashimori A, Yokoi Y. Use of Indigo Carmine angiography to qualitatively assess adequate distal perfusion after endovascular revascularization in critical limb ischemia. *J Endovasc Ther*. 2015; 22(3): 352–355.

[45] Montero-Baker MF, Au-Yeung KY, Wisniewski NA, et al. The first-in-man "Si Se Puede" study for the use of micro-oxygen sensors (MOXYs) to determine dynamic relative oxygen indices in the feet of patients with limb-threatening ischemia during endovascular therapy. *J Vasc Surg.* 2015; 61: 1501–1510.

[46] Bell PRF, Charlesworth D, DePalma RG, et al. The definition of critical ischemia of a limb. Working Party of the International Vascular Symposium. *Br J Surg.* 1982; 69(Suppl): S2.

[47] Mills JL Sr, Conte MS, Armstrong DG, et al. The society for vascular surgery lower extremity threatened classification system: risk stratification based on Wound, Ischemia, and foot Infection (WIfI). *J Vasc Surg.* 2014; 59: 220–234.

[48] Abu Dabrh AM, Steffen MW, Undavalli C, et al. The natural history of untreated severe or critical limb ischemia. *J Vasc Surg.* 2015; 62: 1642–1651.

[49] Vallabhaneni R, Kalbaugh CA, Kouri A, et al. Current accepted hemodynamic criteria for critical limb ischemia do not accurately stratify patients at high risk for limb loss. *J Vasc Surg.* 2016; 63: 105–113.

[50] Bollinger A, Breddin K, Hess H, et al. Semiquantitative assessment of lower limb atherosclerosis from routine angiographic images. *Atherosclerosis.* 1981; 38: 339–46.

[51] Dormandy JA, Rutherford RB. Management of peripheral arterial disease (PAD). TASC Working Group: TransAtlantic Inter-Society Consensus (TASC). *J Vasc Surg.* 2000; 31(Suppl): S1–S296.

[52] Rutherford RB, Baker JD, Ernst C, et al. Recommended standards for reports dealing with lower extremity ischemia: revised version. *J Vasc Surg.* 1997; 26: 517–38.

[53] Setacci C, Ricco JB, Apelqvist J, et al. Management of critical limb ischemia and diabetic foot. *Eur J Vasc Endovasc Surg.* 2011; 42(S2): S1–S90.

[54] Graziani L, Silvestro A, Bertone V, et al. Vascular involvement in diabetic subjects with ischemic foot ulcer: a new morphologic categorization of disease severity. *Eur J Vas Endovasc Surg.* 2007; 33: 453–460.

[55] Toursarkissian B, D'Ayala M, Stefanidis D, et al. Angiographic scoring of vascular occlusive disease in the diabetic foot: relevance to bypass graft patency and limb salvage. *J Vasc Surg.* 2002; 35(3): 494–500.

[56] Mustapha JA, Heaney CM. A new approach to diagnosing and treating CLI. *Endovasc Today.* 2010; 9: 41–50.

[57] Lepantalo M, Apelqvist J, Setacci C, et al. Chapter V: diabetic foot. *Eur J Vasc Endovasc Surg.* 2011; 42(52): S60–S74.

[58] Ndip A, Jude EB. Emerging evidence for neuroischemic diabetic foot ulcers: model of care and how to adapt practice. *Int J Low Ext Wounds.* 2009; 8: 82–94.

[59] O'Neal LW. Surgical pathology of the foot and clinicopathologic correlations. In: *Levin and O'Neal's The Diabetic Foot*. 2008. Philadelphia: Mosby Elsevier: 367–401.

[60] Waltenberg J. Impaired collateral vessel development in diabetes: potential cellular mechanisms and therapeutic implications. *Cardiovasc Res*. 2001; 49: 554–560.

[61] Dangwal S, Stratmann B, Bang C, et al. Impairment of wound healing in patients with type 2 diabetes mellitus influences circulating. micro RNA patterns via inflammatory Cytokines. *Arterioscler Thromb Vasc Biol*. 2015; 35(6): 1480–1488.

[62] Alexandrescu VA, Van Espen D. Threatening inferior limb ischemia: when to consider fasciotomy and what principles to apply? *ISRN Vasc Med*. 2014; 21: 1–9.

[63] Defraigne JO. A central pathophysiological mechanism explaining diabetic complications? *Rev Med Liege*. 2005; 60(5–6): 472–478.

[64] Wagner FW Jr. The dysvascular foot: a system for diagnosis and treatment. *Foot Ankle*. 1981; 2: 64–122.

[65] Schaper NC. Diabetic foot ulcer classification system for research purposes: a progress report on criteria for including patients in research studies. *Diabet Metab Res Rev*. 2004; 20: S90–S95.

[66] Armstrong DG, Lavery LA, Harkless LB. Validation of a diabetic wound classification system. The contribution of depth, infection, and ischemia to risk of amputation. *Diabetes Care*. 1998; 21: 855–859.

[67] Macfarlane RM, Jeffcoate WJ. Classification of diabetic foot ulcers: the S(AD) SAD system. *Diabetic Foot*. 1999; 2: 123–31.

[68] Beckert S, Witte M, Wicke C, et al. A new wound-based severity score for diabetic foot ulcers: a prospective analysis of 1000 patients. *Diabetes Care*. 2006; 29: 988–992.

[69] Beckert S, Pietsch AM, Küper M, et al. M.A.I.D.: a prognostic score estimating probability of healing in chronic lower extremity wounds. *Ann Surg*. 2009; 249: 677–681.

[70] Martinez-de Jesús FR. A checklist to score healing progress of diabetic foot ulcers. *Int J Low Extrcm Wounds*. 2010; 9: 74–83.

[71] Alexandrescu VA, Hubermont G. Does peripheral neuropathy have a clinical impact on the endovascular approach as a primary treatment for limb-threatening ischemic foot wounds in diabetic patients? *J Diab Metab*. 2012; S5: 006.

[72] Azuma N, Uchida H, Kokubo T, et al. Factors influencing wound healing of critical ischaemic foot after bypass surgery: is the angiosome important in selecting bypass target artery? *Eur J Vasc Endovasc Surg*. 2012; 43(3): 322–328.

[73] Jens S, Conijn AP, Koelemay MJ, et al. Randomized trials for endovascular treatment of infrainguinal arterial disease: systematic review and meta-analysis (Part 2: Below the knee). *Eur J Vasc Endovasc Surg*. 2014; 47(5): 536–544.

[74] Park SW, Kim JS, Yun IJ, et al. Clinical outcomes of endovascular treatments for critical limb ischemia with chronic total occlusive lesions limited to below-the-knee arteries. *Acta Radiol.* 2013; 54(7): 785–789.

[75] Pernès JM, Auguste M, Borie H, et al. Infrapopliteal arterial recanalization: a true advance for limb salvage in diabetics. *Diagn Interv Imaging.* 2015; 96(5): 423–434.

[76] Brochado-Neto FC, Cury MV, Bonadiman SS, et al. Vein bypass to branches of pedal arteries. *J Vasc Surg.* 2012; 55(3): 746–752.

[77] Good DW, Al Chalabi H, Hameed F, et al. Popliteo-pedal bypass surgery for critical limb ischemia. *Ir J Med Sci.* 2011; 180(4): 829–835.

[78] Hughes K, Domenig CM, Hamdan AD, et al. Bypass to plantar and tarsal arteries: an acceptable approach to limb salvage. *J Vasc Surg.* 2004; 40(6): 1149–1157.

[79] Abu Dabrh AM, Steffen MW, Asi N, et al. Bypass surgery versus endovascular interventions in severe or critical limb ischemia. *J Vasc Surg.* 2016 Jan; 63(1):244-53.e11. doi: 10.1016/j.jvs.2015.07.068. Epub 2015 Sep 11. Review.

[80] Jaff MR, White CJ, Hiatt WR, et al. An update on methods for revascularization and expansion of the TASC lesion classification to include below-the-knee arteries: a supplement to the Inter-Society Consensus for the management of peripheral arterial disease (TASC II). *J Endovasc Surg.* 2015; 22(5): 663–677.

[81] Taneja M, Tay KH, Dewan A, et al. Bare nitinol stent enabled recanalization of long-segment, chronic total occlusion of superficial femoral and adjacent proximal popliteal artery in diabetic patients presenting with critical limb ischemia. *Cardiovasc Revasc Med.* 2010; 11(4): 232–235.

[82] Spiliopoulos S, Theodosiadou V, Katsanos K, et al. Long-term clinical outcomes of infrapopliteal drug-eluting stent placement for critical limb ischemia in diabetic patients. *J Vasc Interv Radiol.* 2015; 26(10): 1423–1430.

[83] Laird JR, Schneider PA, Tepe G, et al. Durability of treatment effect using a drug-coated balloon for femoropopliteal lesions: 24-month results of IN.PACT SFA. *J Am Coll Cardiol.* 2015; 66(21): 2329–2338.

[84] Cioppa A, Stabile E, Popusoi G, et al. Combined treatment of heavy calcified femoro-popliteal lesions using directional atherectomy and a paclitaxel coated balloon: one-year single centre clinical results. Cardiovasc Revasc Med. 2012; 13(4): 219–223.

[85] Zeller T, Rastan A, Macharzina R, et al. Novel approaches to the management of advanced peripheral artery disease: perspectives on drug-coated balloons, drug-eluting stents, and bioresorbable scaffolds. *Curr Cardiol Rep.* 2015; 17(9): 624–627.

[86] Baerlocher MO, Kennedy SA, Rajebi MR, et al. Meta-analysis of drug-eluting balloon angioplasty and drug-eluting stent placement for infrainguinal peripheral arterial disease. *J Vasc Interv Radiol.* 2015; 26(4): 459–473.

[87] Rorive M, Scheen AJ, Diagnostic approach of the pathophysiological triad leading to a diabetic foot. *Rev Med Liege*. 2015; 70(9): 465–471.

[88] Alexandrescu VA, Hubermont G, Coessens V, et al. Why a multidisciplinary team may represent a key factor for lowering the inferior limb loss rate in diabetic neuro-ischaemic wounds: application in a departmental institution. *Acta Chir Belg*. 2009; 109: 79–86.

[89] Dosluoglu HH, Lall P, Cherr GS, Harris LM, Dryjski ML. Role of simple and complex hybrid revascularization procedures for symptomatic lower extremity occlusive disease. *J Vasc Surg*. 2010; 51(6): 1425–1435.

[90] Bazan HA, Le L, Donovan M, et al. Retrograde pedal access for patients with critical limb ischemia. *J Vasc Surg*. 2014; 60(2): 375–381.

[91] Alexandrescu V, Vincent G, Azdad K, et al. A reliable approach to diabetic neuroische-mic foot wounds: below-the-knee angiosome-oriented angioplasty. *J Endovasc Ther*. 2011; 18: 376–387.

[92] Biancari F, Juvonen T. Angiosome-targeted lower limb revascularization for ischemic foot wounds: systematic review and meta-analysis. *Eur J Vasc Endovasc Surg*. 2014; 47(5): 517–522.

[93] Neville RF, Attinger CE, Bulan EJ, et al. Revascularization of a specific angiosome for limb salvage: does the target artery matter? *Ann Vasc Surg*. 2009; 23(3): 367–73.

[94] Houlind K, Christensen JK, Jepsen JM. Vein arterialization for lower limb revasculari-zation. *J Cardiovasc Surg (Torino)*. 2016; 57(2): 266–272.

[95] Alexandrescu VA. Is limb loss always inevitable for critical neuro- ischemic foot wounds in diabetic patients with end stage rénal disease and unfit for vascular reconstructions? In: Sahay M, ed.: *Diseases of Renal Parenchyma*. 2012. Rijeka, Croatia: InTech Open Science: 228–246.

[96] Spillerova K, Biancari F, Leppäniemi A, et al. Differential impact of bypass surgery and angioplasty on angiosome-targeted infrapopliteal revascularization. *Eur J Vasc Endovasc Surg*. 2014; 49(4): 412–419.

[97] Alexandrescu VA. Myths and proofs of angiosome applications in CLI: where do we stand? *J Endovasc Ther*. 2014; 21: 616–624.

[98] Iida O, Takahara M, Soga Y, et al. Impact of angiosome-oriented revascularization on clinical outcomes in critical limb ischemia patients without concurrent wound infection and diabetes. *J Endovasc Ther*. 2014; 21(5): 607–615.

[99] Huang TY, Huang TS, Wang YC, et al. Direct revascularization with the angiosome concept for lower limb ischemia: a systematic review and meta-analysis. *Medicine (Baltimore)*. 2015; 94(34): 1427.

[100] Spillerova K, Sörderström M, Albäck A, et al. The feasibility of angiosome-targeted endovascular treatment in patients with critical limb ischaemia and foot ulcer. *Ann Vasc Surg*. 2015; 30: 270–276.

[101] Bouchet A, Cuilleret J. Topographic anatomy of the inferior limb. In: *Topographic Anatomy of the Human Body*. 3rd Ed. 1995. Masson, Paris: Simep Publ.: 26–97.

[102] Williams PL, Warwick R, Dyson M, et al. Angiology, blood vessels. In: *Gray's Anatomy*. 1996. Churchill Livingstone, New York: 682–694.

[103] Macchi C, Catini C, Giannelli F, et al. Collateral circulation in distal occlusion of lower limb arteries: an anatomical study and statistical research in 40 elderly subjects by echo-color-Doppler method. *Ital J Anat Embryol*. 1996; 101(4): 221–227.

[104] Lehoux S, Lévi BI. Collateral artery growth: making the most of what you have. *Circ Res*. 2006; 99: 567–569.

[105] Schaper W. Collateral circulation, past and present. *Basic Res Cardiol*. 2009; 104(1): 5–21.

[106] Ziegler MA, Distasi MR, Bills RG, et al. Marvels, mysteries and misconceptions of vascular compensation to peripheral artery occlusion. *Microcirculation*. 2010; 17(1): 3–20.

[107] Kropman RH, Kiela G, Moll FL, et al. Variations in the anatomy of the popliteal artery and its side branches. *Vasc Endovasc Surg*. 2011; 45(6): 536–540.

[108] Abou-Foul AK, Borumandi F. Anatomical variations of lower limb vasculature and implications for free fibula flap: systematic review and critical analysis. *Microsurgery*. 2016; 36(2): 165–172.

[109] Ovcharenko DV, Kaputin MI, Voronkov AA, et al. Angiographic assessment of the incidence rate of atypical variants of the development of crural and plantar arteries. *Angiol Sosud Khir*. 2012; 18(1): 57–60.

[110] Kim D, Orron DE, Slillman JJ. Surgical significance of popliteal arterial variants. A unified angiographic classification. *Ann Surg*. 1989; 210(6): 776–781.

[111] Yamada T, Gloviczki P, Bower TC, et al. Variations of the arterial anatomy of the foot. *Am J Surg*. 1993; 166(2): 130–135.

[112] Lee JH, Dauber W. Anatomic study of the dorsalis pedis-first dorsal metatarsal artery. Ann Plast Surg. 1997; 38(1): 50–55.

[113] Singh BN, Burmeister W, Machado K, et al. Variations of the origin of the arcuate artery. *J Am Podiatr Med Assoc*. 2013; 103(3): 181–184.

[114] Gabrielli C, Olave E, Mandiola E, et al. The deep plantar arch in humans: constitution and topography. *Surg Radiol Anat*. 2001; 23(4): 253–258.

[115] Karacagil S, Almgren B, Lorelius LE, et al. Angiographic runoff patterns in patients undergoing lower limb revascularization. *Acta Chir Scand*. 1989; 155(1): 19–24.

[116] Ciavarella A, Silletti A, Mustacchio A, et al. Angiographic evaluation of the anatomic pattern of arterial obstructions in diabetic patients with critical limb ischemia. *Diabetes Metab*. 1993; 19(6): 586–589.

[117] Santos VP, Alves CA, Fidelis C, et al. Arteriographic findings in diabetic and non-diabetic with critical limb ischemia. *Rev Assoc Med Bras*. 2013; 59(6): 557–562.

[118] Acin F, Varela C, de Maturana IL, et al. Results of infrapopliteal endovascular procedures performed in diabetic patients with critical limb ischemia and tissue loss from the perspective of an angiosome-oriented revascularization strategy. *Intern J Vasc Med*. 2014; 10: 2–15.

[119] Jörneskog G. Why critical limb ischemia criteria are not applicable to diabetic foot and what the consequences are. *J Scan Surg*. 2012; 101(2): 114–118.

[120] Hingorani A, LaMuraglia GM, Henke P, et al. The management of the diabetic foot: a clinical practice guideline by the Society for Vascular Surgery in collaboration with the American Podiatric Medical Association and the Society for Vascular Medicine. *J Vasc Surg*. 2016; 63: 3S–21S.

[121] Apelqvist J, Bakker K, van Houtum WH, et al. Practical guidelines on the management and prevention of the diabetic foot: based upon the International Consensus on the Diabetic Foot (2007) Prepared by the International Working Group on the Diabetic Foot. *Diabetes Metab Res Rev*. 2008; 24(Suppl. 1): S181–S187.

[122] Van Acker K. Importance of multidisciplinary surveillance after topographic arterial treatment for limb salvage. In: *Angiosomes Applications in Critical Limb Ischemia: In Search for Relevance*. 2012. Torino: Minerva Medica: 87–95.

[123] Van Acker K. Importance of multidisciplinary surveillance after topographic arterial treatment for limb salvage. In: *Angiosomes Applications in Critical Limb Ischemia: In Search for Relevance*. Editor : Alexandrescu VA, 2012. Torino: Minerva Medica: 87–95.

[124] Aydin K, Isildak M, Karakaya J, et al. Change in amputation predictors in diabetic foot disease: effect of multidisciplinary approach. *Endocrine*. 2010; 38: 87–92.

[125] Christman AL, Selvin E, Margolis DJ, et al. Hemoglobin A1c predicts healing rate in diabetic wounds. *J Invest Dermatol*. 2011; 131: 2121–2127.

[126] Yazdanpanah L, Nasiri M, Adarvishi S. Literature review on the management of diabetic foot ulcer. *World J Diab*. 2015; 6(1): 37–53.

[127] Elraiyah T, Apostolos T, Prutsky G, et al. A systematic review and meta-analysis of adjunctive therapies in diabetic foot ulcers. *J Vasc Surg*. 2016; 63: 46S–58S.

[128] Elraiyah T, Domecq JP, Prutsky G, et al. A systematic review and meta-analysis of debridement methods for chronic diabetic foot ulcers. *J Vasc Surg*. 2016; 63: 37S–45S.

[129] Lew EJ, Mills JL Sr, Armsrong DG. The deterioration of DFU: prioritising the risk factors to avoid amputation. *J Wound Care*. 2015; 24(5 Suppl. 2): 31–37.

5

Physical Modalities in the Management of Wound(s)

Amir Feily, Fatemeh Moeineddin and
Shadi Mehraban

Abstract

Wound is caused by disruption of the integrity of body skin as a result of environmental or medical factors. Managing chronic and refractory wounds is a significant dilemma physicians are facing. Large varieties of treatment modalities have been used to enhance wound healing among which were different medicines, surgical procedures, physical therapy, hyperbaric oxygen therapy, and physical modalities such as laser and shockwave. In this chapter, the authors discuss physical modalities that are most used in the management of wound healing with a focus on lasers, shockwaves, photodynamic therapy, UVB therapy, and lights and describe some important experimental and clinical trials that have been done in this regard with an attempt to explain their mechanisms.

Keywords: wound healing, low-level lasers, shockwave, photodynamic therapy, phototherapy, CO_2 laser

1. Introduction

Wound is caused by disruption of the integrity of body skin as a result of environmental or medical factors. Managing chronic and refractory wounds represents a significant dilemma that physicians are facing. Wound healing is a complex cascade of events that restores skin integrity by replacing damaged cells and tissues which consists of four phases: hemostasis, inflammation, proliferation, and remodeling. In the first phase, hemostatic changes result in a reduced blood flow and clot formation. Activated platelets as well as the injury itself attract inflammatory agents, neutrophils, and predominantly macrophages, which clear the apoptotic cells. By releasing growth factors, these leukocytes trigger proliferation of fibroblasts, epithelial and endothelial cells in the trauma site forming the granulation tissue. Turnover of collagen from type III to I restores skin integrity in the remodeling phase. Various factors can influence the quality of wound healing including nutrition, vitamin deficiencies, smoking, sex hormones, oxygenation, age, stress, diabetes, alcoholism, and medications such as glucocorticoid steroids, chemotherapeutic agents, and nonsteroidal antiinflammatory drugs [1].

Large varieties of treatment modalities have been used to enhance wound healing such as different medicines, surgical procedures, physical therapy, hyperbaric oxygen therapy, and physical modalities such as laser and shockwave. Some substances like honey have also proved to be beneficial in wound healing as a result of antiinflammatory and antibacterial features [2]. The ideal physical therapy modality is chosen based on the patient's factors, type of wound, previous therapies, and clinician's preference.

Electrical stimulation is another method of physical therapy used for accelerating wound healing. Electrotherapy works by stimulating cell migration, cell proliferation rate, and growth factor secretion via creating an electrical current. The anode attracts macrophages, neutrophils, and keratinocytes. The cathode attracts activated neutrophils, fibroblasts, myofibroblasts, and endothelial cells [3].

Low-level laser therapy (LLLT) is also a novel approach for treating wounds. Greatest benefits have been achieved through wavelengths of 632–1000 nm. The mechanism of action of LLLT is defined through wound contraction which accelerates the wound healing process [4].

Pulsed radiofrequency energy also promotes chronic wound healing by contracting the wound [5]. It has minimum side effects as well as the advantage of reducing wound pain.

Light-emitting diode (LED) has somewhat similar effects as light amplification by stimulated emission of radiation (LASER) in expediting the process of wound healing by increasing fibroblasts and collagens and decreasing inflammatory cells in the trauma site [6].

Shockwaves have also proved to be beneficial in overcoming chronic and intractable wounds such as diabetic ones with minimal adverse effects and long-lasting results. The mechanism through which they work remains unknown; however, several factors are considered to be effective in this procedure including stimulation of microcirculation and metabolism, reduction of inflammatory cells, release of growth factors, and stimulation of stem cells [7].

Photodynamic therapy (PDT) has also proved to be effective in wound healing. However, it seems to display best results when used in conjunction with lasers [8].

The effect of ultraviolet therapy on wound healing seems not promising and may even delay the process as it has shown to affect focal adhesion dynamics [9]. On the other hand, there are studies which suggest that ultraviolet C can be beneficial in expediting wound healing with antibacterial effects [10].

In this chapter, the authors tend to discuss physical modalities that are most used in the management of wound healing with a focus on lasers, shockwaves, photodynamic therapy, UVB therapy, and lights.

2. Low-level laser and wound healing

In the recent years, it has been shown that the laser therapy had the potential to improve wound healing and reduce pain and inflammation [11].

The main indications of low-reactive-level laser therapy (LLLT) are reduction of pain and inflammation. It amplifies tissue repair, enhances regeneration of different nerves and tissues, and prevents tissue injury in situations where it is likely to occur [12, 13].

Low-reactive-level laser therapy (LLLT) enhances the activation of intracellular or extracellular chromophores and the initiation of cellular signaling by exposing cells or tissue to low levels of red and near infrared (NIR) light [11]. The biological effects of LLLT are decreased inflammatory cells, increased fibroblast reproduction and angiogenesis, and stimulation of granulation tissue and augmented collagen synthesis [14].

LLLT assumes the use of photons at a nonthermal irradiation to alter biological activity. LLLT is composed of two sources: coherent light and noncoherent light sources (lasers) consisting of filtered lamps or light-emitting diodes (LED) or, on occasion, a combination of both [13, 14].

The reason of the term "low level" is the use of low-power contents compared to the other forms of laser therapy such as cutting, ablation, and thermally coagulating tissue.

The mechanism of LLLT on wound healing is not yet fully understood nevertheless it appears that LLLT has a wide area of effects at all the levels of molecular, cellular, and tissue ingredients. The main biological mechanism behind the effects of LLLT is proposed to be absorption of red and NIR light by mitochondrial components, in particular cytochrome c oxidase (CCO) which is concluded in the respiratory chain located within the mitochondria [15–17], and also in the plasma membrane of cells. Accordingly, a chain of events and various process carries out in the mitochondria [18] leading to wound healing.

Although LLLT is now used as a portable minimally invasive, easy-to-use, and cost-effective modality to promote wound healing, it is also employed for treatment of diabetic lower extremity ulcer. However, it remains controversial in this therapy for two reasons. First, there are uncertainties about the basic molecular and cellular mechanisms responsible for appropriate biological effects on the affected tissue. Second, there are significant variations in terms of parameters measuring: wavelength, irradiation or power density, pulse structure, coherence, polarization, energy, fluence, irradiation time, contact versus noncontact application, and repetition regimen. Lower level parameters can result in lower impact of the treatment and higher ones can lead to tissue injury [12, 14].

Inappropriate choice of light source and dosage can be the cause of negative results of many of the published studies on LLLT. In addition, eventual mismatch of the patient's skin to the application of LLLT were described, such as: improper preparation and oily debris that can interfere with the influence of the light source, and cause failure to account for skin pigmentation [19]. Unsuitable maintenance of the LLLT devices can reduce its efficiency and interfere with clinical results as well. It is important to notice that there is an optimal dose of light for any particular issues [14].

Nevertheless, many systematic reviews point that LLLT is an effective therapeutic modality on wound healing and diabetic foot ulcer recovery [20], but additional clinical studies must be performed in order to find out the best parameters of wavelength, dosage, and methodology and especially appropriate treatment protocol.

3. Relative contraindications/precautions

3.1. Relative contraindications

3.1.1. Cancer

Do not use LLLT over any known malignant lesions unless: for pain relief during the terminal stages of the illness, and for cancer therapy side effects (e.g., oral mucositis, radiation dermatitis, etc.).

3.1.2. Pregnancy

There is no evidence of harm to an unborn baby; however, there are no safety tests either, so for medico legal reasons it is recommended to not treat directly over the developing fetus.

3.1.3. Thyroid

Although relatively low intensity is far less likely to trigger any adverse events when treating that region of the neck, we suggest not applying lasers directly over the thyroid.

4. Photodynamic therapy and wound healing

Photodynamic therapy (PDT) as a photochemistry process can kill cancer cells, inactivate infected pathogens, and demolish target tissue. In PDT process, one special material called photosensitizer or nontoxic dyes absorbs visible light and produces excited singlet state such as singlet oxygen and hydroxyl radicals that are able to attack to target cells [21]. Administration of photosensitizer either topically or systemically in combination with irradiation appropriate wavelength laser is a promising treatment modality in wound healing especially for chronic pressure and decubitus wounds frequently encountered in diabetic and disable patients. The healing of chronic wounds and venous stasis ulcers of the leg is compromised by infection, yet PDT has an antimicrobial action [22]. Bacterial burden in chronic ulcer decreases by treatment with infrared radiation. A radiation via endogenous protoporphyrin (and/or protoporphyrin IX [PpIX] of bacteria) is virtually similar to a mild PDT [23]. It appears that PDT with suitable PS together with suitable laser parameters represents effective treatment modalities in promoting wound healing. PSs associates with three main groups of agents: azine dyes, macrocyclic dyes, and metallated derivatives [24–27]. An extensive range of PSs from different groups including azines, porphyrins, phthalocyanines, and chlorophyll derivatives have been described in eradication of many pathogens such as a variety of bacteria, parasites, viruses, and fungi [22].

Several types of first- and second-generation PSs have been used at minimal doses with laser irradiation performed at wavelengths ranging from 630 to 690 nm, and showed that PDT of acute wounds can lead to an improvement of healing outcomes. Interestingly in one study, the healing of skin flaps after being subjected to ischemia was impaired by PDT treatment, although only one PS (Photofrin) was tested. Further animal model and human wound studies are required to find the main process of enhancement of reepithelization and granulation tissue formation with PDT.

In photodynamic therapy, irradiation of cells with low dosage or small energy may incite proliferation. In using PDT clinically, it is essential to use the suitable doses of both the PS and the activating light source in order to achieve cell death for cancer therapy, or regeneration for wound healing [23]. The newest generations of PSs allowing a faster clearance time of normal tissues are more selective for tumor cells. Although PDT may be nontraumatic but in comparison with nature of lower laser therapy it is almost always traumatic and can cause burns, swelling, pain, and scarring in nearby normal tissue [28].

4.1. Contraindication

Cutaneous hypersensitivity, porphyria, known allergies to porphyrins.

Both Aminolevulinic acid (ALA) and Methyl aminolevulinate (MAL) are in FDA pregnancy category C; reproduction studies have not been performed on animals.

Photodynamic therapy is not approved for use in children.

5. Phototherapy (UV irradiation) and wound healing

New contemporary research shows that controlled UV exposure might have some eventual benefit in wound healing and cutaneous homeostasis. The effectiveness of UV energy in enhancing biological changes depends on the chosen irradiation parameters, with maximal effective wavelength and lowest irradiation level [29]. The main mechanism of phototherapy is related to the depth of penetration. UVA, for example, has the longest wavelength and penetrates to the upper part of dermis in human skin, and UVB only penetrates down to the basal layer; however, UVC only reaches the upper part of the epidermis [30].

UV has bactericidal effect and its radiation to the skin can increase blood flow, producing erythema and epidermal hyperplasia [31]. The induced erythema via vasodilatation and inflammatory response represents the first phase of healing. In addition, UV light irradiation increases cellular proliferation in the stratum corneum [32], which can be a protective mechanism against further sunlight damage.

Although UV protection and antisolars are commonly advised during and after wound healing, it is possible that UV also affects the melanocyte redistribution and prevents the normal cutaneous response to injury [33].

It has been shown that UVC light *per se* could stimulate wound healing. UVC light enhances fibronectin and growth factors release leading to increase healing cascade and wound contraction [34, 35]. UV can promote endothelial cell proliferation [36] and augment epidermal thickness and reepithelialization or desquamation of the leading edge of periulcer epidermal cells [31].

UVC (200–280 nm) has a significant antimicrobial effect and can be used as efficient bactericide agent for treatment of acute wound infections and killing pathogens without undesirable injury to host tissue. UVB (280–315 nm) irradiation to the wound has wound healing stimulating effect and extracorporeal UVB irradiation of blood adds immune system stimulating effects too. Although UVA (315–400 nm) has specific effects on cell biologic events, it has not yet been extensively applied to wound treatment [31].

An interesting study compared the efficacy of phototherapy on wound healing in rats under the normal and high-fat diets and revealed increased wound healing by regulating oxidative stress in rats with metabolic disorders under a high-fat diet [37]. The efficacy of UV therapy on pressure ulcer is not clear due to eventual bias and limited number of trials available for consideration. Further research is recommended to determine possible benefit or drawbacks of this treatment [38].

While low level laser (or light) and photodynamic therapy both have considerable applications in wound care, but penetration of UV light into tissues and its efficacy is restricted. UVC and UVB can damage DNA in host cells and chronic exposure to UV can be carcinogenic. Accordingly, additional study of cellular signaling that occurs after UV exposure of tissue is needed to better indicate the risk and benefits of UV irradiation in wound healing.

5.1. Contraindication of phototherapy

- Childhood

- Pregnancy and breastfeeding (PUVA)

- Immobility or inability to stand unassisted for 10 min or longer

- Very fair skin (skin type 1 and 2, especially PUVA)

- Past excessive exposure to natural sun light or phototherapy

- Immunosuppressive medication

- Photosensitizing creams or medications

- Past skin cancer, especially melanoma [39]

6. Shock wave and wound healing

Although hearing extracorporal shock wave brings the treatment of urinary stones in the mind [40–43] but it also has some benefits in the treatment of acute and chronic wounds [44]. Shock waves are biphasic high-energy acoustic waves that can be produced by electrohy-draulics. Although the exact mechanisms of shock wave therapy are not entirely elucidated, it may harbor eventual immunomedulatory effects, acting by transient micromechanical forces in altering various biologic activities. Shock wave therapy increased expression of macromo-lecules in wound healing such as VEGF, proliferating cell nuclear antigen, and endothelial nitric oxide synthesis. Because of the considerable experience in using shock wave in the treatment of urolithiasis and other conditions in humans, it appears to be a safe technology. The clinical effect of this technology in various wound types and the particular mechanisms of action are now beginning to be understood. Shock waves may also stimulate sensory nerve fibers and decrease pain. Clinical studies of shock wave therapy in wound healing suggest that many factors such as wound cause, size, and duration may impact response to shock wave therapy. However, the actual administration of shock wave therapy in current clinical studies varies in type (unfocused versus focused). Primary studies suggest that unfocused shock wave therapy is more effective than focused one in the treatment of superficial soft tissue defects yet, without direct comparison between unfocused and focused shock wave therapy in clinical trials to date [33]. Importantly, additional basic science studies along with randomized controlled trials will be necessary to determine the optimal shock wave therapy settings. Currently, the U.S. Food and Drug Administration has approved devices that administer shock wave therapy for the treatment of plantar fasciitis and lateral epicondylitis. Application of such devices for treatment of acute and chronic wounds has not been approved yet. We look forward to future innovation in this field to find out the accurate mechanisms of action and optimal treatment of specific wound types.

6.1. Contraindications

6.1.1. Absolute

Lungs: Treatments must not be performed across or directed to the lungs and heart.

Eyes: Tissue of the eye could be adversely affected by shock wave.

Brain: The destructive forces seen at transitions could damage and destroy brain matter.

Major blood vessels: Both the major blood vessels in the neck and thigh should be avoided to prevent damage and potential catastrophic bleeding.

Major nerves: Superficial major nerves like the brachial plexus, ulna/radial nerve should not be treated directly (treatment around these areas is acceptable just not directly to the nerve).

Open wounds/postsurgical wounds with or without stabilization (glue, stitches, steristrips): Shock wave damages tissues and local circulation. This could lead to degradation of the wound, further bleeding, and delayed healing.

Implanted devices or hormones.

Epiphysis: Open growth plates could potentially be damaged by shock wave either by using settings that create more growth and close them too quickly or by using settings that delay growth.

6.1.2. Relative

Genitals; pregnancy; clotting disorders/anticoagulants; joint replacements, certain settings have been used to loosen previously implanted joints ready for a new implant; infection; and cancer.

Corticosteroid injection: Generally people recommend waiting 1 month before application [45].

7. CO_2 laser and wound healing

There are some anecdotal reports of CO_2 laser and wound healing. In an interesting case series two pediatric patients with chronic wounds within scars showed rapid healing with a single-pass treatment by fractionated carbon dioxide (CO_2) laser [46]. In another case series done by Phillips et al., CO_2 laser was used in the treatment of posttraumatic slow healing wounds in three elderly patients. In their report each wound was healed by 60% or greater within 3 weeks [47]. In an interesting article reepithelialization and accelerated wound healing within 4 weeks was reported in one recessive dystrophic epidermolysis bullosa (RDEB) patient with CO_2 laser without blistering or other adverse effects [48]. Although there are no considerable reports of the efficacy of fractional carbon dioxide laser on wound healing, it seems that it has a promising effect on chronic wound without remarkable complications.

7.1. Contraindication

Isotretinoin use within the previous 6 months, active cutaneous bacterial or viral infection in the area to be treated, history of keloid formation or hypertrophic scarring, ongoing ultraviolet exposure, prior radiation therapy to treatment area, collagen vascular disease, chemical peel, and dermabrasion [49].

8. Conclusion

Managing chronic and refractory wounds represents a significant dilemma that physicians are facing and needs invention of new treatment modalities. Wide ranges of the above physical modalities have been introduced and used in wound-healing treatment with different efficacies, but most of them, to some extent, are strange for patients and physicians. Although additional clinical studies must be performed in order to find out the best modalities and the best parameters of wavelength, dosage, and methodology, and especially appropriate treatment protocols, we think these modalities need more attention to be paid and should be kept in mind for treating persistent ulcers.

Author details

Amir Feily[1*], Fatemeh Moeineddin[1] and Shadi Mehraban[2]

*Address all correspondence to: dr.feily@yahoo.com

1 Skin and Stem Cell Research Center, Tehran University of Medical Sciences, Tehran, Iran

2 Jahrom University of Medical Sciences, Jahrom, Iran

References

[1] Guo S, Dipietro LA. Factors affecting wound healing. J Dent Res. 2010 Mar;89(3):219–229.

[2] Pazyar N, Yaghoobi R, Rafiee E, Mehrabian A, Feily A. Skin wound healing and phytomedicine: a review. Skin Pharmacol Physiol. 2014;27(6):303–310.

[3] Walter C, Chua MD. Advanced wound care modalities for the treatment of pressure ulcers. PVA Summit. 2011; 2011:35–37.

[4] Hopkins JT, McLoda TA, Seegmiller JG, David Baxter G. Low-level laser therapy facilitates superficial wound healing in humans: a triple-blind, Sham-controlled study. J Athl Train. 2004 Jul–Sep; 39(3):223–229.

[5] Li Q, Kao H, Matros E, Peng C, Murphy GF, Guo L. Pulsed radiofrequency energy accelerates wound healing in diabetic mice. Plast Reconstr Surg. 2011 Jun;127(6):2255–2262.

[6] de Abreu Chaves ME, de Araújo AR, Piancastelli ACC, Pinotti M. Effects of low-power light therapy on wound healing: LASER×LED. An Bras Dermatol. 2014 Jul–Aug; 89(4): 616–623.

[7] Kuo YR, Wang CT, Wang FS, Chiang YC, Wang CJ. Extracorporeal shock-wave therapy enhanced wound healing via increasing topical blood perfusion and tissue regeneration in a rat model of STZ-induced diabetes. Wound Repair Regen. 2009 Jul–Aug; 17(4): 522–530.

[8] Jayasree RS, Gupta AK, Rathinam K, Mohanan PV, Mohanty M. The influence of photodynamic therapy on the wound healing process in rats. J Biomater Appl. 2001 Jan;15(3):176–186.

[9] Liu H, Yue J, Lei Q, Gou X, Chen SY, He YY, Wu X. Ultraviolet B inhibits skin wound healing by affecting focal adhesion dynamics. Photochem Photobiol. 2015 Jul–Aug; 91(4):909–916.

[10] Thai TP, Houghton PE, Campbell KE, Woodbury MG. Ultraviolet light C in the treatment of chronic wounds with MRSA: a case study. Ostomy Wound Manage. 2002 Nov;48(11):52–60.

[11] Kushibiki T, Hirasawa T, Okawa S, Ishihara M. Low reactive level laser therapy for mesenchymal stromal cells therapies. Stem Cells Int. 2015;2015:974864.

[12] Chung H, Dai T, Sharma SK, Huang YY, Carroll JD, Hamblin MR. The nuts and bolts of low-level laser (light) therapy. Ann Biomed Eng. 2012 Feb;40(2):516–533.

[13] Gupta A, Avci P, Sadasivam M, et al. Shining light on nanotechnology to help repair and regeneration. Biotechnol Adv. Biotechnol Adv. 2013 Sep–Oct;31(5):607–631.

[14] Avci P, Gupta A, Sadasivam M, Vecchio D, Pam Z, Pam N, Hamblin MR. Low-level laser (light) therapy (LLLT) in skin: stimulating, healing, restoring. Semin Cutan Med Surg. 2013 Mar;32(1):41–52.

[15] Karu TI, Kolyakov SF. Exact action spectra for cellular responses relevant to photo-therapy. Photomed Laser Surg. 2005 Aug;23(4):355–361.

[16] Greco M, Guida G, Perlino E, Marra E, Quagliariello E. Increase in RNA and protein synthesis by mitochondria irradiated with helium-neon laser. Biochem Biophys Res Commun. 1989 Sep 29;163(3):1428–1434.

[17] Karu TI, Pyatibrat LV, Kalendo GS. Photobiological modulation of cell attachment via cytochrome c oxidase. Photochem Photobiol Sci. 2004 Feb;3(2):211–216.

[18] Oron U. Light therapy and stem cells: a therapeutic intervention of the future? Interven Cardiol. 2011;3(6):627–629.

[19] Posten W, Wrone DA, Dover JS, Arndt KA, Silapunt S, Alam M. Low-level laser therapy for wound healing: mechanism and efficacy. Dermatol Surg. 2005 Mar;31(3):334–340.

[20] Tchanque-Fossuo CN, Ho D, Dahle SE, Koo E, Li CS, Rivkah Isseroff R, Jagdeo J. A systematic review of low-level light therapy for treatment of diabetic foot ulcer. Wound Repair Regen. 2016; 24:418–26.

[21] Silva ZS Jr, Bussadori SK, Fernandes KP, Huang YY, Hamblin MR. Animal models for photodynamic therapy (PDT). Biosci Rep. 2015; 28;35(6), pii:e00265.

[22] O'Riordan K, Akilov OE, Hasan T. The potential for photodynamic therapy in the treatment of localized infections. Photodiagnosis Photodyn. Ther. 2005;2:247–262.

[23] Peplow PV, Chung TY, Baxter GD. Photodynamic modulation of wound healing: a review of human and animal studies. Photomed Laser Surg. 2012 Mar;30(3):118–148.

[24] Malik Z, Hanania J, Nitzan Y. Bactericidal effects of photoactivated porphyrins – an alternative approach to antimicrobial drugs. J Photochem Photobiol B. 1990 May;5(3–4):281–293.

[25] Wainwright M. Photodynamic antimicrobial chemotherapy (PACT). J Antimicrob Chemother. 1998;42:13–28.

[26] Ali H, van Lier JE. Metal complexes as photo and radio-sensitizers. Chem Rev. 1999;99:2379–2450.

[27] Josefsen LB, Boyle RW. Photodynamic therapy and the development of metal-based photosensitisers. Met Based Drugs. 2008;2008:276109.

[28] Vrouenraets MB, Visser GW, Snow GB, van Dongen GA. Basic principles, applications in oncology and improved selectivity of photodynamic therapy. Anticancer Res. 2003 Jan–Feb;23(1B):505–522.

[29] Nussbaum EL, Biemann I, Mustard B. Comparison of ultrasound/ultraviolet-C and laser for treatment of pressure ulcers in patients with spinal cord injury. Phys Ther. 1994;74:812.

[30] Ennis WJ, Lee C, Meneses P. A biochemical approach to wound healing through the use of modalities. Clin Dermatol. 2007;25:63.

[31] Gupta A, Avci P, Dai T, Huang YY, Hamblin MR. Ultraviolet radiation in wound care: sterilization and stimulation. Adv Wound Care (New Rochelle). 2013 Oct;2(8):422–437.

[32] Sauder DN, Stanulis-Praeger BM, Gilchrest BA. Autocrine growth stimulation of human keratinocytes by epidermal cell-derived thymocyte-activating factor: implications for skin aging. Arch Dermatol Res.1988;280:71.

[33] Rennekampff HO, Busche MN, Knobloch K, Tenenhaus M. Is UV radiation beneficial in postburn wound healing? Med Hypotheses. 2010;75:436.

[34] Morykwas M, Marks M. Effects of ultraviolet light on fibroblast fibronectin production and lattice contraction. Wounds. 1998;10:111.

[35] James LC, Moore AM, Wheeler LA, Murphy GM, Dowd PM, Greaves MW. Transforming growth factor alpha: in vivo release by normal human skin following UV irradiation and abrasion. Skin Pharmacol.1991;4:61.

[36] Eaglstein WH, Weinstein GD. Prostaglandin and DNA synthesis in human skin: possible relationship to ultraviolet light effects. J Invest Dermatol. 1975;64:386.

[37] Leite SN, Leite MN, Caetano GF, Ovidio PP, Jordão Júnior AA, Frade MA. Phototherapy improves wound healing in rats subjected to high-fat diet. Lasers Med Sci. 2015 Jul; 30(5):1481–1488.

[38] Chen C, Hou WH, Chan ES, Yeh ML, Lo HL. Phototherapy for treating pressure ulcers. Cochrane Database Syst Rev. 2014 Jul 11;7:CD009224.

[39] Schaden W, Fischer A, Sailler A. Extracorporeal shock wave therapy of nonunion or delayed osseous union. Clin Orthop Relat Res. 2001;387:90–94.

[40] Contrandication of phototherapy. http://www.dermnetnz.org/doctors/scaly-rashes/phototherapy.html#contra. Accessed at 7 May, 2016.

[41] Wang CJ, Liu HC, Fu TH. The effects of extracorporeal shockwave on acute high-energy long bone fractures of the lower extremity. Arch Orthop Trauma Surg. 2007;127:137–142.

[42] Wang CJ, Chen HS, Chen CE, Yang KD. Treatment of nonunions of long bone fractures with shock waves. Clin Orthop Relat Res. 2001;387:95–101.

[43] Elster EA, Stojadinovic A, Forsberg J, Shawen S, Andersen RC, Schaden W. Extracorporeal shock wave therapy for nonunion of the tibia. J Orthop Trauma 2010;24:133–141.

[44] Qureshi AA, Ross KM, Ogawa R, Orgill DP. Shock wave therapy in wound healing. Plast Reconstr Surg. 2011;128:721e-7e.

[45] Contrandication of shock wave therapy. http://www.shockwavetherapy.education/index.php/theory/contraindications. Accessed at 7 May, 2016.

[46] Krakowski AC, Diaz L, Admani S, Uebelhoer NS, Shumaker PR. Healing of chronic wounds with adjunctive ablative fractional laser resurfacing in two pediatric patients. Lasers Surg Med. 2016 Feb;48(2):166–169.

[47] Phillips TJ, Morton LM, Uebelhoer NS, Dover JS. Ablative fractional carbon dioxide laser in the treatment of chronic, posttraumatic, lower-extremity ulcers in elderly patients. JAMA Dermatol. 2015 Aug;151(8):868–871.

[48] Krakowski AC, Ghasri P. Case report: rapidly healing epidermolysis bullosa wound after ablative fractional resurfacing. Pediatrics. 2015 Jan;135(1):e207-10.

[49] Krupa Shankar DS, Chakravarthi M, Shilpakar R. Carbon dioxide laser guidelines. J Cutan Aesthet Surg. 2009 Jul–Dec;2(2):72–80.

6

Topical Wound Oxygen Versus Conventional Compression Dressings in the Management of Refractory Venous Ulcers

Sherif Sultan, Wael Tawfick, Edel P Kavanagh and Niamh Hynes

Abstract

Topical wound oxygen (TWO$_2$) proposes an innovative therapy option in the management of refractory non-healing venous ulcers (RVU) that aims to accelerate wound healing. TWO$_2$ accelerates epithelialisation. This leads to the development of a higher tensile strength collagen, which lessens scarring and the risk of recurrence. Sixty-seven limbs with 67 ulcers were managed using TWO$_2$ therapy, and 65 limbs with 65 ulcers were managed using conventional compression dressings (CCD). The proportion of ulcers completely healed by 12 weeks was 76% in patients managed with TWO$_2$, compared to 46% in patients managed with CCD ($p < 0.0001$). The mean reduction in ulcer surface area at 12 weeks was 96% in the TWO$_2$ therapy group, compared to 61% in patients managed with CCD. The median time to full ulcer healing was 57 days in the TWO$_2$ group, in contrast to 107 days in patients managed with CCD ($p < 0.0001$). TWO$_2$ patients had a significantly improved Quality-Adjusted Time Spent Without Symptoms of disease and Toxicity of treatment (Q-TWiST) compared to CCD patients, denoting an improved outcome ($p < 0.0001$). TWO$_2$ reduces the time needed for RVU healing and is successful in pain alleviation and MRSA elimination. TWO$_2$ therapy radically degrades recurrence rates. Utilising diffused oxygen raises the capillary partial pressure of oxygen (Po$_2$) levels at the wound site, stimulating epithelialisation, and granulation of new healthy tissue. Taking the social and individual aspects of chronic venous ulceration into account, the use of TWO$_2$ can provide an overwhelmingly improved quality of life for long-time sufferers of this debilitating disease.

Keywords: topical wound oxygen, conventional compression dressings, refractory venous ulcers, MRSA, epithelialisation

1. Introduction

Chronic venous ulceration is a common disease. Its prevalence is 1% of the total population, with 20% of venous ulcers presented in octogenarians [1–5]. Refractory venous leg ulceration is a common basis of morbidity [6, 7] and leads to a reduced quality of life [8], especially in the elderly population [4, 5]. It causes a considerable amount of work incapacity, social exclusion and lack of self-esteem [4]. There is a probable underestimation of the true extent of venous leg ulceration in the general population due to its underreporting [7]. Venous ulcers are characterised by a recurring pattern of healing and subsequent 70% recurrence rate at one year [9–14]. Venous ulceration places a huge monetary burden on the healthcare system [15]. The cost of managing venous ulcers accrues to £400 million sterling per year in the UK [16].

Ambulatory venous hypertension is one of the leading causes of chronic reperfusion injury. This in turn provokes venous ulceration with its habitual history of chronicity and recurrence [1]. Over the past 40 years, compression bandaging has been the gold standard form of therapy for treatment of venous ulceration. We have learned that compression will both improve perfusion and enhance healing [2, 17, 18]. Nevertheless, active healthy tissue granulation can take upwards to 3 weeks to cultivate [19]. Therefore, the following question is posed: How can we speed up epithelial coverage in a granulating wound?

1.1. Topical wound oxygen

Topical wound oxygen (TWO_2) proposes an innovative therapy option in the management of refractory non-healing venous ulcers (RVU) that aims to accelerate wound healing. The application of positive pressure oxygen to manage open wounds has been studied extensively and has demonstrated promising clinical results [20–28]. The systemic complications associated with the use of a full-body hyperbaric chamber have been overcome by the application of topical wound pure oxygen at an appropriate cycled pressure to only the specific wound site. This maximizes the beneficial wound healing effects and minimizes the negative systemic side effects [29].

Delivered through a targeted delivery system, a Hyper-Box, TWO_2 accelerates epithelialisation and eliminates MRSA within 72 h. This leads to the development of a higher tensile strength collagen, which lessens scarring and the risk of recurrence [29–32]. Hyperbaric oxygen promotes angiogenesis and increases the expression of angiogenesis-related growth factors [33, 34]. It promotes leukocyte function with enhanced bactericidal activity [35–40]. The intermittent cycled pressure, under which TWO_2 is delivered, stimulates circulation, reduces oedema and provides a sealed humidified environment essential for healing [41].

2. Materials and methods

The aim of this study is to scrutinise the use of TWO_2 when compared to conventional compression dressings (CCD) for managing RVU, with reference to technical and clinical outcomes from our tertiary referral leg ulcer clinic.

A 5-year study of TWO_2 versus CCD for chronic RVU was carried out at our tertiary referral leg ulcer clinic [42, 43]. This parallel group observational comparative study aimed at examining the safety and efficacy of TWO_2 in managing RVU in the short-term (12 weeks), and the mid-term (36 months).

Ethical approval was obtained from the local research ethics committee. Patients with chronic RVU, with an ulcer of more than two years duration, were recruited from the vascular unit. All patients must show no sign of improvement of the ulcer over the past 12 months, despite acceptable compliance with a suitable treatment, provided by community-based leg ulcer clinics. All patients were managed on an intention to treat basis and were given the choice of receiving CCD or TWO_2 therapy. Patients were informed on both CCD and TWO_2 therapies, and the treatment choice was discussed with their primary care physician and local tissue viability nurse. Treatment allocation was based on each patient's choice. All patients signed an informed consent form prior to beginning therapy.

2.1. Technical and clinical endpoints

The end points of this study were the proportion of ulcers healed at 12 weeks and recurrence rates at 36 months. Secondary end-points were time taken for full healing, percentage of reduction in the ulcer size at 12 weeks, methicillin-resistant *Staphylococcus aureus* (MRSA) elimination, pain reduction, recurrence rates and Quality-Adjusted Time Spent Without Symptoms of disease and Toxicity of treatment (Q-TWiST).

2.2. Inclusion criteria

Informed written consent was required from patient's aged ≥ 18 years.

The patients must be treated at a dedicated veins unit with $C_{6,s}$ in the Clinical, Etiological, Anatomical, and Pathophysiological (CEAP) classification [44, 45]. The venous ulcer must have been present for more than 2 years, with no improvement over the past 12 months despite adequate treatment at the veins unit. The patients must also have a normal ankle-brachial index (ABI) with a normal digital pressure.

2.3. Exclusion criteria

Patients who are bedridden, have ischemic or malignant ulcers, or osteomyelitis in the treated limb were primarily excluded. Patients with ischemic diabetic ulcers were excluded; however, it should be noted that diabetes in isolation was not considered an exclusion criterion. A prior study has shown that the AOTI Hyper-Box (AOTI Ltd., Galway, Ireland) is not sufficient in ischemic diabetic ulcers. It may induce iatrogenic deterioration of the affected diabetic limb due to the cyclic pressure of the Hyper-Box [46, 47].

2.4. Statistical analysis

Data was collected and analysed using SPSS 18 software (SPSS Inc., Chicago, IL). An independent sample t-test was used for continuous variables, while the Mann-Whitney U test was used to compare unpaired, non-parametric data. Categorical proportions were examined using the chi-squared test. Time for healing was examined using Kaplan-Meier with log-rank comparison.

2.5. Quality-Adjusted Time Spent Without Symptoms of disease and Toxicity of treatment (Q-TWiST)

The survival time for patients was divided into three separate phases: the time spent with toxicity of the disease or severe adverse events prior to disease progression known as Toxicity (TOX); the time spent without any symptoms of disease progression or toxicity of treatment known as TWiST; and finally the time spent with progression of the disease known as Progression (PROG). Ulcer recurrence in fully healed ulcers or an increase of size in ulcers that had not fully healed was defined as progression of disease. The Kaplan Meier method was used to determine the mean time spent in each of the TOX, TWiST and PROG periods for each treatment group. Mean Q-TWiST was calculated for each treatment.

2.6. Techniques

The anatomical location and duration of the ulcer, signs of infection, slough, and cellulitis, as well as any other vascular risk factors were observed in each patient. The leg ulcers were swabbed for culture as well as for level of sensitivity. Prior to therapy, a numerical rating scale in regards to pain was used. This was then repeated every three days. To record surface area, maximum length and maximum width of the ulcer, the ulcers were cleaned, debrided and digitally photographed using a Visitrak system (Smith & Nephew Ltd., Hull, United Kingdom). For all patients, ABI with big toe digital pressure measurement and punch biopsy were performed, as well as venous duplex ultrasound scan for full CEAP assessment [44, 45]. Venous Clinical Severity Score was recorded for each patient [48, 49].

2.6.1. TWO$_2$ therapy

Sixty-seven ulcers were treated with TWO$_2$ therapy. The limb was placed in the Hyper-Box for twice daily for a duration of 180 min and under pressure of 50 mbar. Oxygen supplied at 10 L/min with continuous humidification. Between each session, wounds were washed and left exposed with no dressings or compression. Wounds were cleaned, debrided and re-measured twice weekly [42, 46, 47].

2.6.2. Compression therapy

Sixty-five ulcers were treated with compression therapy. Full compression was performed using Profore ◊ multilayer compression bandage system with underlying non-adherent Profore◊ wound contact layer dressings (Profore◊, Smith & Nephew plc., London, United Kingdom). Dressings were applied by a wound care specialist nurse and changed as required, one to three times per week, depending on the amount of exudates.

Treatment was continued for 12 weeks or until complete healing of the ulcer or whichever can be first. As soon as the ulcer is healed, the leg was fitted with a class 3, closed toe, below knee elastic stocking during the day [50]. Patients were advised to revitalise the skin by soaking the leg with tap water, baby oil or olive oil to prevent itching and dry cracked skin. Patients were followed up at 3 monthly intervals following the end of the therapy. Patients without full healing of their ulcer by 12 weeks were considered failures of treatment. They were managed with CCD and continued to be seen on a weekly basis.

3. Results

Over the course of 5 years at our tertiary referral leg ulcer clinic, 1460 patients were diagnosed of chronic venous ulcers (**Figure 1**). Following application of the inclusion and exclusion criteria, 431 patients were enrolled in this study, but only 148 patients were eligible. One hundred and thirty-two patients consented to join the study, of which 67 limbs with 67 ulcers were treated using TWO_2 therapy, and 65 limbs with 65 ulcers were treated with CCD. Fifty-seven percent of the patients treated with TWO_2 were males ($n = 38$), and 54% of the patients treated with CCD were males ($n = 35$). Risk factors, such as age, gender, the presence of diabetes mellitus, smoking, hypertension and MRSA, were similar, with no statistical significance between each group. There was no significant difference between both the groups in the anatomical distribution of ulcers, size of the ulcers or the duration of the ulcer.

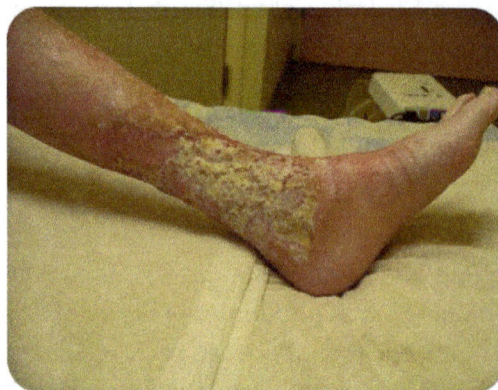

Figure 1. Patient with a chronic venous leg ulcer prior to therapy.

Twenty-four patients (36%) in the TWO_2 group and 19 patients (28%) in the CCD group were MRSA positive. Following treatment, MRSA was eliminated in 11 patients (46%), while zero cases of MRSA were eliminated in the CCD group.

The proportion of ulcers completely healed by 12 weeks was 76% ($n = 51/67$) in patients managed with TWO_2 compared to 46% ($n = 30/65$) in patients managed with CCD ($P < 0.0001$). The mean reduction in ulcer surface area at 12 weeks was 96% in the TWO_2 therapy group (**Figure 2**) compared to 61% in patients managed with CCD. The median time to full ulcer healing was 57 days in the TWO_2 group in contrast to 107 days in patients managed with CCD ($P < 0.0001$). Healing time for patients managed with TWO_2 was not affected by the extent of time of the ulcer and its size. In fact, ulcers managed with TWO_2 had a considerably shorter healing time, when compared to CCD ulcers, regardless of duration ($P < 0.0001$) or ulcer size ($P < 0.0001$). TWO_2 patients had a significantly improved Q-TWiST compared to CCD patients, denoting an improved outcome ($p < 0.0001$).

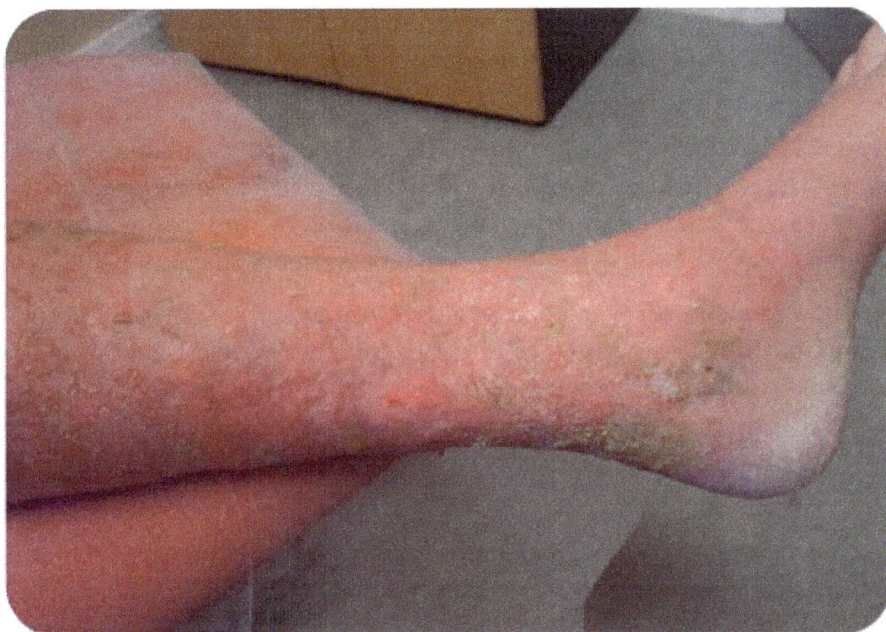

Figure 2. Significant healing and decrease in ulcer surface area post 9 weeks of TWO_2 therapy.

In all, three of the patients managed with TWO_2 were referred to our facility for primary amputation following the failure of other treatment modalities, including skin grafting. These three ulcers fully healed with no need for amputation in any case. After 36 months of follow-up, 14 of the 30 healed CCD ulcers showed recurrence compared to three of the 51 TWO_2-healed ulcers. Two CCD-managed ulcers that had not completely healed showed signs of deterioration and increase in surface area ($P < 0.0001$). All the cases that healed with TWO_2 showed reversed gradient healing phenomena where the ulcer healed from the centre to the periphery. This might be the reason for the absence of scarring and recurrence.

4. Discussion

The socio-economic consequences of management of RVU, merged with high recurrence rates, have encouraged the development of a disruptive technology innovative therapy, such as TWO_2 therapy. Compression therapy within the setup of a leg ulcer clinic is widely recognised as the main modality for managing venous leg ulcers [17, 18, 51, 52]. A previous study mentioned that contemporary dressing materials do not stimulate healing, and expenses are not clinically justified as they have no proven efficacy [19]. After 30 years of research, there is no data to defend using anything other than a simple, inexpensive, low-adherence dressing under multilayer compression [19].

The first publication on the use of TWO_2 was by Fischer in 1969 [20]. Fischer noted that lesions became aseptic and enhanced granulation was witnessed two days after TWO_2. In a prospective randomised study by Heng et al. red granulation tissue was present one week after TWO_2 [27]. Heng noted an absence of clinical scarring and most ulcers healed within 2–16 weeks. Gordillo et al. conducted a study on full-body hyperbaric oxygen (HBO) therapy versus TWO_2. Topical oxygen treatment showed a significant reduction in wound size and was associated with higher vascular endothelial growth factor (VEGF)165 expression in healing wounds [53].

Blackman et al. explored the efficacy of topical oxygen therapy as an adjunctive modality in repairing diabetic ulcers that failed to heal by best practice standard wound care. The healing rate after 12 weeks of topical wound oxygen therapy was 82.4%, and the mean time to complete healing was reduced. Patients also showed very low recurrence rates after 18 months [54].

Results from the Venous ULcer Cost-effectiveness of Antimicrobial dressings (VULCAN) trial showed that it took 101 days to heal 3-cm ulcers, while there was a 1-year recurrence rate of 14% in 86% of small ulcers [55], using silver dressings. These types of dressings are now rarely seen in a standard tertiary vein unit. In our unit, we have abandoned the use of silver dressing in any form as it showed a higher incidence of contacting eczema and an increase in the chronicity of the wounds.

Oxygen plays a major role in the promotion of vascular endothelial cell proliferation, collagen synthesis [56, 57] and infection control [58] by providing a direct microbial growth inhibitory effect [59] and also by activating neutrophils [60]. TWO_2 therapy evades the consequences of a full-body hyperbaric chamber [61], such as grand mal seizures and pulmonary oxygen toxicity [61, 62]. There is also the high associated cost of acquiring and maintaining a chamber to consider.

Utilising diffused oxygen raises the capillary partial pressure of oxygen (Po_2) levels at the wound site, stimulating epithelialisation and granulation of new healthy tissue [29, 32]. Oxygen generates reactive oxygen species at the wound site, acting as signalling substances, which increase the production of VEGF [63, 64]. Repeated treatment therefore accelerates wound closure.

TWO_2 therapy enhances both polymorph nuclear function and bacterial clearance and is fatal to anaerobic bacteria [35–37]. It reduces neutrophil adherence based on hindering the β-2 integrin function [38]. Eleven patients (46%) with MRSA were negative at the end of treatment with TWO_2. This informs us of its effectiveness against MRSA infection in comparison to CCD. TWO_2 therapy supports and strengthens antibiotic distribution for aminoglycosides, cephalosporins, quinilones and amphotericin [39, 40].

While TWO_2 therapy has been available for many years, there is paucity in clinical evidence for its safety and efficacy. Experience from our clinic shows that TWO_2 therapy is effective and valuable in managing RVU. Our course of therapy accomplished enhanced wound healing time, without complications, in a relatively large number of patients. TWO_2 therapy drastically reduced the time required for RVU healing and recurrence rates when compared to CCD. Quality of time spent without symptoms or toxicity of the disease was significantly improved in TWO_2 managed patients compared to CCD patients ($p < 0.0001$).

5. Conclusion

TWO_2 therapy is practical, effective and valuable in managing RVU without the risks associated with full-body hyperbaric chambers. TWO_2 therapy requires no further specialist skills by the primary care physician or local tissue viability nurse. It is therefore readily available for application under most circumstances, even for domiciliary use. The treatment has an extremely low risk of systemic complications when compared to HBO, and single-use devices greatly reduce the possibility of secondary infections.

TWO_2 slashes the time needed for RVU healing and is successful in pain alleviation, MRSA elimination and management. Utilising diffused oxygen raises the capillary partial Po_2 levels at the wound site, stimulating epithelialisation and granulation of new healthy tissue. TWO_2 therapy radically degrades recurrence rates. Taking the social and individual aspects of chronic venous ulceration into account, the use of TWO_2 can provide an overwhelmingly improved quality of life for long-time sufferers of this debilitating disease.

Author details

Sherif Sultan[1,2*], Wael Tawfick[1], Edel P Kavanagh[2] and Niamh Hynes[2]

*Address all correspondence to: sherif.sultan@hse.ie

1 Department of Vascular and Endovascular Surgery, Western Vascular Institute, University College Hospital Galway, Galway, Ireland

2 Department of Vascular and Endovascular Surgery, Galway Clinic, Doughiska, Galway, Ireland

References

[1] Trent JT, Falabella A, Eaglstein WH, Kirsner RS. Venous ulcers: pathophysiology and treatment options. Ostomy/Wound Management. 2005 May;51(5):38–54.

[2] O'Meara S, Cullum NA, Nelson EA. Compression for venous leg ulcers. Cochrane Database Systematic Review. 2009 Jan 21;1:CD000265.

[3] Moffatt CJ, Franks PJ, Doherty DC, Martin R, Blewett R, Ross F. Prevalence of leg ulceration in a London population. QJM. 2004 Jul 1;97(7):431–7.

[4] Graham ID, Harrison MB, Nelson EA, Lorimer K, Fisher A. Prevalence of lower-limb ulceration: a systematic review of prevalence studies. Advances in Skin & Wound Care. 2003 Nov 1;16(6):305–16.

[5] Margolisa DJ, Bilkerb W, Santannab J. Venous leg ulcer: incidence and prevalence in the elderly. Journal of the American Academy of Dermatology. 2002 Mar 31;46(3):381–6.

[6] Anand SC, Dean C, Nettleton R, Praburaj DV. Health-related quality of life tools for venous-ulcerated patients. British Journal of Nursing. 2003 Jan 9;12(1):48–59.

[7] Phillips TJ. Chronic cutaneous ulcers: etiology and epidemiology. Journal of Investigative Dermatology. 1994 Jun 1;102(6):38S–41S.

[8] Persoon A, Heinen MM, Van Der Vleuten CJ, De Rooij MJ, Van De Kerkhof P, Van Achterberg T. Leg ulcers: a review of their impact on daily life. Journal of Clinical Nursing. 2004 Mar 1;13(3):341–54.

[9] Armstrong SA. Compression hosiery. Professional Nurse (London, England). 1997 Apr; 12(7 Suppl):S10–1.

[10] Moffatt CJ, Dorman MC. Recurrence of leg ulcers within a community ulcer service. Journal of Wound Care. 1995 Feb;4(2):57–61.

[11] Monk BE, Sarkany I. Outcome of treatment of venous stasis ulcers. Clinical and Experimental Dermatology. 1982 Jul 1;7(4):397–400.

[12] Lees TA, Lambert D. Prevalence of lower limb ulceration in an urban health district. British Journal of Surgery. 1992 Oct 1;79(10):1032–4.

[13] Callam MJ, Ruckley CV, Harper DR, Dale JJ. Chronic ulceration of the leg: extent of the problem and provision of care. British Medical Journal (Clinical Research ed). 1985 Jun 22;290(6485):1855–6.

[14] Nelzen O, Bergqvist D, Lindhagen A. Venous and non-venous leg ulcers: Clinical history and appearance in a population study. British Journal of Surgery. 1994 Feb 1;81(2):182–7.

[15] Ragnarson Tennvall G, Hjelmgren J. Original research articles—clinical science: annual costs of treatment for venous leg ulcers in Sweden and the United Kingdom. Wound Repair and Regeneration. 2005 Jan 1;13(1):13–8.

[16] Ruckley CV. Socioeconomic impact of chronic venous insufficiency and leg ulcers. Angiology. 1997 Jan 1;48(1):67–9.

[17] Palfreyman SJ, Lochiel R, Michaels JA. A systematic review of compression therapy for venous leg ulcers. Vascular Medicine. 1998 Nov 1;3(4):301–13.

[18] Cullum N, Nelson EA, Fletcher AW, Sheldon TA. Compression for venous leg ulcers. Cochrane Database Syst Rev. 2001;(2):CD000265.

[19] Sultan MJ, McCollum C. Don't waste money when dressing leg ulcers. British Journal of Surgery. 2009 Oct 1;96(10):1099–100.

[20] Fischer B. Topical hyperbaric oxygen treatment of pressure sores and skin ulcers. The Lancet. 1969 Aug 23;294(7617):405–9.

[21] Olejniczak S. Employment of low hyperbaric therapy in management of leg ulcers. Michigan Medicine. 1966 Dec;65(12):1067–8.

[22] Gruber RP, Heitkamp DH, Billy LJ, Amato JJ. Skin permeability to oxygen and hyperbaric oxygen. Archives of Surgery. 1970 Jul 1;101(1):69–70.

[23] Fischer BH. Treatment of ulcers on the legs with hyperbaric oxygen. The Journal of Dermatologic Surgery and Oncology. 1975 Oct 1;1(3):55–8.

[24] Kalliainen LK, Gordillo GM, Schlanger R, Sen CK. Topical oxygen as an adjunct to wound healing: a clinical case series. Pathophysiology. 2003 Jan 31;9(2):81–7.

[25] Edsberg LE, Brogan MS, Jaynes CD, Fries K. Topical hyperbaric oxygen and electrical stimulation: exploring potential synergy. Ostomy/Wound Management. 2002 Nov; 48(11):42–50.

[26] Edsberg LE, Brogan MS, Jaynes CD, Fries K. Reducing epibole using topical hyperbaric oxygen and electrical stimulation. Ostomy/Wound Management. 2002 Apr;48(4):26.

[27] Heng MC, Harker J, Csathy G, Marshall C, Brazier J, Sumampong S, Paterno GE. Angiogenesis in necrotic ulcers treated with hyperbaric oxygen. Ostomy/Wound Management. 2000 Sep;46(9):18–28.

[28] Leslie CA, Sapico FL, Ginunas VJ, Adkins RH. Randomized controlled trial of topical hyperbaric oxygen for treatment of diabetic foot ulcers. Diabetes Care. 1988 Feb 1;11(2): 111–5.

[29] Heng MC. Topical hyperbaric therapy for problem skin wounds. The Journal of Dermatologic Surgery and Oncology. 1993 Aug 1;19(8):784–93.

[30] Prost-Squarcioni C, Fraitag S, Heller M, Boehm N. Functional histology of dermis. Annales de Dermatologie et de Venereologie 2008 Jan; 135(1 Pt 2):1S5–20.

[31] Wirthner R, Balamurugan K, Stiehl DP, Barth S, Spielmann P, Oehme F, Flamme I, Katschinski DM, Wenger RH, Camenisch G. Determination and modulation of prolyl-4-hydroxylase domain oxygen sensor activity. Methods in Enzymology. 2007 Dec 31;435:43–60.

[32] Upson AV. Topical hyperbaric oxygenation in the treatment of recalcitrant open wounds. A clinical report. Physical Therapy. 1986 Sep 1;66(9):1408–12.

[33] Knighton DR, Silver IA, Hunt TK. Regulation of wound-healing angiogenesis-effect of oxygen gradients and inspired oxygen concentration. Surgery. 1981 Aug;90(2):262–70.

[34] Scott G. Topical oxygen alters angiogenesis-related growth factor expression in chronic diabetic foot ulcers. Irish Journal of Medical Science. 2007;176:S2.

[35] Kaufman T, Alexander JW, Nathan P, Brackett KA, MacMillan BG. The microclimate chamber: the effect of continuous topical administration of 96% oxygen and 75% relative humidity on the healing rate of experimental deep burns. Journal of Trauma and Acute Care Surgery. 1983 Sep 1;23(9):806–15.

[36] Park MK, Myers RA, Marzella L. Oxygen tensions and infections: modulation of microbial growth, activity of antimicrobial agents, and immunologic responses. Clinical Infectious Diseases. 1992 Mar 1;14(3):720–40.

[37] Mandell GL. Bactericidal activity of aerobic and anaerobic polymorphonuclear neutrophils. Infection and Immunity. 1974 Feb 1;9(2):337–41.

[38] Thom SR. Effects of hyperoxia on neutrophil adhesion. Undersea & Hyperbaric Medicine. 2004 Apr 1;31(1):123.

[39] Mirhij NJ, Roberts RJ, Myers MG. Effects of hypoxemia upon aminoglycoside serum pharmacokinetics in animals. Antimicrobial Agents and Chemotherapy. 1978 Sep 1;14(3):344–7.

[40] Keck PE, Gottlieb SF, Conley J. Interaction of increased pressures of oxygen and sulfonamides on the in vitro and in vivo growth of pathogenic bacteria. Undersea Biomedical Research. 1980 Jun;7(2):95–106.

[41] Olejniczak S, Zielinski A. Topical oxygen promotes healing of leg ulcers. Medical Times. 1976 Dec;104(12):114–21.

[42] Tawfick W, Sultan S. Does topical wound oxygen (TWO 2) offer an improved outcome over conventional compression dressings (CCD) in the management of refractory venous ulcers (RVU)? A parallel observational comparative study. European Journal of Vascular and Endovascular Surgery. 2009 Jul 31;38(1):125–32.

[43] Tawfick WA, Sultan S. Technical and clinical outcome of topical wound oxygen in comparison to conventional compression dressings in the management of refractory nonhealing venous ulcers. Vascular and Endovascular Surgery. 2012 Dec 5:1538574412467684.

[44] Eklöf B, Rutherford RB, Bergan JJ, Carpentier PH, Gloviczki P, Kistner RL, Meissner MH, Moneta GL, Myers K, Padberg FT, Perrin M. American Venous Forum International Ad Hoc Committee for Revision of the CEAP Classification. Revision of the CEAP classification for chronic venous disorders: consensus statement. Journal of Vascular Surgery. 2004 Dec;40(6):1248–52.

[45] Meissner MH, Gloviczki P, Bergan J, Kistner RL, Morrison N, Pannier F, Pappas PJ, Rabe E, Raju S, Villavicencio JL. Primary chronic venous disorders. Journal of Vascular Surgery. 2007 Dec 31;46(6):S54–67.

[46] Tawfick W, Sultan S. Early results of topical wound oxygen (TWO2) therapy in the management of refractory nonhealing venous ulcers: superior role over conventional compression dressings. Vascular. 2008;16(Suppl 2):S156e7.

[47] Tawfick W, Sultan S. Topical wound oxygen versus conventional compression dressings in the management of refractory venous ulcers: a parallel observational pivotal study. Irish Journal of Medical Science. 2007;176(1):S2.

[48] Meissner MH, Moneta G, Burnand K, Gloviczki P, Lohr JM, Lurie F, Mattos MA, McLafferty RB, Mozes G, Rutherford RB, Padberg F. The hemodynamics and diagnosis of venous disease. Journal of Vascular Surgery. 2007 Dec 31;46(6):S4–24.

[49] Ricci MA, Emmerich J, Callas PW, Rosendaal FR, Stanley AC, Naud S, Vossen C, Bovill EG. Evaluating chronic venous disease with a new venous severity scoring system. Journal of Vascular Surgery. 2003 Nov 30;38(5):909–15.

[50] Nelson EA, Harper DR, Prescott RJ, Gibson B, Brown D, Ruckley CV. Prevention of recurrence of venous ulceration: randomized controlled trial of class 2 and class 3 elastic compression. Journal of Vascular Surgery. 2006 Oct 31;44(4):803–8.

[51] Ghauri AS, Taylor MC, Deacon JE, Whyman MR, Earnshaw JJ, Heather BP, Poskitt KR. Influence of a specialized leg ulcer service on management and outcome. British Journal of Surgery. 2000 Aug 1;87(8):1048–56.

[52] Fletcher A, Cullum N, Sheldon TA. A systematic review of compression treatment for venous leg ulcers. British Medical Journal. 1997 Sep 6;315(7108):576–80.

[53] Gordillo GM, Roy S, Khanna S, Schlanger R, Khandelwal S, Phillips G, Sen CK. Topical oxygen therapy induces vascular endothelial growth factor expression and improves closure of clinically presented chronic wounds. Clinical and Experimental Pharmacology and Physiology. 2008 Aug 1;35(8):957–64.

[54] Blackman E, Moore C, Hyatt J, Railton R, Frye C. Topical wound oxygen therapy in the treatment of severe diabetic foot ulcers: a prospective controlled study. Ostomy/Wound Management. 2010 Jun 1;56(6):24.

[55] Michaels JA, Campbell B, King B, Palfreyman SJ, Shackley P, Stevenson M. Randomized controlled trial and cost-effectiveness analysis of silver-donating antimicrobial dress-

ings for venous leg ulcers (VULCAN trial). British Journal of Surgery. 2009 Oct 1;96(10): 1147–56.

[56] Rodriguez PG, Felix FN, Woodley DT, Shim EK. The role of oxygen in wound healing: a review of the literature. Dermatologic Surgery. 2008 Sep 1;34(9):1159–69.

[57] Schreml S, Szeimies RM, Prantl L, Karrer S, Landthaler M, Babilas P. Oxygen in acute and chronic wound healing. British Journal of Dermatology. 2010 Aug 1;163(2):257–68.

[58] Asano S. Leukocyte. In: Uchiyama T, eds. Miwa Hematology 3rd edn, 292–5, Hakuhodo, Tokyo, 2006.

[59] McAllister TA, Stark JM, Norman JN, Ross RM. Inhibitory effects of hyperbaric oxygen on bacteria and fungi. The Lancet. 1963 Nov 16;282(7316):1040–2.

[60] Hohn DC. Host resistance of infection. In: Hunt TK, ed. Wound healing and wound infection. 264–80, Appleton-Century Crofts, New York, 1980.

[61] Leach RM, Rees PJ, Wilmshurst P. Hyperbaric oxygen therapy. British Medical Journal. 1998 Oct 24;317(7166):1140–3.

[62] Kindwall EP. A history of hyperbaric medicine. Hyperbaric medicine practice. Best Publishing Company, Arizona. 1994:2–16.

[63] Sheikh AY, Gibson JJ, Rollins MD, Hopf HW, Hussain Z, Hunt TK. Effect of hyperoxia on vascular endothelial growth factor levels in a wound model. Archives of Surgery. 2000 Nov 1;135(11):1293–7.

[64] Roy S, Khanna S, Nallu K, Hunt TK, Sen CK. Dermal wound healing is subject to redox control. Molecular Therapy. 2006 Jan 1;13(1):211–20.

7

Antimicrobial Dressings for Improving Wound Healing

Omar Sarheed, Asif Ahmed, Douha Shouqair and
Joshua Boateng

Abstract

Wound healing occurs by a series of interrelated molecular events which work together to restore tissue integrity and cellular function. These physiological events occur smoothly in normal healthy individual and/or under normal conditions. However, in certain cases, these molecular events are retarded resulting in hard-to-heal or chronic wounds arising from several factors such as poor venous return, underlying physiological or metabolic conditions such as diabetes as well as external factors such as poor nutrition. In most cases, such wounds are infected and infection also presents as another complicating phenomenon which triggers inflammatory reactions, therefore delaying wound healing. There has therefore been recent interests and significant efforts in preventing and actively treating wound infections by directly targeting infection causative agents through direct application of antimicrobial agents either alone or loaded into dressings (medicated). These have the advantage of overcoming challenges such as poor circulation in diabetic and leg ulcers when administered systemically and also require lower amounts to be applied compared to that required via oral or iv administration. This chapter will review and evaluate various antimicrobial agents used to target infected wounds, the means of delivery, and current state of the art, including commercially available dressings. Data sources will include mainly peer-reviewed literature, clinical trials and reports, patents as well as government reports where available.

Keywords: antimicrobial, bioburden, dressings, infection, wounds, wound healing, bacterial resistance

1. Introduction

A wound may be defined as a disruption to the physiological arrangement of the skin cells and a disturbance to its function in connecting and protecting underlying tissues and organs. It may be primary caused by accidental cut, tear, scratch, pressure, extreme temperatures, chemicals, and electrical current, or secondary to surgical intervention or disease (i.e., diabetes, ulcers, or carcinomas) [1]. It ranges from superficial (affecting the epidermis) to partial-thickness (affecting both epidermis and parts of the dermis) and full-thickness (including subcutaneous fat and bones) wounds [2]. Wound healing is a physiological process, by which the living body repairs tissue damages, restores its anatomical integrity, and regains the functionality of the injured parts. A wound can be closed by primary intention or left to heal by secondary intention, and in both ways the healing process occurs through a series of overlapping events and is influenced by a number of intrinsic and extrinsic factors [3].

1.1. Acute wounds

Acute wounds can heal within a limited amount of time, usually show no complications, and are characterized by the loss of skin integrity (injury) that occurs suddenly. The injured tissue heals in a predictable manner where platelets, keratinocytes, immune surveillance cells, microvascular cells, and fibroblasts play major roles in the restoration of tissue integrity [4]. These wounds are either surgical or traumatic [5].

1.2. Chronic wounds

Chronic wounds are wounds that do not heal within normal period and are associated with predisposing factors that weaken the integrity of dermal and epidermal tissues. Those factors either disrupt the balance between wound bioburden and the patient's immune system or impair the wound healing cycle. In terms of duration, if the wound fails to heal or shows no sign of recovery within 12 weeks, it is considered a chronic wound. Predisposing factors may affect the tissue perfusion causing chronic wounds such as vascular ulcers, associated with metabolic disorders such as diabetes causing diabetic foot ulcers [6]. They can be identified by criteria such as delayed healing and friable granulation tissue, prolonged inflammatory phase, persistent infection, and presence of resistant microorganisms [7–10].

1.3. Wound healing

The repair (wound healing) process involves four overlapping biochemical, physiological, and molecular phases.

I. Hemostasis

> This stage is characterized by microvascular injury and release of blood components at the wound site. Platelets come into contact with and adhere to the wall of the injured blood vessels. This adherence activates the platelets to release cytokines, growth factors, and numerous pro-inflammatory mediators, resulting in platelet aggregation and triggering the intrinsic and extrinsic coagulation path-

ways to form a fibrin clot which limits further blood loss. Growth factors produced by the platelets initiate the healing cascade [11, 12].

II. Inflammatory phase

The inflammatory phase starts at the same time as hemostasis sometime between a few minutes after injury up to 24 h and lasts for about 3 days. Aggregated platelets store vasoactive amines such as prostaglandins and histamine while other amines from granules released by mast cells, in response to injury, result in increased microvascular permeability and vasodilation, leading to exudation of fluid into the extravascular space [13]. This allows the migration of monocytes and protein-rich exudate into the wound and surrounding tissue, resulting in edema. These are typical signs of the inflammation process, and patients start complaining about pain at the site of injury within 24 h.

III. Proliferative phase

This phase commences after the inflammatory phase wanes. The remaining inflammatory cells produce growth factors to initiate angiogenesis, which is important to keep adequate blood supply within the wound bed [14]. Newly formed blood vessels will contribute to granulation tissue (composed of collagen and extracellular matrix) formation and provide the required nutrients.

IV. Maturation phase

This commences when the wound is superficially sealed. It involves the re-epithelialization and remodeling of newly formed tissues in the proliferative phase and restoration of epidermal integrity [15]. It also involves transferring collagen III to collagen I.

1.4. Factors affecting wound healing

Multiple factors affect wound healing and lead to the impairment of healing classified into local and systemic factors [16].

1.4.1. Oxygenation

Oxygen is crucial to wound healing and for resistance to infection, and used for cellular energy production by adenosine triphosphate [17]. It acts on different levels of wound healing by inducing angiogenesis, keratinocytes differentiation, migration, re-epithelialization, fibroblast proliferation, and collagen synthesis, and promotes wound contraction [18]. When injury occurs, temporary hypoxia and oxygen are useful to trigger wound healing by inducing the production of cytokines and growth factors from macrophages, keratinocytes, and fibroblasts [16]. Chronic wounds are generally hypoxic with oxygen tissue tension of 5–20 mm Hg compared to normal levels of 30–50 mm Hg [19]. Factors predisposing chronic wounds such as advancing age and diabetes can induce poor oxygenation through impaired vascular flow. Interventional revascularization therapies have been used to reverse hypoxic conditions in diabetic foot ulcers [20]. However, it has also been reported that such procedures can cause adverse effects to diabetic patients [21]. Recently, some topical foam dressings containing dissolved oxygen were developed to increase oxygen perfusion into the chronic wound area [22]. Results showed that dissolved oxygen from topical foam dressing penetrates into skin layers compared to topical gaseous oxygen.

1.4.2. Wound bioburden and infection

1.4.2.1. Bioburden

The intact skin acts to control the microbial population on the skin surface itself [23]. Once the integrity is lost through injury, the subcutaneous tissue becomes exposed, providing an environment for colonization and growth of microbes. However, this does not necessarily lead to an infection as there is a balance between the wound bioburden and the immune system [24].

1.4.2.2. Wound infection

Skin microflora is present to about 10^5 colonies without any clinical problems [25]. However, if the balance is disrupted, microorganisms will proliferate and start a microbiological chain of events by invading tissues resulting in an inflammatory response which may lead to tissue damage and delayed healing [7]. Once it causes damage to the host tissue, infection will arise. One of the consequences of infection is the prolonged inflammation due to prolonged elevation of pro-inflammatory cytokines, which causes the wound to enter the chronic stage and fail to heal within the expected 8–12 weeks [26]. This prolonged inflammation is also associated with increased levels of matrix metalloproteases which are capable of degrading the extracellular matrix which is the key component of proliferative phase of wound healing [9]. This increase in protease levels happens at the expense of the naturally occurring protease inhibitor levels that are decreased. From a microbiological perspective, wound infection is described as the presence of replicating microorganisms at the wound site overwhelming the host's immune system. It delays wound healing due to the release of toxins and exhibits active signs and symptoms of infections.

1.4.2.3. Common bacterial species present in chronic wounds

Generally, most infected wounds are polymicrobial and are commonly contaminated by pathogens found in the immediate environment, the endogenous microbes living in the mucous membranes, and the microflora on adjacent skin. Bacteria are the main cause of wound infection among other microorganisms present in the skin, though other microorganisms such as fungi have been implicated in certain mixed infections. In the initial stages of chronic wound formation, Gram-positive organisms such as *Staphylococcus aureus* and *Escherichia coli* are predominant [9]. In the later stages, Gram-negative *Pseudomonas* species are common and tend to invade deeper layers in the wound causing significant tissue damage [27]. Other aerobes implicated include *Staphylococci* and *Streptococci* species as well as anaerobic bacteria and are estimated in 50% of chronic wounds [28, 29].

1.4.3. Chronic wounds and biofilm

Biofilm is defined as "a microbially derived sessile community characterized by cells that are irreversibly attached to a substratum or interface or to each other, are embedded in a secreted matrix of extracellular polymeric substances (EPSs), and exhibit an altered phenotype with respect to growth rate and gene transcription" [30]. Firstly, conditioning film forms and is composed of proteins and polysaccharide molecules adsorbed onto the solid surface. This makes the surface ready to receive the first cells of the insipient biofilm. Secondly, bacteria will start to approach and attach onto the surface by forces such as van der Waals forces and the negative electrostatic charges of bacterial surface [31]. The attached bacteria become encased in a polymeric matrix called extracellular polymeric substance (EPS). This bacterial attachment induces a phenomenon called quorum sensing, which is responsible for "the regulation of gene expression in response to fluctuations in cell population density" [32]. This causes the bacteria within biofilm to alter their phenotypes resulting in the production of more virulent factors in response to signals from other bacteria within biofilm. These factors with barrier made from EPS contribute to the increased resistance to antibiotics. It has been suggested that EPS can interact with antibiotics spontaneously thereby preventing them reaching the bacteria to exert their antimicrobial activity [33]. The biofilm also protects the bacteria from host defenses by the covering of glycocalyx while bacteria secrete products within the film which makes phagocytic penetration poor [34].

This understanding is of great importance for intervention modalities in chronic wounds especially the use of antimicrobial wound dressing. For example macrolides can have inhibitory effect on the film formation or induce phagocytic invasion into biofilms [35]. Furthermore, in clinical wound management, it is always essential to promptly clean the wound and remove necrotic tissue and foreign material (e.g. bacteria and biofilms) from areas around the wound to improve the chances of enhanced wound healing, and this is known as debridement [1]. This is important because the presence of necrotic tissue increases the risk of infection and sepsis, which prolongs the inflammatory phase. Several approaches are employed including surgical removal, wound irrigation (e.g. saline and antiseptics such as chlorhexidine), autolytic rehydration using hydrogel dressings, applying enzymes such as collagenases or streptokinase preparations as well as using maggots to selectively dissolve necrotic and infected tissue (including biofilms) without destroying healthy or newly formed tissue [1].

2. Wound dressings

Wound dressings can maintain a moist environment in the wound which helps in proliferation and migration of fibroblast and keratinocytes. Moisture in the wound serves as a transporter for enzymes, growth factors, and hormones, thus inducing cell growth. Moist wound dressings promote collagen synthesis and decrease scar formation [36] which help wounds to heal faster [37]. Modern moist wound dressings can be classified depending on their materials (synthetic and natural polymers) and physical forms (hydrogels, hydrocolloids, films, and wafers).

Hydrogels consist of hydrated polymers which make them hydrophilic in nature. Water content is higher than 95%, and as a result they cannot absorb much exudate and cause maceration. But, this dressing is very useful in dry wound which can maintain moisture within wounds [36]. A Cochrane Review [38] of hydrogel dressings for healing diabetic foot ulcers suggests that hydrogel dressings are more effective than basic wound contact dressing. Hydrogels have advantages of autolytic debridement of slough and necrotic tissue and do not support bacterial growth [39, 40]. Hydrocolloid dressings are occlusive and can absorb wound exudate into the matrix to help improve healing. It can work for a sustained period of time, thus reducing the frequency of dressing changes. It also assists autolysis of necrotic materials [40]. Due to its extra absorbent nature, it is widely used in the treatment of cavity wounds [41]. A Cochrane Review [42] reported that any type of hydrocolloid and other dressings have no difference in efficacy. Foam dressings are highly absorptive, protective, and comfortable to the body surface. They promote thermal insulation, angiogenesis, and autolysis [43]. Film dressings are adhesive, transparent, durable, comfortable, and cost effective. Due to their transparency, the wound bed can be monitored without removing the dressing. However, films are suitable for superficial pressure wounds. The disadvantage of film dressing is maceration of wound exudate [36]. Lyophilized wafers are one of the most recent moist dressings proposed for wound care. Due to their highly porous nature, they can absorb high amounts of exudate rapidly which improves wound healing. Wafers can carry both antibacterial and anti-inflammatory drugs at the same time which give dual effects of inhibiting bacteria and reducing inflammation [44]. Wafers have good adhesion and diffusion properties [45] while Labovitiadi et al. [46] reported that wafers are a compatible delivery system for both insoluble and soluble antimicrobial drugs that exhibit better antimicrobial activity.

3. Antimicrobial wound dressings

3.1. Need for antimicrobial wound dressing

The major need for antimicrobial dressing is drug resistance to bacteria. Zubair et al. [47] isolated bacteria from diabetic foot ulcer patients and their resistance to different classes of drugs with the penicillins showing highest susceptibility to resistance followed by cephalosporins (54%), quinolones and fluoroquinolones (52.8%), aminoglycosides (38.5%), beta lactams (32.2%), and carbapenems (18.4%). Further, most chronic wound sufferers such as older patients and diabetics with leg and foot ulcers suffer from complications of poor circulation at the lower extremities, which makes oral and IV antibiotics ineffective. In addition, topical dressings are able to avoid the adverse effects of systemic administration (oral and IV) of high antibiotic doses including nausea, vomiting, diarrhea, allergic reactions, leukocyturia, insomnia, headache, and vaginosis, when only small doses above the minimum inhibitory concentration are required at the infected wound site. Finally, production costs of most dressings are less than those of IV or oral products.

3.2. Advanced medicated antimicrobial wound dressings

Antimicrobial dressings can be broadly classified into two groups as antiseptic or antibiotic dressings. Antiseptic dressings have broad spectrum activity which can kill or inhibit bacteria, fungus, protozoa, viruses, and prions [48]; however, some antiseptic dressings often show dose-dependent cytotoxicity to the host cells including keratinocytes, fibroblasts, and leuko-cytes [49, 50]. The concentration of povidone iodine greater than 0.004 and 0.05% is completely toxic to keratinocytes and fibroblasts, respectively [51]. Cadexomer iodine is reported to be nontoxic to fibroblasts *in vitro* at concentrations of up to 0.45% [52]. Chlorhexidine also shows dose-dependent toxicity to fibroblasts at concentrations between 0.2 and 0.001% [53, 54]. Moreover, silver-impregnated dressings have been reported to be more cytotoxic to epidermal keratinocytes and dermal fibroblasts than honey-based dressings [55]. On the other hand,

Dressing type	Polymers	Drug	Reference
Pads	Bovine serum albumin	Ciprofloxacin	[58]
Nanofibers patch	PVA/sodium alginate	Ciprofloxacin	[59]
Hydrogel	Polyethylene glycol	Ciprofloxacin	[60]
Sponges	Alginate/chitosan	Ciprofloxacin	[61]
Films	Chitosan/gelatin	Ciprofloxacin	[62]
Nanofibers	PVA/regenerated silk fibroin	Ciprofloxacin	[63]
Nanofiber mats	Polyurethane/dextran	Ciprofloxacin	[64]
Nanofiber mats	PVA/poly(vinyl acetate)	Ciprofloxacin	[65]
Films	Poly (2-hydroxymethacrylate)	Ciprofloxacin	[66]
Films	PVA/aminophenylboronic acid	Ciprofloxacin	[67]
Collagen dressing	Collagen	Ciprofloxacin	[68]
Hydrogels	Keratin	Ciprofloxacin	[69]
Films	Sodium carboxymethyl cellulose/gelatin	Ciprofloxacin	[70]
Scaffolds	Chitosan/polyethylene glycol	Ciprofloxacin	[71]
Hydrogel films	Carboxymethyl chitin	Chlorhexidine gluconate	[72]
Gel	Chitosan	Ofloxacin	[73]
Wafers and films	Polyox/carrageenan	Streptomycin	[74–76]
Films	PVA/sodium alginate	Clindamycin and nitrofurazone	[77, 78]
Films	PVA/dextran	Gentamicin	[79]
Scaffolds	Collagen	Doxycycline	[80]
Microspheres	Gelatin	Doxycycline	[81]
Microspheres	Chitosan	Levofloxacin	[82]
Nanofibrous scaffolds	Chitosan/poly(e-caprolactone)	Levofloxacin	[82]
Hydrogels	Polyvinylalcohol	Nitric oxide	[83]
Hydrogels	poly(2-hydroxyethyl methacrylate)	Nitric oxide	[84]
Hydrogels	S-Nitrosothiol	Nitric acid	[85]

Table 1. Summary of antibiotic dressings reported in the literature.

antibiotic dressings (**Table 1**) are nontoxic and can work effectively on the target sites without damaging host tissues [49]. The ideal antimicrobial dressing should have broad spectrum activity against all major microorganisms, be nonallergic and nontoxic to host cells, have the ability to drain exudate and maintain a moist wound environment, should release drugs rapidly in a sustained manner, should reduce malodor, and be cost effective [56, 57].

3.3. Silver-based dressings

Silver is a natural broad spectrum antibiotic, and its dressings have not yet shown any bacterial resistance. Silver exists in different forms such as silver oxide, silver nitrate, silver sulfate, silver salt, silver zeolite, silver sulfadiazine (SSD), and silver nanoparticles (AgNPs). Before the eighteenth century, silver nitrate was used for leg ulcers, epilepsy, acne, and venereal infections [86]. Currently different forms of silver are widely used in acute wound (burns, partial-thickness burns, freshly grafted burns, second-degree burns, surgical/traumatic wounds, colorectal surgical wounds, pilonidal sinus, and donor site), and chronic wound (pressure ulcers, leg ulcers, and diabetic foot ulcers) healing [87].

3.3.1. Antimicrobial activity of silver dressings

Antimicrobial activity of silver dressings depends on the amount and rate of silver release and its toxicity to bacterial, fungal, and algal cells. Silver works by interacting with thiol groups present in bacterial cells thus stop their respiration process. In the case of *E. coli*, silver prevents phosphate uptake and catalysation of disulfide bonds with silver tending to change the nature of protein structure in *E. coli*. The degenerative changes in cytosolic protein cause cell death [86, 88]. Feng et al. [89] reported antibacterial mechanism of action of silver ions on *E. coli* and *S. aureus* and showed that silver ions penetrate into bacterial cells and condense DNA molecules which inhibit their replication capabilities leading to cell death. Matsumura et al. [90] introduced two bactericidal mechanism actions of silver zeolite on *E. coli*. Firstly, silver ions released from silver zeolite come into contact with cells and penetrate into cells, altering the cellular functions that cause cell death. Secondly, silver ions inhibit respiration process through the generation of reactive oxygen molecules. Silver zeolite has also been reported against oral microorganisms (*Streptococcus mutans, Lactobacillus casei, Candida albicans, and S. aureus*) [91].

Silver nanoparticles show the most efficient antimicrobial activity amongst all forms of silver. The bactericidal effects of AgNPs depend on the size, shape, surface characteristics, and their dose [88, 92–101]. It has been reported that 75 μg ml^{-1} of AgNPs having 1–100 nm particle size inhibits all bacterial strains (specifically, *E. coli, Vibrio cholerae, Salmonella typhi, and Pseudomonas aeruginosa*). It has also been reported nanoparticles having particle size ~1–10 nm have higher affinity of attaching to the surface of the cell membrane as compared to larger nanoparticles. Because of this nature, AgNPs can attach to the larger surface area of bacterial cell membrane and cause native membrane porations which cause cell damage [92]. Ivask et al. [93] examined toxicity of silver nanoparticles to bacteria (*E. coli*), yeast (*Saccharomyces cerevisiae*), algae (*Pseudokirchneriella subcapitata*), crustacean (*Daphnia magna*), and mammalian cells (murine fibroblast) according to their particle sizes ranging from 10 to 80 nm. They confirmed that the smaller-sized nanoparticles showed highly toxic effect. The review of Rai et al. [88] and Rizzello et al. [92] explained that truncated triangular nanoparticles are the strongest biocidal active products compared to spherical- and rod-shaped nanoparticles. 1 μg of truncated triangular nanoparticles shows greater activity than 12.5 μg of spherical-shaped nanoparticles and 50–100 μg of rod-shaped nanoparticles due to the enhancement of electrostatic interaction with bacterial cells (**Table 2**).

Dressing type	Brand name	Silver form
Contact layer dressings	Restore contact layer	Silver sulfate
	Acticoat Flex 3; Acticoat Flex 7	Elemental silver
	KerraContact Ag	Silver salt
	SilverDerm 7	Ionic silver
	Silverlon Wound & Burn Contact Dressings	Ionic silver
	Therabond 3D with Silvertrak™ Technology	Silver
Foams	RTD	Silver zirconium phosphate
	Acticoat Moisture Control	Elemental silver
	Allevyn Ag	Silver sulfadiazine
	Aquacel Ag	Ionic silver
	Biatain Ag Adhesive	Silver
	HydraFoam/Ag	Silver
	MediPlus Comfort Border Foam Ag+	Silver
	Mepilex Ag	Silver
	Optifoam Ag Adhesive	Ionic silver
	PolyMem MAX Silver Non-Adhesive Dressing	Silver
	Silverlon Negative Pressure	Ionic silver
	UrgoCell Silver/Cellosorb Ag	Silver salts
	V.A.C GranuFoam Silver	Silver
	Silverlon Acute Burn Glove	Silver
	Silvercel	Elemental silver
Fibers/clothes/mats /pads/others	Tegaderm Ag Mesh Dressing	Silver sulfate
	Absorbent Dermanet Ag+ Border	Silver
	Acticoat	Elemental silver
	Allevyn Ag Non-Adhesive	Silver sulfadiazine
	Durafiber Ag	Ionic silver
	Exsalt SD7	Silver

Dressing type	Brand name	Silver form
	Gentell Calcium Alginate Ag	Silver
	Silverlon Calcium Alginate	Silver
	Simpurity Silver Alginate Pads	Silver particles
	Urgotul SSD	Silver sulfadiazine
	Vliwaktiv Ag	Silver
	Acticoat 7	Elemental silver
	Arglaes film	Silver
Films/meshes	Avance	Silver
	Acticoat Absorbent	Elemental silver
	Algicell Ag	Silver
Alginate based	Algidex Ag	Ionic silver
	Biatain Alginate Ag	Silver
	CalciCare	Silver zirconium
	DermaGinate/Ag	Silver
	Dermanet Ag+	Silver
	Maxorb ES Ag+	Silver
	Maxorb Extra Ag+	Silver zirconium phosphate
	McKesson Calcium Alginate with Antimicrobial Silver	Silver
	Opticell Ag+	Ionic silver
	Restore Calcium Alginate Dressing with Silver	Ionic silver
	Sofsorb Ag	Silver
	Sorbalgon Ag	Ionic silver
	Suprasorb A + Ag Calcium Alginate	Silver
	Askina Calgitrol Ag	Silver alginate
	Invacare Silver Alginate	Silver sodium hydrogen zirconium phosphate
	Melgisorb Ag	Silver
	SeaSorb Ag	Ionic silver
	Silvasorb	Ionic silver
	Sorbsan Silver	Silver Sorbsan
	Algidex Ag	Ionic silver
	Urgotul SSD/S.Ag	Silver sulfadiazine

Dressing type	Brand name	Silver form
Gauze	Aquacel Ag	Ionic silver
	Arglaes Powder	Silver
Hydrofiber	Cardinal Health Hydrogel +Ag	Silver
Powder	DermaSyn/Ag	Ionic silver
Hydrogel	Elta Silver Gel	Silver
	ExcelGinate Ag	Silver
	Gentell Hydrogel Ag	Silver sulfadiazine
	SilvaSorb Antimicrobial Silver Dressing	Ionic silver
	Silver-Sept Silver Antimicrobial Skin & Wound Gel	Silver
	SilverMed Amorphous Hydrogel	Silver
	Silverseal	Silver
	SilvrSTAT Gel	Silver nanoparticles
	Viniferamine Hydrogel Ag	Silver
	Silverseal	Silver oxide
	Silver-Sept Antimicrobial Gel	Silver salt
	DermaCol Ag Collagen Matrix	Silver
	Puracol Plus Ag+ MicroScaffold Collagen	Silver
Collagen based	SilvaKollagen Gel	Silver
	Silverlon Adhesive Strips	Silver
	Contreet Hydrocolloid	Silver
Adhesive strips	Silverseal Hydrocolloid	Silver
Hydrocolloid	SilverMed Antimicrobial Wound Cleanser	Silver microparticles

Table 2. List of selected commercially available antimicrobial silver-containing dressings [22, 102, 103].

3.3.2. Silver dressings in wound healing

AgNPs (~11 to ~12 nm) containing gelatin fiber mats were prepared by electrospinning process and inhibited major microorganisms present in wounds [104]. Lin et al. [105] compared silver-containing carbon-activated fibers with commercially available silver-containing dressings and showed the silver-containing carbon-activated fibers to exhibit antibacterial activity and biocompatibility and promoting granulation and collagen deposition. A novel chitosan–hyaluronic acid composite with nanosilver was reported as a potential antimicrobial wound healing dressing for diabetic foot ulcers possessing high porosity, swelling, water uptake abilities, and biodegradable and potential blood clotting ability. The authors proved the inhibitory effects on *S. aureus, E. coli,* MRSA, *P. aeruginosa,* and *Klebsiella pneumoniae* [106].

In a related study, chitosan incorporated with polyphosphate and AgNPs was studied. The polyphosphate acts as a procoagulant which boosts blood clotting, platelet adhesion, and thrombin generation [107]. A similar scaffold dressing was developed by incorporating silver nanoparticles with chitin and showed antibacterial and blood clotting activity [108]. In another study, AgNPs containing hydrogel without any cytotoxicity but with antibacterial activity were reported [109]. Various inorganic forms of silver including silver zeolite, silver zirconium phosphate silicate, and silver zirconium phosphate demonstrate antimicrobial activity against oral microorganisms [91]. Pant et al. [110] stated AgNPs containing nylon-6 nanofibers prepared by one-step electrospinning process could be an effective antimicrobial wound dressing to kill both Gram-negative *E. coli* and Gram-positive *S. aureus*. Archana et al. [111] evaluated chitosan-blended polyvinyl pyrrolidone (PVP)–nano silver oxide (CPS) as an effective wound dressing *in vitro* and *in vivo*.

Lansdown et al. [112] investigated two forms of silver-containing dressings (Contreet foam and Contreet hydrocolloid) and found these promoted healing in chronic venous leg ulcers and diabetic foot ulcers. Polyvinylpyrolidone and alginate-based hydrogel-containing nanosilver has been functionally evaluated for efficient fluid handling capacity and strong antimicrobial activity against all major microorganisms such as *Pseudomonas, Staphylococcus, Escherichia, and Candida* [113]. Jodar et al. [114] demonstrated silver sulfadiazine-impregnated hydrogel for antimicrobial topical application for wound healing. Silver sulfadiazine (SSD)-impregnated hydrogel was prepared by polyvinyl alcohol (PVA) and dextran blending. Boateng et al. [115] formulated an ideal lyophilized wafer dressing composed of alginate and gelatin containing silver sulfadiazine for wound healing and showed the controlled release of SSD over 7 h and expected to diminish microbial load in the wound area. A novel SSD-loaded bilayer chitosan membrane was prepared with sustained release of silver which inhibits the growth of *P. aeruginosa and S. aureus* [116]. Shanmugasundaram et al. [117] formulated SSD-impregnated collagen-based scaffold with strong antibacterial activity *in vitro*. Ammons et al. [118] formulated dressings by combining commercial silver dressings (Acticoat™ Absorbent, Aquacel® Ag, and Tegaderm™Ag) with lactoferrin and xylitol and demonstrated greater efficacy against MRSA and *P. aeruginosa*.

There are several clinical studies with silver-containing dressings in the treatment of infected wounds to enhance wound healing, and the reader is referred to these [119–125].

3.4. Iodine and other antiseptics

Iodine is an old agent used in the treatment of chronic wounds and was used by soldiers during wars. The antibacterial activity of iodine was first investigated by Davaine in 1880 [126]. Iodine penetrates into the cell wall of microorganisms and damages the cell membrane by blocking hydrogen bond. This phenomenon alters the structure and function of cell proteins and enzymes, leading to cell death [127]. Iodine is active against a broad spectrum of microorganisms including *S. aureus, E. coli, Pseudomonas, Streptococcus, Salmonella, Candida, Enterobacter, Klebsiella, Clostridium, Corynebacterium, and Mycobacterium* [126]. Iodine dressings can be found in two preparations as povidone iodine and cadexomer iodine, and the various commercial formulations are summarized in **Table 3**.

Polyhexamethylene biguanide (PHMB) is an another antiseptic and widely used as antimicrobial dressing in wound healing. PHMB is known to be effective against *E. coli. S. aureus* and *S. epidermidis*. PHMB also works like iodine as it attaches to the bacterial cells and disrupts cell membrane resulting in leakage of potassium ions and cytosolic components that lead to cell death [128]. A study by Eberlein et al. [129] confirmed that PHMB containing biocellulose wound dressings were more effective than silver-containing dressing in retarding microbial loads present in locally infected wounds. Loke et al. [130] developed a two-layer dressing with sustained release of chlorhexidine which showed activity against *S. aureus* and *P. aeruginosa in vitro*.

Dressing type	Product name	Antiseptic
Pad	Iodoflex 0.9% Cadexomer Iodine Pad	Cadexomer iodine
Foam	IodoFoam	Iodine
Fibers	**Inadine**	Povidone iodine
Colloidal ointment base	Braunovidon ointment/ointment gauze	Povidone
Hydrogel dressing	Iodozym	Iodine
Liposome hydrogel	Repithel	Povidone
Foam	Kerlix AMD	PHMB
Sponges	Telfa AMD	PHMB
Foam	Kendall AMD	PHMB
Gauzes sponges	Curity AMD Antimicrobial Gauze Sponges	PHMB

Table 3. List of other commercially available antiseptics [36, 127].

3.5. Honey dressings

Honey has been used as wound dressing over centuries [131]. Honey has been reported in several clinical studies for treating chronic diabetic foot ulcers [132–135] and has antimicrobial and anti-inflammatory activity [136–138]. It is reported that honey can inhibit around 60 species of bacteria including *Alcaligenes faecalis, Citrobacter freundii, E. coli, Enterobacter aerogenes, Klebsiella pneumoniae, Mycobacterium phlei, Salmonella california, Salmonella enteritidis, Salmonella typhimurium, Shigella sonnei, S. aureus, and Staphylococcus epidermidis* [139]. In addition, it is reported Manuka honey and Cameroonian honey have an effect on *Pseudomonas aeruginosa*, methicillin-resistant *S. aureus* (MRSA), and vancomycin-resistant *Enterococcus* species [137, 140]. The antimicrobial properties of honey are ascribed to its low pH, hygroscopic nature, and peroxide-containing compounds [141]. The rich contents of sugar in honey generate high osmotic pressure and present an unsuitable environment to bacterial growth and cell proliferation [139]. Van den Berg et al. [142] investigated the anti-inflammatory properties of different types of honey *in vitro* by testing reactive oxygen species (ROS) inhibition capability and found American buckwheat honey exhibits high ROS inhibition ability. Many clinical studies have been performed on the basis of the antimicrobial effect of honey [143–145]. Clinical studies and bioactivity demonstrate the efficiency of honey in wound healing, maintaining a moist environment, promoting drainage of wound exudate and autolytic debridement [144]. It has been reported in minimizing malodour and scar formation of the wound [145] as well as angiogenic activity [146].

Sasikala et al. [147] developed a chitosan-based film dressing loaded with Manuka honey. They identified chitosan–lactic acid with 6% honey showed ideal dressing properties in terms of water vapor transmission rate, water absorption, tensile strength, elongation, and antibacterial activity against *E. coli* and *S. aureus*. **Table 4** summarizes the commercially available honey-based dressings currently sold on the market.

Dressing type	Product Name	Honey type
Hydrocolloid	MediHoney	Leptospermum honey
Alginate-based	MediHoney	Leptospermum honey
Fibers	MANUKAhd	Manuka honey
Pure honey	Surgihoney	Bioengineered honey
Foam	Ligasano	Honeycomb
Pure honey	MGO Manuka Honey	Manuka honey
Sterile Manuka honey	ManukaFill	Manuka honey
Honey-impregnated gauze	Manuka IG	Manuka honey
Sheets, ribbon, gel	TheraHoney	Manuka honey
Knitted viscose mesh dressing, pure honey	Activon	Manuka honey
Alginate ribbon and dressing	Algivon	Manuka honey
Composite, foam/silicone dressings	Actilite	Manuka honey
Nonadherent gauze fibers	MelDra	Buckwheat honey

Table 4. List of selected commercially available honey dressings used in wound healing [22, 148, 149].

3.6. Polymer-based antimicrobial dressings

Natural and synthetic polymers are widely used in acute and chronic wound healing due to their biodegradability, biocompatibility, and wound exudate handling capacity. However, some polymers themselves have an antimicrobial activity [150]. The combination of polymers and antimicrobial drugs provides effective dressings to improve wound healing. Biazar et al.

[151] evaluated a synthetic polymer-based hydrogel dressing that exhibits biocompatible and antimicrobials activity. In another study, synthetic polyvinyl alcohol was blended with calcium alginate to produce nano fiber matrix by electrospinning technique. *In vitro* antibacterial test showed the rate of inhibition of *S. aureus* depends on the concentration of calcium alginate [152]. Chitosan is a cationic polymer whose positive charge interacts with a negative charge of the microbial cell membrane, resulting in disruption and agglutination [153]. Carboxymethyl chitosan has been reported as a broad spectrum antibiofilm agent which can prevent biofilm formation for *E. coli and S. aureus* by 81.6 and 74.6%, respectively [154].

4. Summary

In this chapter, wound healing processes and types of dressings incorporating antimicrobial agents have been briefly discussed. Antimicrobials loaded into dressings for direct application to infected wound sites are becoming more popular worldwide in terms of safety, efficacy, cost effective, and convenience. The key antimicrobial agents ranging from antiseptics such as iodine, metals such as silver, antibiotics such as cephalosporins and aminoglycosides as well as natural products such as honey have been covered. In addition, the driving forces behind the developing of advanced therapeutic dressings have been reviewed. Furthermore, this review has demonstrated different and wide range of antimicrobial-loaded dressings, and a few clinical studies and commercially available antimicrobial dressings have been highlighted. Given the wide range of scientific studies and commercial products publicly available, it is evident that more evidence-based clinical trials are required to select appropriate dressings for the patients. It is also important to note the interdisciplinary fields (including formulation technology, biopharmaceutics, microbiology, materials and polymer chemistry and molecular biology) required for developing an effective antimicrobial dressing able to treat infection and also contribute towards enhanced wound healing.

Author details

Omar Sarheed[1*], Asif Ahmed[2], Douha Shouqair[1] and Joshua Boateng[2*]

*Address all correspondence to: sarheed@rakmhsu.ac.ae and j.s.boateng@gre.ac.uk

1 RAK College of Pharmaceutical Sciences, RAK Medical and Health Sciences University, Ras Al Khaiamah, United Arab Emirates

2 Department of Pharmaceutical, Chemical and Environmental Sciences, Faculty of Engineering and Science, University of Greenwich, Kent, UK

References

[1] Boateng JS, Matthews KH, Stevens HN, Eccleston GM. Wound healing dressings and drug delivery systems: a review. J Pharm Sci. 2008;97(8):2892–2923.

[2] Flanagan M. Wound care. Assessment criteria. Nurs Times. 1994;90(35):76–88.

[3] Hutchinson J. The Wound Programme. Centre for Medical Education: Dundee; 1992.

[4] Singer AJ, Clark RA. 1999. Cutaneous wound healing. N Engl J Med. 1999;341:738–746.

[5] Gottrup F, Melling A, Hollander DA. An overview of surgical site infections: aetiology, incidence and risk factors. EWMA J. 2005;5(2):11–15.

[6] Alavi A, Sibbald RG, Phillips TJ, Miller OF, Margolis DJ, Marston W, Woo K, Romanelli M, Kirsner RS. What's new: management of venous leg ulcers: approach to venous leg ulcers. J Am Acad Dermatol. 2016;74(4):627–640.

[7] Moffatt C. Identifying criteria for wound infection. EWMA Position document: 1–5 [Internet]. 2005. http://ewma.org/fileadmin/user_upload/EWMA/pdf/Position_Documents/2005__Wound_Infection_/English_pos_doc_final.pdf. [Accessed 17 Mar 2016].

[8] Eming SA, Krieg T, Davidson JM. Inflammation in wound repair: molecular and cellular mechanisms. J Invest Dermatol. 2007;127(3):514–525.

[9] Edwards R, Harding KG. Bacteria and wound healing. Curr Opin Infect Dis. 2004;17:91–96.

[10] Wolcott RD, Rhoads DD, Dowd SE. Biofilms and chronic wound inflammation. J Wound Care. 2008;17(8):333–341.

[11] Weyrich AS, Zimmerman GA. Platelets: signaling cells in the immune continuum. Trends Immunol. 2004;25(9):489–495.

[12] Reinke JM, Sorg H. Wound repair and regeneration. Eur Surg Res. 2012;49(1):35–43.

[13] Singer AJ, Clark RA. Cutaneous wound healing. N Engl J Med. 1999;341:738–746.

[14] Li J, Zhang YP, Kirsner RS. Angiogenesis in wound repair: angiogenic growth factors and the extracellular matrix. Microsc Res Tech. 2003;60(1):107–114.

[15] Steed, DL. The role of growth factors in wound healing. Surg Clin North Am. 1997;77(3): 575–586.

[16] Guo S, Dipietro LA. Factors affecting wound healing. J Dent Res. 2010;89(3): 219–229.

[17] Gottrup F. Oxygen in wound healing and infection. World J Surg. 2004;28(3):312–315.

[18] Rodriguez PG, Felix FN, Woodley DT, Shim EK. The role of oxygen in wound healing: a review of the literature. Dermatol Surg. 2008;34(9):1159–1169.

[19] Tandara AA, Mustoe TA. Oxygen in wound healing—ore than a nutrient. World J Surg. 2004;28(3):294–300.

[20] Faries PL, Teodorescu VJ, Morrissey NJ, Hollier LH, Marin ML. The role of surgical revascularization in the management of diabetic foot wounds. Am J Surg. 2004;187(5):S34–S37.

[21] Smith SC, Faxon D, Cascio W, Schaff H, Gardner T, Jacobs A, et al. Prevention conference VI: diabetes and cardiovascular disease: writing group VI: revascularization in diabetic patients. In: Proceeding of the American Heart Association; 18–20 January 2001; Circulation. 2002;105(18). p. 165–169.

[22] Boateng JS, Catanzano O. Advanced therapeutic dressings for effective wound healing —a review. J Pharm Sci. 2015;104(11):3653–3680.

[23] Bowler PG, Duerden BI, Armstrong DG. Wound microbiology and associated approaches to wound management. Clin Microbiol Rev. 2011;14 (2):244–269.

[24] Sue E. Gardner, Rita A. Frantz. Wound bioburden and infection-related complications in diabetic foot ulcers. Biol Res Nurs. 2008;10(1): 44–53.

[25] Noble WC. Ecology and Host Resistance in Relation to Skin Disease. 5th ed. New York: McGraw-Hill; 1999. p. 184–191.

[26] Menke NB, Ward KR, Witten TM, Bonchev DG, Diegelmann RF. Impaired wound healing. Clin Dermatol. 2007;25(1):19–25.

[27] Dow G, Browne A, Sibbald RG. Infection in chronic wounds: controversies in diagnosis and treatment. Ostomy Wound Manage. 1999;45(8):23–7, 29–40; quiz 41–2.

[28] Sun Y, Smith E, Wolcott R, Dowd SE. Propagation of anaerobic bacteria within an aerobic multi-species chronic wound biofilm model. J Wound Care. 2009;18(10):426–431.

[29] Stephens P, Wall IB, Wilson MJ, Hill KE, Davies CE, Hill CM, Harding KG, Thomas DW. Anaerobic cocci populating the deep tissues of chronic wounds impair cellular wound healing responses in vitro. Br J Dermatol. 2003;148(3):456–66.

[30] Donlan RM1, Costerton JW. Biofilms: survival mechanisms of clinically relevant microorganisms. Clin Microbiol Rev. 2002;15(2):167–193.

[31] Garrett TR, Bhakoo M, Zhang Z. Bacterial adhesion and biofilms on surfaces. Prog Natl Sci. 2008;18(9):1049–1056.

[32] Miller MB, Bassler BL. Quorum sensing in bacteria. Annu Rev Microbiol. 2001;55:165–199.

[33] Song C, Sun XF, Xing SF, Xia PF, Shi YJ, Wang SG. Characterization of the interactions between tetracycline antibiotics and microbial extracellular polymeric

substances with spectroscopic approaches. Environ Sci Pollut Res Int. 2014;21(3): 1786–1795.

[34] Costerton JW, Stewart PS, Greenberg EP. Bacterial biofilms: a common cause of persistent infections. Science. 1999;284(5418):1318–1322.

[35] Yamasaki O, Akiyama H, Toi Y, Arata J. A combination of roxithromycin and imipenem as an antimicrobial strategy against biofilms formed by *Staphylococcus aureus*. J Antimicrob Chemother. 2001;48(4):573–577.

[36] Moura LI, Dias AM, Carvalho E, de Sousa HC. Recent advances on the development of wound dressings for diabetic foot ulcer treatment—a review. Acta Biomater. 2013;9(7):7093–7114.

[37] Harding KG, Jones V, Price P. Topical treatment: which dressing to choose. Diabetes Metab Res Rev. 2000;16: S47–S50.

[38] Dumville JC, O'Meara S, Deshpande S, Speak K. Hydrogel dressings for healing diabetic foot ulcers. Cochrane Database Syst Rev. 2011;9:CD009101.

[39] Fonder M., Lazarus G, Cowan D, Aronson-Cook B, Kohli A, Mamelak A. Treating the chronic wound: a practical approach to the care of nonhealing wounds and wound care dressings. J Am Acad Dermatol. 2008;58(2):185–206.

[40] Hilton JR, Williams DT, Beuker B, Miller DR, Harding KG. Wound dressings in diabetic foot disease. Clin Infect Dis. 2004;39(Suppl 2):S100–S103.

[41] Lloyd LL, Kennedy JF, Methacanon P, Paterson M, Knill CJ. Carbohydrate polymers as wound management aids. Carbohydr Polym. 1998;37(3):315–322.

[42] Dumville JC, Deshpande S, O'Meara S, Speak K. Hydrocolloid dressings for healing diabetic foot ulcers. Cochrane Database Syst Rev. 2013; 8:CD009099.

[43] Skórkowska-Telichowska K, Czemplik M, Kulma A, Szopa J. The local treatment and available dressings designed for chronic wounds. J Am Acad Dermatol. 2013;68(4):117–126.

[44] Pawar HV, Boateng JS, Ayensu I, Tetteh J. Multifunctional medicated lyophilised wafer dressing for effective chronic wound healing. J Pharm Sci. 2014;103(6):1720–1733.

[45] Boateng JS, Pawar HV, Tetteh J. Evaluation of in vitro wound adhesion characteristics of composite film and wafer based dressings using texture analysis and FTIR spectroscopy: a chemometrics factor analysis approach. RSC Adv. 2015;5(129): 107064–107075.

[46] Labovitiadi O, Lamb AJ, Matthews KH. In vitro efficacy of antimicrobial wafers against methicillin-resistant *Staphylococcus aureus*. Ther Deliv. 2012; 3(4):443–55.

[47] Zubair M, Malik A, Ahmad J. Clinico-microbiological study and antimicrobial drug resistance profile of diabetic foot infections in North India. Foot (Edinburgh, Scotland). 2011;21(1):6–14.

[48] Gethin G. Role of topical antimicrobials in wound management. J Wound Care. 2009;Nov:4–8.

[49] Lipsky BA, Hoey C. Topical antimicrobial therapy for treating chronic wounds. Clin Infect Dis. 2009;49(10):1541–1549.

[50] Drosou A, Falabella A, Kirsner RS. Antiseptics on wounds: an area of controversy. Wounds Compend Clin Res Pract. 2003;15(5):149–166.

[51] Burks RI. Povidone-iodine solution in wound treatment. Phys Ther. 1998;78(2):212–218.

[52] Zhou LH, Nahm WK, Badiavas E, Yufit T, Falanga V. Slow release iodine preparation and wound healing: in vitro effects consistent with lack of in vivo toxicity in human chronic wounds. Br J Dermatol. 2002;146(3):365–374.

[53] Mirhadi H, Azar MR, Abbaszadegan A, Geramizadeh B, Torabi S, Rahsaz M. Cytotoxicity of chlorhexidine-hydrogen peroxide combination in different concentrations on cultured human periodontal ligament fibroblasts. Dent Res J. 2014;11(6):645–648.

[54] Severyns AM, Lejeune A, Rocoux G, Lejeune G. Non-toxic antiseptic irrigation with chlorhexidine in experimental revascularization in the rat. J Hosp Infect. 1991;17(3): 197–206.

[55] Du Toit, DF, Page BJ. An in vitro evaluation of the cell toxicity of honey and silver dressings. J Wound Care. 2009;18:383–389.

[56] Vowden K, Vowden K, Carville K. Antimicrobials made easy. Wounds Int. 2011;2(1):1–6.

[57] Cutting K. Wound dressings: 21st century performance requirements. J Wound Care. 2010;19(Suppl 1):4–9.

[58] Phoudee W, Wattanakaroon W. Development of protein-based hydrogel wound dressing impregnated with bioactive compounds. Nat Sci. 2015;49(1):92–102.

[59] Kataria K, Gupta A, Rath G, Mathur RB, Dhakate SR. In vivo wound healing performance of drug loaded electrospun composite nanofibers transdermal patch. J Pharm Sci. 2014;469(1):102–110.

[60] Shi Y, Truong V, Kulkarni K, Qu Y, Simon G, Boyd R. Light-triggered release of ciprofloxacin from an in situ forming click hydrogel for antibacterial wound dressings. J Mater Chem B. 2015;3(45):8771–8774.

[61] Öztürk E, Ağalar C, Keçeci K, Denkba E. Preparation and characterization of cipro-floxacin-loaded alginate/chitosan sponge as a wound dressing material. J Appl Polym Sci. 2006;101(3):1602–1609.

[62] Hima Bindu, TVL, Vidyavathi M, Kavitha K, Sastry T P, Kumar RVS. Preparation and evaluation of chitosan-gelatin composite films for wound healing activity. Trends Biomater Artif Organs. 2010;24(3):122–130.

[63] El-Shanshory A, Chen W, Mei M. Preparation of antibacterial electrospun PVA/ regenerated silk fibroin nanofibrous composite containing ciprofloxacin hydrochloride as a wound dressing. J Donghua Univ. 2014;31(5):566–571.

[64] Unnithan AR, Barakat NA, Pichiah PB, Gnanasekaran G, Nirmala R, Cha YS, Jung CH, El-Newehy M, Kim HY. Wound-dressing materials with antibacterial activity from electrospun polyurethane–dextran nanofiber mats containing ciprofloxacin HCl. Carbohydr Polym. 2012;90(4):1786–1793.

[65] Jannesari M, Varshosaz J, Morshed M, Zamani M. Composite poly(vinyl alcohol)/ poly(vinyl acetate) electrospun nanofibrous mats as a novel wound dressing matrix for controlled release of drugs. Int J Nanomed. 2011;6:993–1003.

[66] Tsou TL, Tang ST, Huang YC, Wu JR., Young JJ, Wang HJ. Poly(2-hydroxyethyl methacrylate) wound dressing containing ciprofloxacin and its drug release studies. J Mater Sci Mater Med. 2005;16(2):95–100.

[67] Manju S, Antony M, Sreenivasan K. Synthesis and evaluation of a hydrogel that binds glucose and releases ciprofloxacin. J Mater Sci. 2010;45(15):4006–4012.

[68] Puoci F, Piangiolino C, Givigliano F, Parisi OI, Cassano R, Trombino S, Curcio M. Ciprofloxacin–collagen conjugate in the wound healing treatment. J Funct Biomater. 2012;3(2):361–371.

[69] Roy DC, Tomblyn S, Burmeister DM, Wrice NL, Becerra SC, Burnett LR., Saul J. Ciprofloxacin-loaded keratin hydrogels prevent infection and support healing in a porcine full-thickness excisional wound. Adv Wound Care. 2015;4(8):457–468.

[70] Okoye EI, Okolie TA. Development and in vitro characterization of ciprofloxacin loaded polymeric films for wound dressing. Int J Health Allied Sci. 2015;4(4): 234–42.

[71] Sinha M, Banik RM, Haldar C, Maiti P. Development of ciprofloxacin hydrochloride loaded poly(ethylene glycol)/chitosan scaffold as wound dressing. J Porous Mater. 2013;20:799–807.

[72] Loke WK, Lau SK, Yong LL, Khor E, Sum CK. Wound dressing with sustained anti-microbial capability. J Biomed Mater Res. 2000;53(1):8–17.

[73] Kota S, Jahangir M, Ahmed M, Kazmi I, Bhavani P, Muheem A, Saleem M. Development and evaluation of ofloxacin topical gel containing wound healing modifiers from natural sources. Sch Res Library. 2015;7(10):226–233.

[74] Boateng JS, Pawar HV, Tetteh J. Polyox and carrageenan based composite film dressing containing anti-microbial and anti-inflammatory drugs for effective wound healing. Int J Pharm. 2013;1–2(441):181–191.

[75] Pawar HV, Boateng JS, Ayensu I, Tetteh, J. Multifunctional medicated lyophilised wafer dressing for effective chronic wound healing. J Pharm Sci. 2014;103(6):1720–1733.

[76] Pawar HV, Tetteh J, Boateng JS. Preparation, optimisation and characterisation of novel wound healing film dressings loaded with streptomycin and diclofenac. Colloid Surf B: Biointerfaces. 2013;102:102–110.

[77] Kim JO, Choi JY, Park JK, Kim JH, Jin SG, Chang SW, Li DX. Development of clinda-mycin-loaded wound dressing with polyvinyl alcohol and sodium alginate. Biol Pharm Bull. 2008;December(31):2277–2282.

[78] Kim JO, Park JK, Kim JH, Jin SG, Yong CS, Li DX, Choi JY. Development of polyvinyl alcohol–sodium alginate gel-matrix-based wound dressing system containing nitro-furazone. Int J Pharm. 2008;1–2(359): 79–86.

[79] Hwang MR, Kim JO, Lee JH, Kim YI, Kim JH, Chang SW, Jin SG. Gentamicin-loaded wound dressing with polyvinyl alcohol/dextran hydrogel: gel characterization and in vivo healing evaluation. AAPS PharmSciTech. 2010;11(3):1092–103.

[80] Adhirajan N, Shanmugasundaram N, Shanmuganathan S, Babu M. Collagen-based wound dressing for doxycycline delivery: in-vivo evaluation in an infected excisional wound model in rats. J Pharm Pharmacol. 2009; 61(12):1617–23.

[81] Adhirajan N, Shanmugasundaram N, Shanmuganathan S, Babu M. Functionally modified gelatin microspheres impregnated collagen scaffold as novel wound dressing to attenuate the proteases and bacterial growth. Eur J Pharm Sci. 2009;36(2–3):235–245.

[82] Guan J, Dong LZ, Huang SJ, Jing ML. Characterization of wound dressing with microspheres containing levofloxacin. In: Proceedings of the International Conference on Information Technology and Scientific Management; 20 December 2010; Tianjin, China: 2010;1–2. p. 344–348.

[83] Bohl MKS, Leibovich SJ, Belem P, West JL, Poole WLA. Effects of nitric oxide releasing poly(vinyl alcohol) hydrogel dressings on dermal wound healing in diabetic mice. Wound Repair Regen. 2002;10(5):286–294.

[84] Halpenny GM, Steinhardt RC, Okialda KA, Mascharak, PK. Characterization of pHEMA-based hydrogels that exhibit light-induced bactericidal effect via release of NO. J Mater Sci Mater Med. 2009;20(11):2353–2360.

[85] Li Y, Lee PI. Controlled nitric oxide delivery platform based on S-nitrosothiol conjugated interpolymer complexes for diabetic wound healing. Mol Pharm. 2010;7(1):254–266.

[86] Lansdown AB. Silver. I: its antibacterial properties and mechanism of action. J Wound Care. 2002;11(4):125–130.

[87] Leaper D. Appropriate use of silver dressings in wounds: international consensus document. Int Wound J. 2012;9(5):461–464.

[88] Rai M, Yadav A, Gade A. Silver nanoparticles as a new generation of antimicrobials. Biotechnol Adv. 2009;27(1):76–83.

[89] Feng QL, Wu J, Chen GQ, Cui FZ, Kim TN, Kim JO. A mechanistic study of the antibacterial effect of silver ions on *Escherichia coli* and *Staphylococcus aureus*. J Biomed Mater. 2000;52(4):662–668.

[90] Matsumura Y, Yoshikata K, Kunisaki SI, Tsuchido T. Mode of bactericidal action of silver zeolite and its comparison with that of silver nitrate. Appl Environ Microbiol. 2003;69(7):4278–4281.

[91] Saengmee-anupharb S, Srikhirin T, Thaweboon B, Thaweboon S, Amornsakchai T, Dechkunakorn S, Suddhasthira T. Antimicrobial effects of silver zeolite, silver zirconium phosphate silicate and silver zirconium phosphate against oral microorganisms. Asian Pac J Trop Biomed. 2013;3(1):47–52.

[92] Rizzello L, Pompa PP. Nanosilver-based antibacterial drugs and devices: mechanisms, methodological drawbacks, and guidelines. Chem Soc Rev. 2014;43(5):1501–18.

[93] Ivask A, Kurvet I, Kasemets K, Blinova I, Aruoja V, Suppi S, Vija H. Size-dependent toxicity of silver nanoparticles to bacteria, yeast, algae, crustaceans and mammalian cells in vitro. PLoS One. 2014;9(7):e1–14.

[94] Sondi I, Salopek-Sondi B. Silver nanoparticles as antimicrobial agent: a case study on *E. coli* as a model for Gram-negative bacteria. J Colloid Interface Sci. 2004;275(1):177–182.

[95] Shrivastava S, Bera T, Roy A, Singh G, Ramachandrarao P, Dash D. Characterization of enhanced antibacterial effects of novel silver nanoparticles. Nanotechnology 2010;18(22):1–9.

[96] Kazachenko A, Legler A, Per'yanova O, Vstavskaya Y. Synthesis and antimicrobial activity of silver complexes with histidine and tryptophan. Pharm Chem J. 2000;34(5):257–258.

[97] Baker C, Pradhan A, Pakstis L, Pochan DJ, Shah SI. Synthesis and antibacterial properties of silver nanoparticles. J Nanosci Nanotechnol. 2005;5(2):244–249.

[98] Morones JR, Elechiguerra JL, Camacho A, Holt K, Kouri JB, Ram JT, Yacaman MJ. The bactericidal effect of silver nanoparticles. Nanotechnology. 2005;16(10):2346–53.

[99]   Panacek A, Kvítek L, Prucek R, Kolar M, Vecerova R., Pizúrova N, Sharma VK. Silver colloid nanoparticles: synthesis, characterization, and their antibacterial activity. J Phys Chem B. 2006;110(33):16248–16253.

[100]   Kim JS, Kuk E, Yu KN, Kim JH, Park SJ, Lee HJ, Kim SH. Antimicrobial effects of silver nanoparticles. Nanomed Nanotechnol Biol Med. 2007;3(1):95–101.

[101]   Gade AK, Bonde P, Ingle AP, Marcato PD, Durán N, Rai MK. Exploitation of *Aspergillus niger* for synthesis of silver nanoparticles. J Biobased Mater Bioenergy. 2008;2(3):1–5.

[102]   Lindsay S. Silver white paper—everything you ever wanted to know about the use of silver in wound therapy [Internet]. 2011. http://www.systagenix.co.uk/cms/uploads/ 1458_Silver_WhitePaperA4_LP3_060.pdf. [Accessed 10 Mar 2016].

[103]   Wound Source [Internet]. http://www.woundsource.com/product-category/dressings/ antimicrobial-dressings. [Accessed 10 Mar 2016].

[104]   Rujitanaroj PO, Pimpha N, Supaphol P. Wound-dressing materials with antibacterial activity from electrospun gelatin fiber mats containing silver nanoparticles. Polymer. 2008;49(21):4723–4732.

[105]   Lin YH, Hsu WS, Chung WY, Ko TH, Lin JH. Evaluation of various silver-containing dressing on infected excision wound healing study. J Mater Sci Mater Med. 2014;25(5): 1375–1386.

[106]   Anisha BS, Biswas R, Chennazhi KP, Jayakumar R. Chitosan–hyaluronic acid/nano silver composite sponges for drug resistant bacteria infected diabetic wounds. Int J Biol Macromol. 2013;62:310–320.

[107]   Ong SY, Wu J, Moochhala SM, Tan MH, Lu J. Development of a chitosan-based wound dressing with improved hemostatic and antimicrobial properties. Biomaterials. 2008;29(32):4323–4332.

[108]   Madhumathi K, Sudheesh Kumar PT, Abhilash S, Sreeja V, Tamura H, Manzoor K, Nair SV. Development of novel chitin/nanosilver composite scaffolds for wound dressing applications. J Mater Sci Mater Med. 2010;21(2):807–813.

[109]   Boonkaew B, Suwanpreuksa P, Cuttle L, Barber PM, Supaphol P. Hydrogels containing silver nanoparticles for burn wounds show antimicrobial activity without cytotoxicity. J Appl Polym Sci. 2014;131(9):40215.

[110]   Pant B, Pant HR, Pandeya DR, Panthi G, Nam KT, Hong ST, Kim CS. Characterization and antibacterial properties of Ag NPs loaded nylon-6 nanocomposite prepared by one-step electrospinning process. Colloid Surf A: Physicochem Eng Aspects. 2012;395:94–99.

[111]   Archana D, Singh BK, Dutta J, Dutta PK. Chitosan-PVP-nano silver oxide wound dressing: in vitro and in vivo evaluation. Int J Biol Macromol. 2015;73(1):49–57.

[112] Lansdown BG, Jensen K, Jensen MQ. Contreet foam and contreet hydrocolloid: an insight into two new silver-containing dressings. J Wound Care. 2003;12(6):205–210.

[113] Singh R., Singh D. Radiation synthesis of PVP/alginate hydrogel containing nanosilver as wound dressing. J Mater Sci Mater Med. 2012;23(11):2649–2658.

[114] Jodar KSP, Balcão VM, Chaud MV, Tubino M, Yoshida VMH, Oliveira JM, Vila MMDC. Development and characterization of a hydrogel containing silver sulfadiazine for antimicrobial topical applications. J Pharm Sci. 2015;104(7):2241–2254.

[115] Boateng JS, Burgos AR, Okeke O, Pawar H. Composite alginate and gelatin based bio-polymeric wafers containing silver sulfadiazine for wound healing. Int J Biol Macromol. 2015;79:63–71.

[116] Mi FL, Wu YB, Shyu SS, Schoung JY, Huang YB, Tsai YH, Hao JY. Control of wound infections using a bilayer chitosan wound dressing with sustainable antibiotic delivery. J Biomed Mater Res. 2002;59(3):438–449.

[117] Shanmugasundaram N, Sundaraseelan J, Uma S, Selvaraj D, Babu M. Design and delivery of silver sulfadiazine from alginate microspheres-impregnated collagen scaffold. J Biomed Mater Res B: Appl Biomater. 2006;77(2):378–388.

[118] Ammons M, Ward L, James G. Anti-biofilm efficacy of a lactoferrin/xylitol wound hydrogel used in combination with silver wound dressings. Int Wound J. 2011;8(3):268–273.

[119] Rayman G, Rayman A, Baker NR, Jurgeviciene N, Dargis V, Sulcaite R., Pantelejeva O. Sustained silver-releasing dressing in the treatment of diabetic foot ulcers. Br J Nurs (Mark Allen Publishing). 2005;14(2):109–114.

[120] Jude EB, Apelqvist J, Spraul M, Martini J, Jones G, Harding K, Benbow S. Prospective randomized controlled study of Hydrofiber® dressing containing ionic silver or calcium alginate dressings in non-ischaemic diabetic foot ulcers. Diabet Med. 2007;24(3):280–288.

[121] Gago M, Garcia F, Gaztelu V, Verdu J, Lopez P, Nolasco A. A comparison of three silver-containing dressings in the treatment of infected, chronic wounds. Wound Res. 2008;20(10):273–278.

[122] Hiro ME, Pierpont YN, Ko F, Wright TE, Robson MC, Payne WG. Comparative evaluation of silver-containing antimicrobial dressings on in vitro and in vivo processes of wound healing. Eplasty. 2012;12:48.

[123] Thomas S, McCubbin P. A comparison of the antimicrobial effects of four silver-containing dressings on three organisms. J Wound Care. 2003;12(3):101–107.

[124] Thomas S, McCubbin P. An in vitro analysis of the antimicrobial properties of 10 silver-containing dressings. J Wound Care. 2003;12(8):305–308.

[125] Gaisford S, Beezer AE, Bishop AH, Walker M, Parsons D. An in vitro method for the quantitative determination of the antimicrobial efficacy of silver-containing wound dressings. Int J Pharm. 2009;1–2(366):111–116.

[126] Sunil KP, Raja BP, Jagadish RG, Uttam A. Povidone iodine—revisited. Indian J Dent Adv. 2011;3(3):617–620.

[127] Sibbald R, Leaper D, Queen D. Iodine made easy. Wounds Int. 2011;2(2):1–6.

[128] Gilliver S. PHMB: a well-tolerated antiseptic with no reported toxic effects. J Wound Care. 2009; Active Health Care Suppl:9–14.

[129] Eberlein T, Haemmerle G, Signer M, Gruber MU, Traber J, Mittlboeck M, Abel M. Comparison of PHMB-containing dressing and silver dressings in patients with critically colonised or locally infected wounds. J Wound Care. 2012;21(1):13–19.

[130] Loke WK, Lau SK, Yong LL, Khor E, Sum CK. Wound dressing with sustained anti-microbial capability. J Biomed Mater Res. 2000;53(1):8–17.

[131] Forrest RD. Early history of wound treatment. J R Soc Med. 1982;75(3):198–205.

[132] Hammouri S. The role of honey in the management of diabetic foot ulcers. JRMS. 2004;11(2):20–22.

[133] Schumacher HH. Use of medical honey in patients with chronic venous leg ulcers after split-skin grafting. J Wound Care. 2004;13(10):451–452.

[134] Molan P, Betts J. Using honey to heal diabetic foot ulcers. Adv Skin Wound Care. 2008;21(7):313–316.

[135] Mclennan ASV, Henshaw FR, Twigg SM. What's the buzz: bee products and their potential value in diabetic wound healing. J Diabet Foot Complic. 2014;6(2):24–39.

[136] Boateng JS, Diunase K. Comparing the antibacterial and functional properties of Cameroonian and Manuka honeys for potential wound healing—have we come full cycle in dealing with antibiotic resistance? Molecules. 2015;20(9):16068–16084.

[137] Subrahmanyam M. A prospective randomised clinical and histological study of superficial burn wound healing with honey and silver sulfadiazine. Burns J Int Soc Burn Inj. 1998;24(2):157–161.

[138] Cooper RA, Halas E, Molan, PC. The efficacy of honey in inhibiting strains of Pseudomonas aeruginosa from infected burns. J Burn Care Rehabil. 2002;23(6):366–370.

[139] Aggad H, Guemour D. Honey antibacterial activity. Med Aromat Plants. 2014;2(3):1–2.

[140] Song JJ, Salcido R. Use of honey in wound care: an update. Adv Skin Wound Care. 2011;24(1):40–4; quiz 45–6.

[141] Karayil S, Deshpande SD, Koppikar GV. Effect of honey on multidrug resistant organisms and its synergistic action with three common antibiotics. J Postgrad Med. 1998;44(4):93–96.

[142] Van den Berg AJ, Van den Worm E, Van Ufford HC, Halkes SB, Hoekstra MJ, Beukelman CJ. An in vitro examination of the antioxidant and anti–inflammatory properties of buckwheat honey. J Wound Care. 2008;17(4):172–174, 176–178.

[143] Gethin G, Cowman S. Bacteriological changes in sloughy venous leg ulcers treated with Manuka honey or hydrogel: an RCT. J Wound Care. 2008;17(6):241–244, 246–247.

[144] Molan P, Betts J. Clinical usage of honey as a wound dressing: an update. J Wound Care. 2004; 13(9):353–356.

[145] Alam F, Islam M, Gan S, Khalil M. Honey: a potential therapeutic agent for managing diabetic wounds. Evidence Based Complement Altern Med. 2014; 2014:Article ID 169130

[146] Rossiter K, Cooper AJ, Voegeli D, Lwaleed BA. Honey promotes angiogeneic activity in the rat aortic ring assay. J Wound Care. 2010;19(10):440, 442–446.

[147] Sasikala L, Durai B, Rathinamoorthy R. Manuka honey loaded chitosan hydrogel films for wound dressing applications. Int J PharmTech Res. 2013;5(4):1774–1785.

[148] Halstead F, Webber M, Rauf M, Burt R, Dryden M, Oppenheim B. In vitro activity of an engineered honey, medical-grade honeys, and antimicrobial wound dressings against biofilm-producing clinical bacterial isolates. J Wound Care. 2016;25(2):93–102.

[149] Molan PC. The evidence and the rationale for the use of honey as a wound dressing. Wound Practice Res. 2011;19(4):204–220.

[150] Mogosanu GD, Grumezescu AM. Natural and synthetic polymers for wounds and burns dressing. Int J Pharm. 2014;463(2):127–136.

[151] Biazar E, Roveimiab Z, Shahhosseini G, Khataminezhad M, Zafari M, Majdi A. Biocompatibility evaluation of a new hydrogel dressing based on polyvinylpyrroli-done/polyethylene glycol. J Biomed Biotechnol. 2012; 2012:Article ID 343989.

[152] Tarun K, Gobi N. Calcium alginate/PVA blended nano fibre matrix for wound dressing. Indian J Fibre Textile Res. 2012;37(2):127–132.

[153] Dai T, Tanaka M, Huang YY, Hamblin MR. Chitosan preparations for wounds and burns: antimicrobial and wound-healing effects. Exp Rev Anti-infect Ther. 2011;9(7): 857–879.

[154] Tan Y, Han F, Ma S, Yu W. Carboxymethyl chitosan prevents formation of broad-spectrum biofilm. Carbohydr Polym. 2011;84(4):1365–1370.

8

Delivery Systems in Wound Healing and Nanomedicine

Lina Fu

Abstract

Introduction: Delivery systems in nanomedicine contribute to the improvements in wound healing, tissue regeneration, and anticancer pharmacological fields. Although various wound dressings have been used in wound care treatments, there is a great challenge in the wound management of ulcers, trauma, chronic wounds, and severe injury and burns, especially infected wounds.

Body: To accelerate wound healing, influence tissue repair, reduce scarring, and control infection, various delivery devices have been developed in wound healing. The application of delivery devices has improved early as well as long-term wound care in delayed healing wounds. Main delivery systems are described, including drugs, bioactive proteins/growth factors, genes, and cells, outlining the advantages and limitations of each carrier in wound healing, as well as the mechanisms and release. This chapter reviews biomaterials and scaffolds that provide the carriers of bioactive agents, which include antimicrobial agents, combinations of cells, growth factors and genes, both scaffolds and cell interactions toward regeneration of skin tissues, vascular reconstructions, as well as transdermal carriers. In addition, the regulations, procedures, and clinical trails for delivery systems for wound healing are discussed.

Conclusion: In the past decades, many wound dressings and skin substitutes have been developed to treat skin loss and wounds. Delivery systems can improve wound healing and tissue regeneration. Looking toward the future, the need for delivery wound healing products for chronic and complex wounds will increase. Functionalized delivery systems will probably be the academic interest and industrial focus on wound healing.

Keywords: wound healing, delivery system, wound dressing, skin regeneration, biomaterials

1. Introduction

Nanomedicine has had a significant impact on delivery system development for pharmacological fields that include controlled-release wound dressings and biocompatible nanocarriers for biomedical applications [1]. As the largest organ in the human body, skin gives the body protection, but in so doing sustains a variety of skin wounds that require immediate repair process [2]. Modern wound dressings have been under development for decades. Although there are a wide array of wound dressings, ointments, and medical devices for clinical use, the time-consuming process of wound management is mainly restricted to wound repair rather than regeneration, which are two distinct definitions [3]. The key problem of skin regeneration is how to restore the native structure and function of the injured organ, including blood capillaries. Recently, biomaterial carriers in nanomedicine have shifted the focus from patient survival to quality of skin regeneration in terms of function, scar reduction, and improved aesthetics for reconstruction surgeries and burns [4]. In the formats of wound dressings and transdermal formulations, delivery systems have been applied to accelerate wound healing and to promote tissue regeneration, as well as to treat skin cancers using nanomedicine.

There are different circumstances in which people may need wound care and management. To meet the challenges of wound treatments for acute wounds and chronic wounds, such as large-area skin loss, burns, ulcers (pressure, diabetic, neuropathic, or ischemic), trauma, and especially infected wounds, which are mostly caused by microbes [5], the accurate delivery of antimicrobial agents is attracting much attention from researchers [6–8]. In addition to antimicrobial wound dressing, delivery systems of bioactive proteins, such as peptides and growth factors (platelet-derived growth factor, PDGF; endothelial growth factor, EGF; and fibroblast growth factor 2, FGF2 or bFGF), have demonstrated their promising effects in wound healing [9]. Cell therapy, including stem cell strategy, provides a novel therapeutic approach to wound healing [10]. Interestingly, mesenchymal stem cells (MSCs) and adipose-derived stem cells (ASCs) have emerged as a new approach in skin tissue engineering to accelerate wound closure, which would be of enormous benefit particularly for those wounds experiencing delayed healing in patients with diabetes and elderly [11, 12]. Gene delivery systems for wound healing have been also developed to transfer deoxyribonucleic acid (DNA) and ribonucleic acid (RNA) to wound sites [13, 14]. The regulations of delivery systems in wound healing can be complicated and vary greatly depending on the specific biomaterials and scaffolds, as well as the clinical use in particular [15]. In the commercialization of delivery wound healing systems, developmental and regulatory challenges are greater than in normal wound dressing and wound healing products. The biomaterials and scaffolds used in delivery systems take advantage of different structures, chemical parameters, and sources and so may require more rigorous development and regulation.

This chapter reviews biomaterials and scaffolds used in the design, characterization, and evaluation of delivery systems for wound healing, which include delivering antimicrobial drugs, combinations of proteins (growth factors and peptides), cells, and genes (**Figure 1**). Specific examples of application are summarized. Regenerations of skin tissues and reconstructions of blood capillaries in the wound care process are covered. In addition, the regulatory considerations for delivery systems in the wound healing field are also explored.

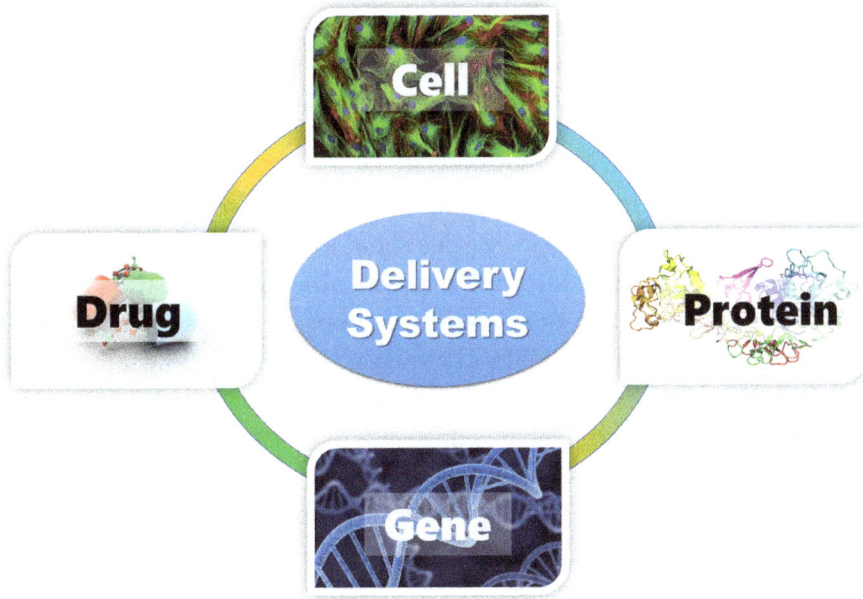

Figure 1. Delivery systems in wound healing.

2. Drug delivery system in wound healing

Chronic wounds and infected wounds currently pose a significant burden worldwide. Drug delivery systems (DDS) in wound healing that release antimicrobial and anti-inflammatory drugs represent a great opportunity to prevent infections or enhance the effectiveness of current commercial drugs. Many biocompatible biomaterials have been extensively investigated to deliver drugs into wound beds and to improve wound healing. Significant efforts have been made to develop DDS using different types of biomaterials, such as polymeric microspheres and nanospheres, lipid nanoparticles, nanofibrous structures, hydrogels, and scaffolds [16].

2.1. Delivery of antibiotics

Wound healing is a complex process that often requires treatment with antibiotics. To optimize and improve the usage of currently available antibiotics, DDS of antibiotics have attracted much attention. Antibiotic drugs used in delivery systems for wound healing are cefazolin [17], gentamicin sulfate [6], ceftazidime pentahydrate [18], ciprofloxacin [19], gentamicin [20], doxycycline hyclate [21], and the anti-inflammatory drug diclofenac [20]. Various biodegradable polymeric scaffolds (electrospun nanofibers, microspheres, composites, and films) were investigated for antibiotic delivery systems, including electrospun nanofibers of poly(lactide-co-glycolide) (PLAGA) [17], composites of a polyglyconate core and a porous poly(DL-lactic-co-glycolic acid) shell [18], chitosan (CS)-gelatin composite films [19], a three-dimensional (3D) polycaprolactone-tricalcium phosphate (PCL-TCP) mesh [6], bacterial cellulose (BC) membranes grafted with RGDC peptides (R for arginine, G for glycine, D for aspartic acid, C for cysteine) [20], poly(vinyl alcohol) (PVA) microspheres sandwiched poly(3-hydroxybutyric acid) (PHB) electrospun fibers [21], and β-cyclodextrin-conjugated hyaluronan hydrogels [22].

Antibiotic agents used in wound healing typically incur adverse effects (e.g., nephrotoxicity for vancomycin, cytotoxicity for ciprofloxacin, and hemolysis for antimicrobial polymers). Loading of antibiotics within polymeric vesicles could attenuate side effects, which has been demonstrated recently [23]. Li et al. reported a general strategy to construct a bacterial strain-selective delivery system for antibiotics based on responsive polymeric vesicles. That was in response to enzymes, including penicillin G amidase (PGA) and β-lactamase (Bla) that are closely associated with drug-resistant bacterial strains. A sustained release of antibiotics enhanced stability and reduced side effects. The results demonstrated that methicillin-resistant *Staphylococcus aureus* (*S. aureus*) (MRSA)-triggered release of antibiotics from Bla-degradable polymeric vesicles *in vitro* inhibited MRSA growth, and enhanced wound healing in an *in vivo* murine model.

2.2. Delivery of silver

To solve the problem of the increased prevalence and growth of multidrug-resistant bacteria, silver is used to reduce and eliminate wound infections using methodologies that limit the ability of bacteria to evolve into further antibiotic-resistant strains. In recent decades, the developments of silver (colloidal silver solution, silver proteins, silver salts, silver sulfadiazine (SSD) and nanosilver)-containing wound dressings for healing promotion and infection reduction have provided promising approaches [24]. The main synthesis approaches of silver monocrystalline silver (nanosilver or silver nanoparticle) include chemical reduction, micro-organism reduction, microwave-assisted photochemical reduction, and laser ablation. Antibacterial wound dressings in the formats of AgNP-embedded poly(vinyl pyrrolidone) (PVP) hydrogels were prepared by γ-irradiation at various doses: 25, 35, and 45 kGy [25]. Antibacterial tests showed that the 1 and 5 mM AgNP-embedded PVP hydrogels were effective, with 99.99% bactericidal activity at 12 and 6 h, respectively. A gamma-irradiated PVA/nanosilver hydrogel was also developed for potential use in burn dressing applications [26]. Interestingly, the wound healing activity of 0.1% w/w AgNPs in Pluronic F127 gels was enhanced to a considerable extent [27]. A new type of high surface area metallic silver in the form of highly porous silver microparticles (AgMPs) was studied [28]. Polylactic acid (PLA) nanofibers were successfully loaded with either highly porous AgMPs or AgNPs. A simulated three-dimensional (3D) coculture system was designed to evaluate human epidermal keratinocytes and *S. aureus* bacteria on the wound dressings. PLA nanofibers containing highly porous AgMPs exhibited steady silver ion release at a greater rate of release than nanofibers containing AgNPs.

Due to its antimicrobial activity, good coagulation and immunostimulating activities, chitosan is one of the native polymers chosen to control infection and enhance wound healing. Chitosan-based wound dressings can be gels, microparticles or nanoparticles, sponges and films [29]. Sacco et al. combined the two antimicrobial agents, silver and chitosan, to develop a silver-containing antimicrobial membrane based on chitosan-tripolyphosphate (TPP) hydrogel for wound treatments. Based on the slow diffusion of TPP, the macroscopic chitosan hydrogels were obtained that included AgNPs stabilized by a lactose-modified chitosan. Besides the good bactericidal properties of the material, the biocompatibility assays on keratinocytes (HaCaT) and fibroblasts (NIH-3T3) cell lines did not prove to have any harmful effects on the viability of cells using the MTT [1-(4,5-dimethylthiazol-2-yl)-3,5-diphenylformazan] method [8]. Chitin was also used to form the composite scaffolds with nanosilver. These chitin/nanosilver composites were found to be bactericidal against *S. aureus* and *Escherichia coli* (*E. coli*) with good blood-clotting ability [30].

Bioelectric wound dressing can also deliver silver to wound beds. *Pseudomonas aeruginosa* (*P. aeruginosa*) is a common bacterium associated with chronic wound infection. An US Food and Drug Administration (FDA)-approved wireless electroceutical dressing (WED), which in the presence of conductive wound exudate is activated to generate an electric field (0.3–0.9 V), was investigated to test its anti-biofilm properties using a pathogenic *P. aeruginosa* strain PAO1. WED markedly disrupted biofilm integrity in a setting where normal silver dressing was ineffective. Biofilm thickness and number of live bacterial cells were decreased in the presence of WED because WED served a spontaneous source of reactive oxygen species [31].

2.3. Delivery of other drugs

Besides silver, other drugs can be used to improve wound healing, for example, the anti-scar drug astragaloside IV [32]. In a rat full-skin excision model, the**** *in vivo* regulation of 9% astragaloside IV-based solid lipid nanoparticles-gel enhanced the migration and proliferation of keratinocytes, increased drug uptake on fibroblasts *in vitro* ($P < 0.01$) through the caveolae endocytosis pathway, and inhibited scar formation *in vivo* by increasing wound closure rate ($P < 0.05$) and by contributing to angiogenesis and collagen regular organization.

Different from most antibiotics that select for resistant bacteria, curcumin acts using multiple mechanisms. Curcumin (diferuloylmethane) is a bioactive and major phenolic component of turmeric derived from the rhizomes of *Curcuma longa linn*. Owing to its antioxidant and anti-inflammatory properties, curcumin plays a significant beneficial and pleiotropic regulatory role not only in cancers, cardiovascular disease, Alzheimer's disease, inflammatory disorders, and neurological disorders but also in wound healing because of its innate antimicrobial properties. However, the clinical implication of native curcumin is hindered due to low solubility, physicochemical instability, poor bioavailability, rapid metabolism, and poor pharmacokinetics, but these issues can be overcome by efficient delivery systems [33]. A biodegradable sponge, made from chitosan (CS) and sodium alginate (SA) with water uptake ability ranging between 1000 and 4300%, was developed to deliver curcumin as a wound dressing material up to 20 days. The *in vivo* animal test using SD rats showed that this CS/SA sponge had a better effect than cotton gauze, and adding curcumin into the sponge enhanced the therapeutic healing effect and improved collagen arrangement [34]. Curcumin nanoparticles (Curc-np) with an average diameter of 222 ± 14 nm were synthesized [35]. Curc-np represent a significant advance for reducing bacterial load. They can inhibit *in vitro* growth of methicillin-resistant *S. aureus* (MRSA) and *P. aeruginosa* in dose-dependent fashion, and so may represent a novel topical antimicrobial and wound healing adjuvant for infected burn wounds and other cutaneous injuries. Bacterial cellulose (BC) can be used for drug loading and controlled release [36]. The topical or transdermal drug delivery systems of two model drugs (lidocaine hydrochloride and ibuprofen) were developed. Diffusion studies with Franz cells showed that the incorporation of lidocaine hydrochloride in BC membranes provided lower permeation rates than those obtained with the conventional formulations [37].

There is a high mortality in patients with diabetes and severe pressure ulcers, resulting from the reduced neovascularization caused by the impaired activity of the transcription factor hypoxia-inducible factor-1 alpha (HIF-1α). To improve HIF-1α activity, Duscher et al. developed the drug delivery system of an FDA-approved small molecule deferoxamine (DFO), which is an iron chelator that increases HIF-1α transactivation in diabetes by preventing iron-catalyzed reactive oxygen stress [38]. The animal study on a pressure-induced ulcer model in diabetic mice showed a significantly improved wound healing using the transdermal delivery of DFO. DFO-treated wounds demonstrated increased collagen density, improved neovascularization, and reduction of free radical formation, leading to decreased cell death.

3. Bioactive protein delivery systems in wound healing

Wound healing in skin is an evolutionarily conserved, complex, multicellular process, which is executed and regulated by an equally complex signaling network involving numerous growth factors, cytokines, and chemokines [39]. Growth factors are soluble secreted proteins capable of affecting a variety of cellular processes important for tissue regeneration. However, the application of growth factors in clinics remains limited due to lack of good delivery systems and carriers. Recently, biomaterial carriers and sophisticated delivery systems such as nanoparticles and nanofibers for delivery of growth factors and peptides related in wound healing are a main focus in this research area [40].

3.1. Delivery of growth factors

EGF, PDGF, FGF2, keratinocyte growth factor (KGF) [41], transforming growth factor-β (TGF-β), insulin-like growth factor (IGF), vascular endothelial growth factor (VEGF), granulocyte macrophage colony stimulating factor (GM-CSF), and connective tissue growth factor (CTGF) are the main growth factors correlated with the wound healing process of skin [16]. Growth factors usually have short half-life time leading to a rapid deactivation at local wound beds in the body and resulting in a low efficacy. In order to enhance the efficacy of growth factor delivery systems, some bioactive and biodegradable matrixes including extracellular matrixes, have been used as carriers [42].

EGF is one of the most common growth factors used for treating skin wounds. Succinoylated dextrin (~85,000 g/mol; ~19 mol% succinoylation), a clinically well-tolerated polymer, was used to deliver EGF and led to sustained release of free recombinant human EGF over time (52.7% release after 168 h) [43]. Using a layer-by-layer assembly technique, EGF was successfully encapsulated using poly(acrylic acid) (PAA)-modified polyurethane (PU) films [44] or chitosan and alginate films [45]. Johnson and Wang treated the full-thickness wounded mice with a heparin-binding epidermal growth factor coacervate delivery system, and the results exhibited the enhanced migration of keratinocytes with retained proliferative potential, forming a confluent layer for regained barrier function within 7 days [46]. Chitosan-based gel formulations containing egg yolk oil and EGF are better alternatives compared to Silverdin® (1% silver sulfadiazine), given their significant difference ($P < 0.05$) treating wounds in Wistar rats [47]. Since the healing rate of wound is an important factor influencing the outcome of clinical treatments, as well as a crucial step in burn wound treatment, and the quality of wound healing has a direct bearing on the life quality of patients, FGF2 clearly has clinical efficacy in a variety of wound managements [48]. Skin flap survival is a major challenge in reconstructive plastic surgery. A sustained delivery system of FGF2 using heparin-conjugated fibrin was used to improve skin flap survival significantly in a rat animal model [49]. A delivery system composed of fibrin hydrogels doped with bFGF-loaded double emulsion increased the proliferation of endothelial cells compared to sham controls, indicating that the released bFGF was bioactive [50]. An injectable delivery system of PDGF using two-component polyurethane scaffolds was reported to achieve a sustained release for up to 21 days. The *in vitro* bioactivity of the released PDGF was largely preserved by a lyophilized powder. The presence of PDGF attracted both fibroblasts and mononuclear cells, significantly accelerating the degradation of the polymer and enhancing the formation of new granulation tissue as early as day 3 [51]. Hyaluronan-based porous nanoparticles were also investigated for the delivery of PDGF [52]. Recombinant human stromal cell-derived factor-1 (SDF-1), a naturally occurring chemokine that is rapidly overexpressed in response to tissue injury, was delivered in an alginate gel to accelerate wound closure and reduce scar formation [53]. SDF-1 delivery systems were evaluated using an acute surgical Yorkshire pig model. Wounds treated with SDF-1 protein ($n = 10$) and plasmid ($n = 6$)-loaded alginate patches healed faster than the sham ($n = 4$) or control ($n = 4$). At day 9, SDF-1-treated wounds significantly accelerated wound closure ($55.0 \pm 14.3\%$ healed) compared to nontreated controls ($8.2 \pm 6.0\%$, $p < 0.05$).

Recently, it has been increasingly recognized that biodegradable and biocompatible scaffolds incorporated with multiple growth factors might serve as the most promising medical devices for skin tissue regeneration. Beyond drug delivery, BC hydrogel is used to deliver bFGF, EGF, and KGF with modifications of different extracellular matrices (ECMs; collagen, elastin, and hyaluronan) [54]. *In vitro* and *in vivo* evaluation of the applicability of a dextran hydrogel loaded with chitosan microparticles (255 ± 0.9 μm) containing EGF and VEGF were performed, and they accelerated wound healing [55]. Moreover, the histological analysis revealed the absence of reactive or granulomatous inflammatory reaction in skin lesions. Multiple epidermal induction factors (EIF), such as EGF, insulin, hydrocortisone, and retinoic acid (RA), were prepared for blended and core-shell electrospinnings with gelatin (gel) and poly(L-lactic acid)-co-poly-(e-caprolactone) (PLLCL) solutions [56]. An initial 44.9% burst release from EIF blended electrospun nanofibers was observed over a period of 15 days. The epidermal differentiation potential of adipose-derived stem cells (ADSCs) was used to evaluate the scaffolds prepared either by core-shell spinning or by blend spinning. After 15 days of cell culture, the proliferation of ADSCs on EIF-encapsulated core-shell nanofibers was the highest. Moreover, a higher percentage of ADSCs were differentiated to epidermal lineages on EIF-encapsulated core-shell nanofibers compared to the cell differentiation of EIF-blended nanofibers, and this can be attributed to the sustained release of EIF from the core-shell nanofibers. A method for coating commercially available nylon wound dressings using the layer-by-layer process was utilized to control the release of VEGF165 and PDGF-BB [57]. Animal evaluation was performed using a db/db mouse model of chronic wound healing. This combination delivery system promotes significant increases in the formation of granulation tissue and/or cellular proliferation when compared to dressings utilizing single growth factor therapeutics.

3.2. Delivery of peptides

Current therapeutic regiments of wounded patients are static and mostly rely on matrices, gels, and engineered skin tissue. Accordingly, there is a need to design next-generation grafting materials to enable biotherapeutic spatiotemporal targeting from clinically approved matrices. Peptides are good candidates for controlling wound infections. A drug carrier system was designed for delivering an insect metalloproteinase inhibitor (IMPI) drug to enable treatment of chronic wound infections [58]. Poly(lactic-co-glycolic acid) (PLGA) supplies lactate that accelerates neovascularization and promotes wound healing. Delivery systems of LL37 peptide encapsulated in PLGA nanoparticles (PLGA-LL37 NP) were evaluated in full-thickness excisional wounds. A significantly higher collagen deposition, re-epithelialized and neovascularized composition were found in PLGA-LL37 NP-treated group. *In vitro*, PLGA-LL37 NP induced enhanced cell migration but had no effect on the metabolism and proliferation of keratinocytes. Interestingly, it displayed antimicrobial activity on *E. coli* [59]. CM11 peptide (WKLFKKILKVL-NH$_2$) (128 mg/L), a short cecropin-melittin hybrid peptide, was delivered by an alginate sulfate-based hydrogel as the antimicrobial wound dressing, and its healing effects were tested on skin infections caused by MRSA (200 µL, 3×10^8CFU/mL) in a mouse model [60]. During 8-day period, the 2% mupirocin treatment group and hydrogel containing peptide treatment groups showed similar levels of wound healing.

4. Cell delivery systems in wound healing

Wound healing involves the coordinated efforts of several cell types, including keratinocytes, fibroblasts, endothelial cells, macrophages, and platelets. The migration, infiltration, proliferation, and differentiation of these cells will culminate in an inflammatory response, the formation of new tissue and ultimately wound closure [39]. Cell-based therapies for wound repair are limited by inefficient delivery systems that fail to protect cells from acute inflammatory environments [61]. Wound dressing of cells laden in biomaterials on wound surfaces might not effectively and timely exert functions on deep or chronic wounds, where insufficient blood supply presents. Therefore, cell delivery systems are the main focus in the cell-based therapeutic field. Cell, including stem cells and other cells, delivered wound dressings have recently shown great promise for accelerating wound healing and reducing scar formation.

4.1. Stem cells

Stem cell therapy offers a promising new technique for aiding in wound healing; however, current findings show that stem cells typically die and/or migrate from the wound site, greatly decreasing the efficacy of the treatment. Most stem cells studied in wound healing delivery systems are mesenchymal stem cells (MSCs), endothelial progenitor cells (EPCs), adipose-derived stem cells (ASCs), umbilical cord perivascular cells (UCPCs), and circulating angio-genic cells (CACs). MSCs have been shown to improve tissue regeneration in several preclinical and clinical trials [62]. MSCs from various sources, such as bone marrow and adipose tissue, have been reported in the delivery systems for wound healing [10, 63].

A 3D membrane (FBMSC-CMM) from a freeze-dried bone marrow mesenchymal stem cells-conditioned medium (FBMSC-CM) can hold over 80% of the paracrine factors, which could significantly accelerate wound healing and enhance the neovascularization as well as epithe-lialization through strengthening the trophic factors in the wound bed [11]. Scaffolds strongly influence key parameters of stem cell delivery, such as seeding efficiency, cellular distribution, attachment, survival, metabolic activity, and paracrine release [64]. Pullulan was used to form a composite with collagen hydrogel for the delivery of MSCs into wounds [65]. Hydrogels induced MSC secretions of angiogenic cytokines and expression of transcription factors associated with the maintenance of pluripotency and self-renewal (Oct4, Sox2, Klf4) when compared to MSCs grown in standard conditions. Engrafted MSCs were found to differentiate into fibroblasts, pericytes, and endothelial cells but did not contribute to the epidermis. Wounds treated with MSC-seeded hydrogels demonstrated significantly enhanced angiogen-esis, which was associated with increased levels of VEGF.

There are other kinds of stem cells that have been used in combination with 3D scaffolds as a promising approach in the field of regenerative medicine. For instance, human umbilical cord perivascular cells (HUCPVC) [66], amniotic fluid-derived stem cells (AFSs) [67], EPCs [68], and circulating angiogenic cells (CACs). CACs are known as early EPCs and are isolated from the mononuclear cell fraction of peripheral blood, and provide a potential topical treatment for nonhealing diabetic foot ulcers. A scaffold fabricated from type 1 collagen facilitates topical cell delivery of CACs to a diabetic rabbit ear wound (alloxan-induced ulcer). Increased angiogenesis and increased percentage wound closure were observed with the treatment of collagen and collagen seeded with CSCs [69].

Compared to MSCs and EPCs, adipose-derived mesenchymal stem cells (ASCs) represent an even more appealing source of stem cells because of their abundance and accessibility. ASCs are autologous, non-immunogenic, plentiful, and easily obtained [70]. An acellular dermal matrix (ADM) scaffold made from cadaveric skins of human donors (AlloDerm, LifeCell Corp., Branchburg, NJ, USA) was served as a carrier for the delivery of ASCs [12]. ASCs-ADM grafts secreted various cytokines, including VEGF, HGF, TGFβ, and bFGF. Novel technology and biocompatible biomaterials have been applied for stem cell delivery. A silk fibroin-chitosan (SFCS) scaffold serving as a delivery vehicle for human adipose-derived stem cells (ASCs) was evaluated in a murine soft tissue injury model [71]. Microvessel density at wound bed biopsy sites at 2 weeks postoperative was significantly higher in the ASC-SFCS group vs. SFCS alone (7.5 ± 1.1 vs. 5.1 ± 1.0 blood vessels per high-power field). A newly developed thermoresponsive poly(ethylene) glycol (PEG)-hyaluronic acid (HA) hybrid hydrogel with multiple acrylate functional groups provides an efficient delivery dressing system for human adipose-derived stem cells (hADSCs) [72]. Although cellular proliferation was inhibited, cellular secretion of growth factors, such as VEGF and PDGF production, increased over 7 days, whereas IL-2 and IFNγ release were unaffected. Injectable gelatin microcryogels (GMs) were used to load human ASCs [73]. The results demonstrated the priming effects of GMs on the upregulation of stemness genes and improved secretion of growth factors of hASCs for potential augmented wound healing. In a full-thickness skin wound model in nude mice, multisite injections and dressings of hASC-laden GMs significantly accelerated the healing compared to free stem cell injection.

4.2. Other cells

Endothelial cells (ECs), keratinocytes, and fibroblasts are the most studied cells in terms of accelerated wound healing and improved skin tissue regeneration. A growing number of studies indicate that endothelial cells (ECs) and endothelial progenitor cells (EPCs) may regulate vascular repair in wound healing via paracrine mechanisms [61]. Using dried reagent patches that incorporate dextran (DEX) and a bulk aqueous phase comprising a cell culture medium containing poly(ethylene) glycol (PEG), Bathany et al. made a micro-patterned localized delivery of fluorescent molecules and enzymes for cell detachment [74]. Keratinocytes were delivered to dermal wounds in mice via cell-adhesive peptides attached to chitosan membranes [75]. Two peptides of 12 or 13 amino acids each that bind to cell surface heparin-like receptors (A5G27 and A5G33) were found to promote strong keratinocyte attachment, whereas the one that binds to integrin (A99) was inactive. Recombinant human collagen III (rhCol-III) gel was used as a delivery vehicle for cultured autologous skin cells (keratinocytes only or keratinocyte-fibroblast mixtures) [76]. Its effect on the healing of full-thickness wounds in a porcine wound-healing model was examined. Two Landrace pigs were used for the study. Fourteen deep dermal wounds were created on the back of each pig with an 8-mm biopsy punch. The scaffold enhanced early granulation tissue formation. Interestingly, fibroblast-containing gel was effectively removed from the wound, whereas gels without cells or with keratinocytes only remained intact.

5. Gene delivery systems in wound healing

Gene delivery is an emerging technology in the field of tissue repair and is being used to promote wound healing. Gene delivery is targeted to develop sustained release, to reduce side effects, and to enable both spatial and temporal control of gene silencing afterward. For example, chemical modifications were used to stabilize and reduce nonspecific effects of siRNA molecules using effective delivery [77]. The controlled delivery of nucleic acids (DNA and RNA) to selected tissues remains an inefficient process are affected by low transfection efficacy, poor scalability because of varying efficiency with cell type and location, and questionable safety as a result of toxicity issues arising from the typical materials (e.g., viral vectors) and procedures employed. Biocompatible materials, in the formats of micro/nanoparticles, scaffolds, hydrogels and electrospun fibers, made from cationic polymers and lipids, have been used as nonviral vectors, which has attracted much attention recently.

5.1. Viral vectors in gene delivery

The TGFβ family plays a critical regulatory role in repair and coordination of remodeling after cutaneous wounding. TGFβ3 has been implicated in an antagonistic role regulating overt wound closure and promoting ordered dermal remodeling. A mutant form of TGFβ3

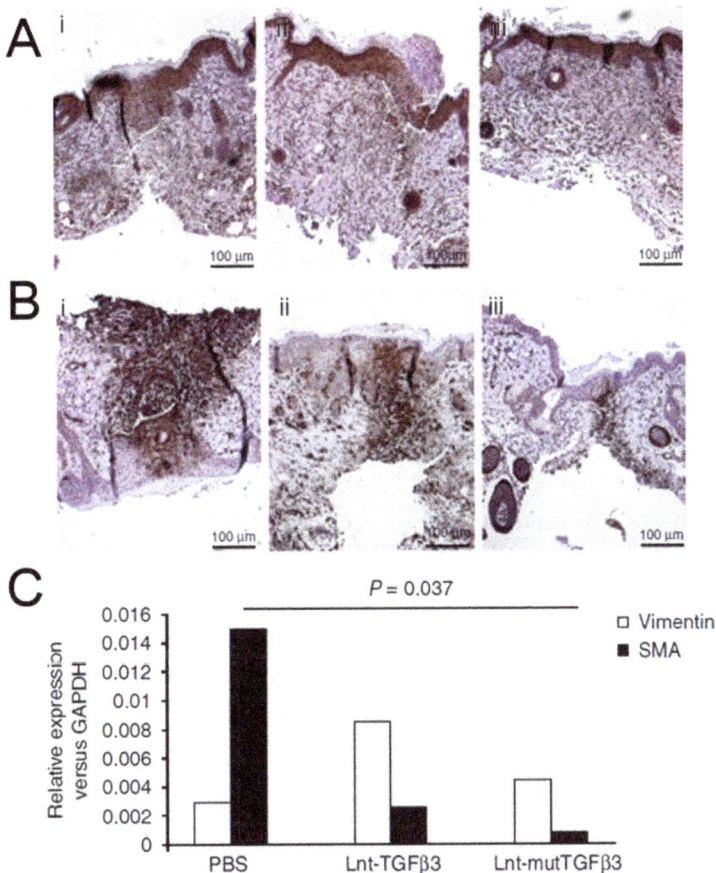

Figure 2. Transgenic overexpression of TGFβ3 decreases fibroblast to myofibroblast differentiation at the site of cutaneous wounding *in vivo*. (A) and (B) wound sections were stained immunohistochemically for fibroblast (a: vimentin) and myofibroblast (b: SMA) markers after treatment with [a and b(i)] PBS, [a and b(ii)] Lnt-TGFβ3, or [a and b(iii)] Lnt-mutTGFβ3. (C) Real-time reverse transcription-PCR showed that both TGFβ3 application groups and the PBS control (n = 4) as well as a significant decrease between the Lnt-mutTGFβ3 and Lnt-TGFβ3 treatment groups. PBS, phosphate-buffered saline; SMA, smooth muscle actin; TGF, transforming growth factor.

(mutTGFβ3) was generated by ablating its binding site for the latency-associated TGFβ-binding protein (LTBP-1) [78]. A localized intradermal transduction using a lentiviral vector expressing the mutTGFβ3 in a mouse skin wounding model was demonstrated to reduce reepithelialization density and fibroblast/myofibroblast trans-differentiation within the wound area. Both of which reduced scar tissue formation (**Figure 2**). Using a noninvasive imaging system, the kinetics of luciferase gene expression was studied when delivered in an adenoviral vector (replication-deficient adenovirus, Ad5). A peak of gene expression occurred at 7 days after delivery [79]. The esophageal cancer-related gene-4 (Ecrg4) delivering a viral-mediated gene was evaluated in a cutaneous wound healing model [80]. Both Ecrg4 mRNA and its protein product were localized to the epidermis, dermis, and hair follicles of healthy mouse skin.

5.2. Nonviral vectors in gene delivery

Gene delivery using adenoviral vectors in tissue regeneration is hindered by a short duration of transgene expression. A fibrin scaffold was used to enhance delivery of the adenovirus to a wound site, precluding the need for high repeated doses [81]. An anti-fibrotic interfering RNA (RNAi) delivery system using exogenous microRNA (miR)-29B was proposed to modulate ECM remodeling following cutaneous injury. A collagen scaffold was used as the carrier of (miR)-29B. The mRNA expressions of collagen type I and collagen type III were reduced up to 2 weeks after fibroblasts culture. *In vivo* evaluation in full-thickness wounds treated with miR-29B delivery revealed that collagen type III/I ratio and matrix metalloproteinase (MMP)-8 to TIMP-1 ratio were improved [82]. Porous (100 and 60 μm) and nonporous (n-pore) hyaluronic acid-MMP hydrogels with encapsulated reporter (pGFPluc) or proangiogenic (pVEGF) plasmids are used as a scaffold-mediated gene delivery [83]. Alginate-DNA gels were used to treat diabetic wounds, which provided sustained release of bioactive factors, such as neuropeptides and VEGF [13]. Silver nanoparticles (AgNPs) can be further augmented for gene delivery applications. The biofunctionalized stable AgNPs with good DNA-binding ability for efficient transfection and minimal toxicity were developed [84]. Polyethylene glycol (PEG)-stabilized chitosan-g-polyacrylamide was used to modify AgNPs. To enhance the efficiency of gene transfection, the Arg-Gly-Asp-Ser (RGDS) peptide was immobilized on the surface of AgNPs. The transfection efficiency of AgNPs increased significantly after immobilization of the RGDS peptide reaching up to $42 \pm 4\%$ and $30 \pm 3\%$ in HeLa and A549 cells, respectively. The transfection efficiency was significantly higher than $34 \pm 3\%$ and $23 \pm 2\%$, respectively, with the use of polyethylenimine (PEI, 25 kDa).

For treating diabetic patients with a threat of limb amputations, genes of various growth factors have been proposed in delivery systems. A simple nonviral gene delivery using minicircle plasmid DNA encoding VEGF was combined with an arginine-grafted cationic dendrimer PAM-RG4 [85]. Mouse ASCs were transfected with DNA plasmid encoding VEGF or green fluorescent protein (GFP) using biodegradable poly (β-amino) esters (PBAE). Cells transfected with Lipofectamine™ 2000, a commercially available transfection reagent, were included as controls. ASCs transfected using PBAEs showed an enhanced transfection efficiency and 12–15-folds higher VEGF production compared with the controls ($*P < 0.05$) [86]. Keratinocyte growth factor-1 (KGF-1) DNA was delivered using NTC8385-VA1 plasmid, a novel minimalized, antibiotic-free DNA expression vector [87].

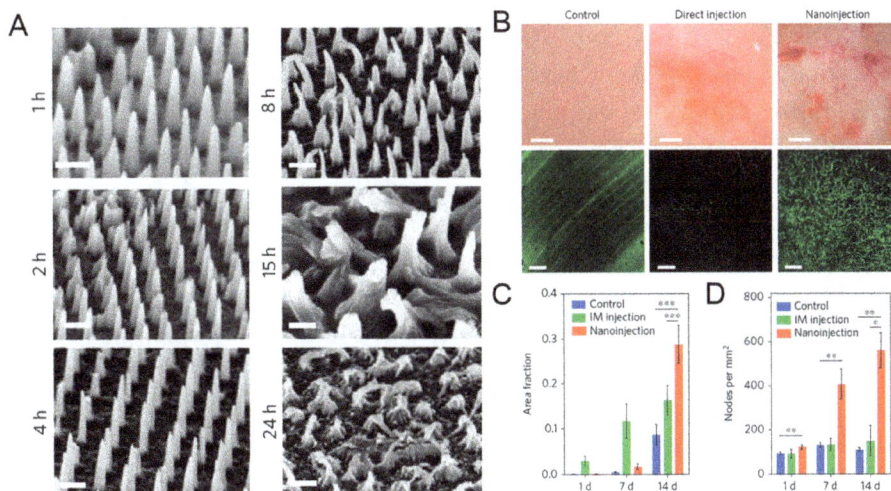

Figure 3. (A) Time course of nanoneedles incubated in cell-culture medium at 37°C. Scale bar = 2 μm. (B) Nanoneedles mediate neovascularization in wound healing. (C) The number of nodes in the vasculature per millimeter square. (D) Within each field of view acquired for untreated control, intramuscular injection (IM), and nanoinjection. $P < 0.05$, $P < 0.01$, $P < 0.001$.

DNA-incorporated electrospun nanofibrous matrix was fabricated to control the release of DNA in response to high concentration of MMPs (matrix metalloproteinases) such as diabetic ulcers [88]. High efficiency and minimal toxicity *in vitro* have been demonstrated that can be used for an intracellular delivery of nucleic acids by using nanoneedles [89]. Biodegradable nanoneedles were fabricated by metal-assisted chemical etching of silicon. These nanoneedles mediated the in situ delivery of an angiogenic gene, VEGF165, and triggered the patterned formation of new blood vessels. The nanoneedles were designed for extremely localized delivery to a few superficial layers of cells (two-dimensional patterning). This gene delivery can access the cytosol to co-deliver DNA and siRNA with an efficiency greater than 90%. *In vivo* studies show that the nanoneedles transfected the VEGF165 gene, improved wound healing and scar-tissue remodeling, and induced sustained neovascularization and a localized sixfold increase in blood perfusion in the target region of the muscle (**Figure 3**). This confined intracellular delivery has the potential to target specific exposed areas within a tissue, further reduce the invasiveness of the injection, and limit the impact on the overall structure of the tissue.

6. Regulatory considerations

The major concerns of commercialization of drug/protein/cell/gene delivery wound dressings are the complicated registration process, specifically regulatory approval, protocol consideration, and clinical trial process. Among all the parameters of delivery wound dressings, the type and source of the materials (e.g., human and animal origin) are critical to the regulatory approval process. A product composed of two or more regulated components, that is, drug/device, biologic/device, drug/biologic, or drug/device/biologic, that are physically, chemically, or otherwise combined or mixed and produced as a single entity is defined as a combination product [90]. The FDA (Food and Drug Administration, United States) regulation of a combination product (e.g., delivery system for wound healing) is mainly determined by the component with the primary mode of action. According to the classification of the product, the clinical trials (for premarket approval, PMA) must provide valid scientific evidence of safety and efficacy to support the indicated use of the wound healing delivery systems. Generally, preclinical studies contain toxicity studies and animal model evaluations. Delivery systems of drugs, bioactive proteins, cells, and genes in wound healing and nanomedicine should test their biocompatibility according to ISO 10993, including dermal irritation, dermal sensitization, cytotoxicity, acute systemic toxicity, hemocompatibility/hemolysis, pyrogenicity, mutagenicity studies, subchronic toxicity, chronic toxicity, and immunogenic potential [91]. Good clinical practices (GCPs) are the standards for designing, conducting, recording, and reporting clinical trials required for Class III medical devices.

For example, autologous stem cells are under clinical trial and are effective in ulcer healing and angiogenesis. However, translating delivery of stem cell application in *in vitro* and *in vivo* experiments from animal models to human clinical trials is still in its infancy. Preclinical studies suggest that cell delivery systems represent an effective and safe therapeutic strategy in the treatment of nonhealing wounds. More clinical studies on human subjects, including better data management of the patients and long-term follow-up of the patients' conditions, are necessary. Improved stem cell delivery vehicles in large-scale human clinical trials may be promising for diabetics with foot ulcers. There are no serious complications or side effects, but its therapeutic mechanisms, effects, and standardization still require further research [92]. While delivery system-based products offer increasingly important strategies for managing complex wounds, potential drawbacks include the risks of infectious agent transfer and immunological rejection. The manufacturing process, transport, and storage of delivery systems in wound healing are major cost implications; thus, their current clinical use remains limited [93]. Many current clinical trials are placing a high emphasis on addressing safety issues in all stem cell therapies, including stem cell delivery in wound healing [94]. The serious adverse effects of stem cell delivery are mainly immune response and tumorigenic potential. Delivery systems used in cell therapy encompass four main approaches, which are systemic administration, injection, topical, and local deliveries. Localized delivery of cells in wound healing is an optimal delivery approach for wound treatments [95]. Nonimmunogenic, nontoxic, biodegradable, and biocompatible biomaterials have been developed as carriers of stem cells that can protect cells and improve wound healing. However, clinical use of stem cells, for example, allogeneic EPCs, is currently inhibited by the risk of immunogenicity and tumorigenicity. To modulate the immune response, mesenchymal stromal cells or umbilical cord blood is already used in clinical trials, but definitive results are still pending. MSCs are known to be hypoimmunogenic [96]. Current challenges are standardized and quality-controlled cell therapy, the differentiation of MSCs to unwanted tissue, and potential tumorigenicity [94]. MSCs have been applied clinically for the treatment of diabetic wounds. Long *in vitro* expansion time and multiple handling procedures are barriers for its clinical application and increase the chances of infection [97]. Autologous induced pluripotent stem cells are nonimmunogenic and can be a promising cell source used in wound healing [98]. By comparison, clinical use of allogeneic cells is more complex and requires additional regulatory, legal, and safety hurdles to be overcome [99]. All things considered, the future prospects for the utilization of both autologous and allogeneic cells in cell delivery systems are bright. In the United States, there are three regulatory processes for the registration of wound healing delivery systems [100]. Only wound dressing with lower complexity and risk that is substantially equivalent to a marketed "predicate" device may be cleared through the 510(k) premarket notification process. In another words, those types of wound dressings are classified as Class I medical device. Clinical data are typically not needed for 510(k) clearance of Class II medical devices. Higher-risk Class III medical devices typically require premarket approval (PMA). In summary, the regulatory processes are depending on multiple factors including the device's classification, the availability of a substantially equivalent predicate, and the level of risk. Before commercialization, investigational devices maybe clinically investigated within the USA through the investigational device exemption (IDE) process, which is a request to conduct clinical research on an investigational device with "significant" risk in the **United States**.

User fees are required with the submissions of 510(k) premarket notifications and PMA application in the **United States**. Recently, Health Canada released a consultation document that discusses the cost recovery (user fee) framework which shows the basis for accountability at Health Canada for the review process [101]. Essentially, the fees "guarantee" a certain level of service from Health Canada—for instance, specifying the target number of days in which Health Canada will process different types of applications. If the targets are not met, that is, if "performance" does not meet the established standard, the entity being charged the user fee will have their future fees reduced by a corresponding amount. Providing a framework for registration approval globally of delivery wound dressings would translate those delivery systems studied from the laboratory investigation stage to clinical use, which will benefit patients' quality of life.

7. Conclusions

In the past few decades, many wound dressings and skin substitutes have been developed to treat skin loss and wounds. Delivery systems have been proven to improve wound healing and skin tissue regeneration. Polymeric microspheres and nanospheres, nanoparticles, nanofibrous structures, hydrogels, and scaffolds have been developed to deliver drugs to wound sites, overcoming the challenges caused by antibiotic-resistant microbial infections. Controlled release of drug delivery systems has been of increasing interest, as well as the applications of nanotechnology and biomaterial scaffolds. Growth factor and peptide delivery systems applied in skin wound healing help in the regeneration of tissue, reduction of scarring, and reconstruction of blood capillaries (neovascularization). Keratinocytes, fibroblasts, endothelial cells, mesenchymal stem cells, adipose-derived stem cells, and endothelial progenitor cells studied in delivery systems have great promise in chronic wounds and diabetic ulcers. Gene therapies now in clinical trials and the discovery of biodegradable polymers, fibrin meshes, and human collagen serving as potential delivery systems may soon be available to clinical wound management. However, regeneration of peripheral nerves is seldom reported. Looking toward the future, these delivery wound healing products may be able to achieve the replacement and regeneration of more normal skin; to gain localized delivery to wound site; to heal severe burns, chronic and complex wounds; to control the release of drugs, growth factors, and cells; and to silence genes.

Author details

Lina Fu

Address all correspondence to: runa0325@gmail.com; lfu28@uwo.ca

Department of Chemical and Biochemical Engineering, Western University, London, Ontario, Canada

Fordham Centre for Biomedical Engineering, London, Ontario, Canada

References

[1] Wan WK, Yang L, Padavan DT. Use of degradable and nondegradable nanomaterials for controlled release. Nanomedicine (Lond). 2007 Aug;2(4):483-509. DOI: 10.2217/17435889.2.4.483

[2] Hurtley S, Hines PJ, Mueller KL, Culotta E. From bench to bedside. Science. 2014 Nov 21; 346(6212):932–3. DOI: 10.1126/science.346.6212.932

[3] Kamolz LP, Griffith M, Finnerty C, Kasper C. Skin regeneration, repair, and reconstruction. BioMed Research International. 2015 Jan 1; 2015. DOI: 10.1155/2015/892031

[4] Orgill DP, Blanco C, editors. Biomaterials for treating skin loss. Cambridge: Woodhead Publishing Limited; 2009 Jan 28.

[5] Gurtner GC, Werner S, Barrandon Y, Longaker MT. Wound repair and regeneration. Nature. 2008 May 15; 453(7193):314–21. DOI:10.1038/nature07039

[6] Teo EY, Ong SY, Chong MS, Zhang Z, Lu J, Moochhala S, Ho B, Teoh SH. Polycapro-lactone-based fused deposition modeled mesh for delivery of antibacterial agents to infected wounds. Biomaterials. 2011 Jan 31; 32(1):279–87. DOI:10.1016/j.biomaterials.2010.08.089

[7] Singh B, Sharma S, Dhiman A. Design of antibiotic containing hydrogel wound dressings: biomedical properties and histological study of wound healing. Interna-

tional Journal of Pharmaceutics. 2013 Nov 30; 457(1):82–91. DOI: 10.1016/j.ijpharm. 2013.09.028

[8]   Sacco P, Travan A, Borgogna M, Paoletti S, Marsich E. Silver-containing antimicrobial membrane based on chitosan-TPP hydrogel for the treatment of wounds. Journal of Materials Science: Materials in Medicine. 2015 Mar 1; 26(3):1–2. DOI: 10.1007/s10856-015-5474-7

[9]   Sun BK, Siprashvili Z, Khavari PA. Advances in skin grafting and treatment of cutaneous wounds. Science. 2014 Nov 21; 346(6212):941–5. DOI: 10.1126/science.1253836

[10] Hanson SE, Kleinbeck KR, Cantu D, Kim J, Bentz ML, Faucher LD, Kao WJ, Hematti P. Local delivery of allogeneic bone marrow and adipose tissue-derived mesenchymal stromal cells for cutaneous wound healing in a porcine model. Journal of Tissue Engineering and Regenerative Medicine. 2013 Feb 1. DOI: 10.1002/term.1700.

[11] Peng Y, Xuan M, Zou J, Liu H, Zhuo Z, Wan Y, Cheng B. Freeze-dried rat bone marrow mesenchymal stem cell paracrine factors: a simplified novel material for skin wound therapy. Tissue Engineering Part A. 2014 Dec 9; 21(5–6):1036–46. DOI: 10.1089/ten.TEA. 2014.0102

[12] Nie C, Zhang G, Yang D, Liu T, Liu D, Xu J, Zhang J. Targeted delivery of adipose-derived stem cells via acellular dermal matrix enhances wound repair in diabetic rats. Journal of Tissue Engineering and Regenerative Medicine. 2015 Mar 1; 9(3):224–35. DOI: 10.1002/term.1622

[13] Tellechea A, Silva EA, Min J, Leal EC, Auster ME, Pradhan-Nabzdyk L, Shih W, Mooney DJ, Veves A. Alginate and DNA gels are suitable delivery systems for diabetic wound healing. The International Journal of Lower Extremity Wounds. 2015 Jun 1:1534734615580018. DOI: 10.1177/1534734615580018

[14] Kobsa S, Kristofik NJ, Sawyer AJ, Bothwell AL, Kyriakides TR, Saltzman WM. An electrospun scaffold integrating nucleic acid delivery for treatment of full-thickness wounds. Biomaterials. 2013 May 31; 34(15):3891–901. DOI: 10.1016/j.biomaterials. 2013.02.016

[15] Narang AS, Chang RK, Hussain MA. Pharmaceutical development and regulatory considerations for nanoparticles and nanoparticulate drug delivery systems. Journal of Pharmaceutical Sciences. 2013 Nov 1; 102(11):3867–82. DOI: 10.1002/jps.23691

[16] Gainza G, Villullas S, Pedraz JL, Hernandez RM, Igartua M. Advances in drug delivery systems (DDSs) to release growth factors for wound healing and skin regeneration. Nanomedicine: Nanotechnology, Biology and Medicine. 2015 Aug 31; 11(6):1551–73. DOI: 10.1016/j.nano.2015.03.002

[17] Katti DS, Robinson KW, Ko FK, Laurencin CT. Bioresorbable nanofiber-based systems for wound healing and drug delivery: optimization of fabrication parameters. Journal

of Biomedical Materials Research Part B: Applied Biomaterials. 2004 Aug 15;70(2):286–96. DOI: 10.1002/jbm.b.30041

[18] Elsner JJ, Zilberman M. Antibiotic-eluting bioresorbable composite fibers for wound healing applications: microstructure, drug delivery and mechanical properties. Acta Biomaterialia. 2009 Oct 31;5(8):2872–83. DOI: 10.1016/j.actbio.2009.04.007

[19] Hima Bindu TV, Vidyavathi M, Kavitha K, Sastry TP, Suresh kumar RV. Preparation and evaluation of ciprofloxacin loaded chitosan–gelatin composite films for wound healing activity. International Journal of Drug Delivery. 2010; 2(2):173–82. DOI: 10.5138/ijdd.2010.0975.0215.02027

[20] Rouabhia M, Asselin J, Tazi N, Messaddeq Y, Levinson D, Zhang Z. Production of biocompatible and antimicrobial bacterial cellulose polymers functionalized by RGDC grafting groups and gentamicin. ACS Applied Materials & Interfaces. 2014 Jan 14;6(3): 1439–46. DOI: 10.1021/am4027983

[21] Nagiah N, Ramanathan G, Sobhana L, Sivagnanam UT, Srinivasan NT. Poly (vinyl alcohol) microspheres sandwiched poly (3-hydroxybutyric acid) electrospun fibrous scaffold for tissue engineering and drug delivery. International Journal of Polymeric Materials and Polymeric Biomaterials. 2014 Jul 24;63(11):583–5. DOI: 10.1080/00914037.2013.854230

[22] Li R, Zhang X, Zhang Q, Liu H, Rong J, Tu M, Zeng R, Zhao J. β-Cyclodextrin-conjugated hyaluronan hydrogel as a potential drug sustained delivery carrier for wound healing. Journal of Applied Polymer Science. 2016 Mar 5;133(9):43072(1–8). DOI: 10.1002/app.43072

[23] Li Y, Liu G, Wang X, Hu J, Liu S. Enzyme-responsive polymeric vesicles for bacterial strain-selective delivery of antimicrobial agents. Angewandte Chemie International Edition England. 2016 Jan 26;55(5):1760-4. DOI: 10.1002/anie.201509401

[24] Atiyeh BS, Costagliola M, Hayek SN, Dibo SA. Effect of silver on burn wound infection control and healing: review of the literature. Burns. 2007 Mar 31;33(2):139–48. DOI: 10.1016/j.burns.2006.06.010

[25] Khampieng T, Brikshavana P, Supaphol P. Silver nanoparticle-embedded poly (vinyl pyrrolidone) hydrogel dressing: gamma-ray synthesis and biological evaluation. Journal of Biomaterials Science, Polymer Edition. 2014 May 24;25(8):826–42. DOI: 10.1080/09205063.2014.910154

[26] Oliveira RN, Rouzé R, Quilty B, Alves GG, Soares GD, Thiré RM, McGuinness GB. Mechanical properties and in vitro characterization of polyvinyl alcohol-nano-silver hydrogel wound dressings. Interface Focus. 2014 Feb 6;4(1):20130049. DOI: 10.1098/rsfs.2013.0049

[27] Shankar S, Jaiswal L, Aparna RS, Prasad RG, Kumar GP, Manohara CM. Wound healing potential of green synthesized silver nanoparticles prepared from *Lansium domesticum*

fruit peel extract. Materials Express. 2015 Mar 1;5(2):159–64. DOI: 10.1166/mex. 2015.1225

[28] Mohiti-Asli M, Pourdeyhimi B, Loboa EG. Skin tissue engineering for the infected wound site: biodegradable PLA nanofibers and a novel approach for silver ion release evaluated in a 3D coculture system of keratinocytes and *Staphylococcus aureus*. Tissue Engineering Part C: Methods. 2014 Mar 17;20(10):790–7. DOI: 10.1089/ten.tec.2013.0458

[29] Patrulea V, Ostafe V, Borchard G, Jordan O. Chitosan as a starting material for wound healing applications. European Journal of Pharmaceutics and Biopharmaceutics. 2015 Nov 30;97:417–26. DOI: 10.1016/j.ejpb.2015.08.004

[30] Madhumathi K, Kumar PS, Abhilash S, Sreeja V, Tamura H, Manzoor K, Nair SV, Jayakumar R. Development of novel chitin/nanosilver composite scaffolds for wound dressing applications. Journal of Materials Science: Materials in Medicine. 2010 Feb 1;21(2):807–13. DOI: 10.1007/s10856-009-3877-z

[31] Banerjee J, Ghatak PD, Roy S, Khanna S, Hemann C, Deng B, Das A, Zweier JL, Wozniak D, Sen CK. Silver-zinc redox-coupled electroceutical wound dressing disrupts bacterial biofilm. PLoS One. 2015 Mar 24;10(3):e0119531. DOI: 10.1371/journal.pone.0119531

[32] Chen X, Peng LH, Shan YH, Li N, Wei W, Yu L, Li QM, Liang WQ, Gao JQ. Astragaloside IV-loaded nanoparticle-enriched hydrogel induces wound healing and anti-scar activity through topical delivery. International Journal of Pharmaceutics. 2013 Apr 15;447(1):171–81. DOI: 10.1016/j.ijpharm.2013.02.054

[33] Yallapu MM, Nagesh PK, Jaggi M, Chauhan SC. Therapeutic applications of curcumin nanoformulations. The AAPS Journal. 2015 Nov 1;17(6):1341–56. DOI: 10.1208/s12248-015-9811-z

[34] Dai M, Zheng X, Xu X, Kong X, Li X, Guo G, Luo F, Zhao X, Wei YQ, Qian Z. Chitosan-alginate sponge: preparation and application in curcumin delivery for dermal wound healing in rat. BioMed Research International. 2009 Nov 11;2009. DOI: 10.1155/2009/595126

[35] Krausz AE, Adler BL, Cabral V, Navati M, Doerner J, Charafeddine RA, Chandra D, Liang H, Gunther L, Clendaniel A, Harper S. Curcumin-encapsulated nanoparticles as innovative antimicrobial and wound healing agent. Nanomedicine: Nanotechnology, Biology and Medicine. 2015 Jan 31;11(1):195–206. DOI: 10.1016/j.nano.2014.09.004

[36] Huang L, Chen X, Nguyen TX, Tang H, Zhang L, Yang G. Nano-cellulose 3D-networks as controlled-release drug carriers. Journal of Materials Chemistry B. 2013;1(23):2976–84. DOI: 10.1039/c3tb20149j

[37] Trovatti E, Freire CS, Pinto PC, Almeida IF, Costa P, Silvestre AJ, Neto CP, Rosado C. Bacterial cellulose membranes applied in topical and transdermal delivery of lidocaine hydrochloride and ibuprofen: in vitro diffusion studies. International Journal of Pharmaceutics. 2012 Oct 1;435(1):83–7. DOI: 10.1016/j.ijpharm.2012.01.002

[38] Duscher D, Neofytou E, Wong VW, Maan ZN, Rennert RC, Inayathullah M, Januszyk M, Rodrigues M, Malkovskiy AV, Whitmore AJ, Walmsley GG. Transdermal deferoxamine prevents pressure-induced diabetic ulcers. Proceedings of the National Academy of Sciences. 2015 Jan 6;112(1):94–9. DOI: 10.1073/pnas.1413445112

[39] Barrientos S, Stojadinovic O, Golinko MS, Brem H, Tomic-Canic M. Growth factors and cytokines in wound healing. Wound Repair and Regeneration. 2008 Sep 1;16(5):585–601. DOI: 10.1111/j.1524-475X.2008.00410.x

[40] Koria P. Delivery of growth factors for tissue regeneration and wound healing. BioDrugs. 2012 Jun 1;26(3):163–75. DOI: 10.2165/11631850-000000000-0000

[41] Geer DJ, Swartz DD, Andreadis ST. Biomimetic delivery of keratinocyte growth factor upon cellular demand for accelerated wound healing in vitro and in vivo. The American Journal of Pathology. 2005 Dec 31;167(6):1575–86. DOI: 10.1016/S0002-9440(10)61242-4

[42] Yao C, Yao P, Wu H, Zha Z. Acceleration of wound healing in traumatic ulcers by absorbable collagen sponge containing recombinant basic fibroblast growth factor. Biomedical Materials. 2006 Mar 15;1(1):33. DOI:10.1088/1748-6041/1/1/005

[43] Hardwicke J, Ferguson EL, Moseley R, Stephens P, Thomas DW, Duncan R. Dextrin–rhEGF conjugates as bioresponsive nanomedicines for wound repair. Journal of Controlled Release. 2008 Sep 24;130(3):275–83. DOI: 10.1016/j.jconrel.2008.07.023

[44] Kulkarni A, Diehl-Jones W, Ghanbar S, Liu S. Layer-by-layer assembly of epidermal growth factors on polyurethane films for wound closure. Journal of Biomaterials Applications. 2014 Aug 1;29(2):278–90. DOI: 10.1177/0885328214523058

[45] Picheth GF, Sierakowski MR, Woehl MA, Ono L, Cofré AR, Vanin LP, Pontarolo R, De Freitas RA. Lysozyme-triggered epidermal growth factor release from bacterial cellulose membranes controlled by smart nanostructured films. Journal of Pharmaceutical Sciences. 2014 Dec 1;103(12):3958–65. DOI: 10.1002/jps.24205

[46] Johnson NR, Wang Y. Controlled delivery of heparin-binding EGF-like growth factor yields fast and comprehensive wound healing. Journal of Controlled Release. 2013 Mar 10;166(2):124–9. DOI: 10.1016/j.jconrel.2012.11.004

[47] Yenilmez E, Basaran E, Arslan R, Berkman MS, Güven UM, Bayçu C, Yazan Y. Chitosan gel formulations containing egg yolk oil and epidermal growth factor for dermal burn treatment. Die Pharmazie: An International Journal of Pharmaceutical Sciences. 2015 Feb 2;70(2):67–73. DOI: 10.1691/ph.2015.4126

[48] Nunes QM, Li Y, Sun C, Kinnunen TK, Fernig DG. Fibroblast growth factors as tissue repair and regeneration therapeutics. PeerJ. 2016 Jan 12;4:e1535. DOI: 10.7717/peerj.1535

[49] Park HJ, Lee S, Kang KH, Heo CY, Kim JH, Yang HS, Kim BS. Enhanced random skin flap survival by sustained delivery of fibroblast growth factor 2 in rats. ANZ Journal of Surgery. 2013 May 1;83(5):354–8. DOI: 10.1111/j.1445-2197.2012.06194.x

[50] Fabiilli ML, Wilson CG, Padilla F, Martín-Saavedra FM, Fowlkes JB, Franceschi RT. Acoustic droplet–hydrogel composites for spatial and temporal control of growth factor delivery and scaffold stiffness. Acta Biomaterialia. 2013 Jul 31;9(7):7399–409. DOI: 10.1016/j.actbio.2013.03.027

[51] Li B, Davidson JM, Guelcher SA. The effect of the local delivery of platelet-derived growth factor from reactive two-component polyurethane scaffolds on the healing in rat skin excisional wounds. Biomaterials. 2009 Jul 31;30(20):3486–94. DOI: 10.1016/j.biomaterials.2009.03.008

[52] Zavan B, Vindigni V, Vezzù K, Zorzato G, Luni C, Abatangelo G, Elvassore N, Cortivo R. Hyaluronan based porous nano-particles enriched with growth factors for the treatment of ulcers: a placebo-controlled study. Journal of Materials Science: Materials in Medicine. 2009 Jan 1;20(1):235–47. DOI: 10.1007/s10856-008-3566-3

[53] Rabbany SY, Pastore J, Yamamoto M, Miller T, Rafii S, Aras R, Penn M. Continuous delivery of stromal cell-derived factor-1 from alginate scaffolds accelerates wound healing. Cell Transplantation. 2010 Apr 1;19(4):399–408. DOI: 10.3727/096368909X481782

[54] Lin YK, Chen KH, Ou KL, Liu M. Effects of different extracellular matrices and growth factor immobilization on biodegradability and biocompatibility of macroporous bacterial cellulose. Journal of Bioactive and Compatible Polymers. 2011 Sep 1;26(5):508–18. DOI: 10.1177/0883911511415390

[55] Ribeiro MP, Morgado PI, Miguel SP, Coutinho P, Correia IJ. Dextran-based hydrogel containing chitosan microparticles loaded with growth factors to be used in wound healing. Materials Science and Engineering: C. 2013 Jul 1;33(5):2958–66. DOI: 10.1016/j.msec.2013.03.025

[56] Jin G, Prabhakaran MP, Kai D, Ramakrishna S. Controlled release of multiple epidermal induction factors through core–shell nanofibers for skin regeneration. European Journal of Pharmaceutics and Biopharmaceutics. 2013 Nov 30;85(3):689–98. DOI: 10.1016/j.ejpb.2013.06.002

[57] Almquist BD, Castleberry SA, Sun JB, Lu AY, Hammond PT. Combination growth factor therapy via electrostatically assembled wound dressings improves diabetic ulcer healing in vivo. Advanced Healthcare Materials. 2015 Oct 1;4(14):2090–9. DOI: 10.1002/adhm.201500403

[58] Eisenhardt M, Dobler D, Schlupp P, Schmidts T, Salzig M, Vilcinskas A, Salzig D, Czermak P, Keusgen M, Runkel F. Development of an insect metalloproteinase inhibitor drug carrier system for application in chronic wound infections. Journal of Pharmacy and Pharmacology. 2015 Nov 1;67(11):1481–91. DOI: 10.1111/jphp.12452

[59] Chereddy KK, Her CH, Comune M, Moia C, Lopes A, Porporato PE, Vanacker J, Lam MC, Steinstraesser L, Sonveaux P, Zhu H. PLGA nanoparticles loaded with host defense

peptide LL37 promote wound healing. Journal of Controlled Release. 2014 Nov 28;194:138–47. DOI: 10.1016/j.jconrel.2014.08.016

[60] Babavalian H, Latifi AM, Shokrgozar MA, Bonakdar S, Mohammadi S, Moghaddam MM. Analysis of healing effect of alginate sulfate hydrogel dressing containing antimicrobial peptide on wound infection caused by methicillin-resistant *Staphylococcus aureus*. Jundishapur Journal of Microbiology. 2015 Sep;8(9). DOI: 10.5812/jjm.28320

[61] Zhang M, Rehman J, Malik AB. Endothelial progenitor cells and vascular repair. Current Opinion in Hematology. 2014 May;21(3):224. DOI: 10.1097/MOH. 0000000000000041.

[62] Xu K, Cantu DA, Fu Y, Kim J, Zheng X, Hematti P, Kao WJ. Thiol-ene Michael-type formation of gelatin/poly (ethylene glycol) biomatrices for three-dimensional mesenchymal stromal/stem cell administration to cutaneous wounds. Acta Biomaterialia. 2013 Nov 30;9(11):8802–14. DOI: 10.1016/j.actbio.2013.06.021

[63] Sánchez-Sánchez R, Brena-Molina A, Martínez-López V, Melgarejo-Ramírez Y, de Dios LT, Gómez-García R, de Lourdes Reyes-Frías M, Rodríguez-Rodríguez L, Garciadiego-Cázares D, Lugo-Martínez H, Ibarra C. Generation of two biological wound dressings as a potential delivery system of human adipose-derived mesenchymal stem cells. Asaio Journal. 2015 Nov;61(6):718. DOI: 10.1097/MAT.0000000000000277

[64] Wahl EA, Fierro FA, Peavy TR, Hopfner U, Dye JF, Machens HG, Egaña JT, Schenck TL. In vitro evaluation of scaffolds for the delivery of mesenchymal stem cells to wounds. BioMed Research International. 2015 Oct 4;2015:1. DOI: 10.1155/2015/108571

[65] Rustad KC, Wong VW, Sorkin M, Glotzbach JP, Major MR, Rajadas J, Longaker MT, Gurtner GC. Enhancement of mesenchymal stem cell angiogenic capacity and stemness by a biomimetic hydrogel scaffold. Biomaterials. 2012 Jan 31;33(1):80–90. DOI: 10.1016/j.biomaterials.2011.09.041

[66] Zebardast N, Lickorish D, Davies JE. Human umbilical cord perivascular cells (HUCPVC) A mesenchymal cell source for dermal wound healing. Organogenesis. 2010 Oct 1;6(4):197–203. DOI: 10.4161/org6.4.12393

[67] Skardal A, Mack D, Kapetanovic E, Atala A, Jackson JD, Yoo J, Soker S. Bioprinted amniotic fluid-derived stem cells accelerate healing of large skin wounds. Stem Cells Translational Medicine. 2012 Nov;1(11):792. DOI: 10.5966/sctm.2012-0088

[68] Kim KL, Han DK, Park K, Song SH, Kim JY, Kim JM, Ki HY, Yie SW, Roh CR, Jeon ES, Kim DK. Enhanced dermal wound neovascularization by targeted delivery of endothelial progenitor cells using an RGD-g-PLLA scaffold. Biomaterials. 2009 Aug 31;30(22):3742–8. DOI: 10.1016/j.biomaterials.2009.03.053

[69] O'Loughlin A, Kulkarni M, Vaughan EE, Creane M, Liew A, Dockery P, Pandit A, O'Brien T. Autologous circulating angiogenic cells treated with osteopontin and delivered via a collagen scaffold enhance wound healing in the alloxan-induced

diabetic rabbit ear ulcer model. Stem cell Research & Therapy. 2013 Dec 1;4(6):1–4. DOI: 10.1186/scrt388

[70] Shingyochi Y, Orbay H, Mizuno H. Adipose-derived stem cells for wound repair and regeneration. Expert Opinion on Biological Therapy. 2015 Sep 2;15(9):1285–92. DOI: 10.1517/14712598.2015.1053867

[71] Altman AM, Yan Y, Matthias N, Bai X, Rios C, Mathur AB, Song YH, Alt EU. IFATS collection: human adipose-derived stem cells seeded on a silk fibroin-chitosan scaffold enhance wound repair in a murine soft tissue injury model. Stem Cells. 2009 Jan 1;27(1): 250–8. DOI: 10.1634/stemcells.2008-0178

[72] Hassan W, Dong Y, Wang W. Encapsulation and 3D culture of human adipose-derived stem cells in an in-situ crosslinked hybrid hydrogel composed of PEG-based hyper-branched copolymer and hyaluronic acid. Stem Cell Research & Therapy. 2013 Mar 21;4(2):32. DOI: 10.1186/scrt182

[73] Zeng Y, Zhu L, Han Q, Liu W, Mao X, Li Y, Yu N, Feng S, Fu Q, Wang X, Du Y. Preformed gelatin microcryogels as injectable cell carriers for enhanced skin wound healing. Acta Biomaterialia. 2015 Oct 1;25:291–303. DOI: 10.1016/j.actbio.2015.07.042

[74] Bathany C, Park J, Cho YK, Takayama S. Dehydrated aqueous two-phase system micro-domains retain their shape upon rehydration to allow patterned reagent delivery to cells. Journal of Materials Chemistry B. 2013;1(44):6020–6. DOI: 10.1039/c3tb21004a

[75] Masuda R, Mochizuki M, Hozumi K, Takeda A, Uchinuma E, Yamashina S, Nomizu M, Kadoya Y. A novel cell-adhesive scaffold material for delivering keratinocytes reduces granulation tissue in dermal wounds. Wound Repair and Regeneration. 2009 Jan 1;17(1):127–35. DOI:10.1111/j.1524-475X.2008.00450.x

[76] Nuutila K, Peura M, Suomela S, Hukkanen M, Siltanen A, Harjula A, Vuola J, Kankuri E. Recombinant human collagen III gel for transplantation of autologous skin cells in porcine full-thickness wounds. Journal of Tissue Engineering and Regenerative Medicine. 2015 Dec 1;9(12):1386–93. DOI: 10.1002/term.1691

[77] Sarett SM, Nelson CE, Duvall CL. Technologies for controlled, local delivery of siRNA. Journal of Controlled Release. 2015 Nov 28;218:94–113. DOI: 10.1016/j.jconrel. 2015.09.066

[78] Waddington SN, Crossley R, Sheard V, Howe SJ, Buckley SM, Coughlan L, Gilham DE, Hawkins RE, McKay TR. Gene delivery of a mutant TGFβ3 reduces markers of scar tissue formation after cutaneous wounding. Molecular Therapy. 2010 Dec 1;18(12): 2104–11. DOI: 10.1038/mt.2010.174

[79] Peterson CY, Shaterian A, Borboa AK, Gonzalez AM, Potenza BM, Coimbra R, Eliceiri BP, Baird A. The noninvasive, quantitative, in vivo assessment of adenoviral-mediated gene delivery in skin wound biomaterials. Biomaterials. 2009 Dec 31;30(35):6788–93. DOI: 10.1016/j.biomaterials.2009.07.069

[80] Shaterian A, Kao S, Chen L, DiPietro LA, Coimbra R, Eliceiri BP, Baird A. The candidate tumor suppressor gene Ecrg4 as a wound terminating factor in cutaneous injury. Archives of Dermatological Research. 2013 Mar 1;305(2):141–9. DOI: 10.1007/s00403-012-1276-7

[81] Breen A, Dockery P, O'Brien T, Pandit A. Fibrin scaffold promotes adenoviral gene transfer and controlled vector delivery. Journal of Biomedical Materials Research Part A. 2009 Jun 15;89(4):876–84. DOI: 10.1002/jbm.a.32039

[82] Monaghan M, Browne S, Schenke-Layland K, Pandit A. A collagen-based scaffold delivering exogenous microRNA-29b to modulate extracellular matrix remodeling. Molecular Therapy. 2014 Apr 1;22(4):786–96. DOI: 10.1038/mt.2013.288

[83] Tokatlian T, Cam C, Segura T. Porous hyaluronic acid hydrogels for localized nonviral DNA delivery in a diabetic wound healing model. Advanced Healthcare Materials. 2015 May 1;4(7):1084–91. DOI: 10.1002/adhm.201400783

[84] Sarkar K, Banerjee SL, Kundu PP, Madras G, Chatterjee K. Biofunctionalized surface-modified silver nanoparticles for gene delivery. Journal of Materials Chemistry B. 2015;3(26):5266–76. DOI: 10.1039/c5tb00614g

[85] Kwon MJ, An S, Choi S, Nam K, Jung HS, Yoon CS, Ko JH, Jun HJ, Kim TK, Jung SJ, Park JH. Effective healing of diabetic skin wounds by using nonviral gene therapy based on minicircle vascular endothelial growth factor DNA and a cationic dendrimer. The Journal of Gene Medicine. 2012 Apr 1;14(4):272–8. DOI: 10.1002/jgm.2618

[86] Nauta A, Seidel C, Deveza L, Montoro D, Grova M, Ko SH, Hyun J, Gurtner GC, Longaker MT, Yang F. Adipose-derived stromal cells overexpressing vascular endothelial growth factor accelerate mouse excisional wound healing. Molecular Therapy. 2013 Feb 1;21(2):445–55. DOI: 10.1038/mt.2012.234

[87] Dou C, Lay F, Ansari AM, Rees DJ, Ahmed AK, Kovbasnjuk O, Matsangos AE, Du J, Hosseini SM, Steenbergen C, Fox-Talbot K. Strengthening the skin with topical delivery of keratinocyte growth factor-1 using a novel DNA plasmid. Molecular Therapy. 2014 Apr;22(4):752. DOI: 10.1038/mt.2014.2

[88] Kim HS, Yoo HS. MMPs-responsive release of DNA from electrospun nanofibrous matrix for local gene therapy: in vitro and in vivo evaluation. Journal of Controlled Release. 2010 Aug 3;145(3):264–71. DOI: 10.1016/j.jconrel.2010.03.006

[89] Chiappini C, De Rosa E, Martinez JO, Liu X, Steele J, Stevens MM, Tasciotti E. Biodegradable silicon nanoneedles delivering nucleic acids intracellularly induce localized in vivo neovascularization. Nature Materials. 2015 May 1;14(5):532–9. DOI: 10.1038/NMAT4249

[90] United States Government Code of Federal Regulations, Title 21 (21CFR), Part 3, Food and Drugs, Office of the Federal Register National Archives and Records Administration, US Government Printing Office, Washington, DC, 2015 April 1.

[91] ISO 10993, Biological Evaluation of Medical Devices. 4th ed. Geneva: International Standards Organization; 2009 October 15.

[92] Dash SN, Dash NR, Guru B, Mohapatra PC. Towards reaching the target: clinical 4 application of mesenchymal stem cells for diabetic foot ulcers. Rejuvenation Research, Mary Ann Liebert, Inc, New Rochelle, New York, United States. 5 2014 Feb 1; 17(1): 40-53. DOI: 10.1089/rej.2013.1467

[93] Chaudhary C, Garg T. Scaffolds: a novel carrier and potential wound healer. Critical Reviews™ in Therapeutic Drug Carrier Systems. 2015;32(4):277–321. DOI: 10.1615/ CritRevTherDrugCarrierSyst.2015011246

[94] Abdi R, Fiorina P, Adra CN, Atkinson M, Sayegh MH. Immunomodulation by mesenchymal stem cells a potential therapeutic strategy for type 1 diabetes. Diabetes. 2008 Jul 1;57(7):1759–67. DOI: 10.2337/db08-0180

[95] Duscher D, Barrera J, Wong VW, Maan ZN, Whittam AJ, Januszyk M, Gurtner GC. Stem cells in wound healing: the future of regenerative medicine a mini-review. Gerontology. 2015 May 29;62(2):216–25. DOI: 10.1159/000381877

[96] Ezquer FE, Ezquer ME, Parrau DB, Carpio D, Yañez AJ, Conget PA. Systemic administration of multipotent mesenchymal stromal cells reverts hyperglycemia and prevents nephropathy in type 1 diabetic mice. Biology of Blood and Marrow Transplantation. 2008 Jun 30;14(6):631–40. DOI: 10.1016/j.bbmt.2008.01.006

[97] Yang M, Sheng L, Zhang TR, Li Q. Stem cell therapy for lower extremity diabetic ulcers: where do we stand?. BioMed Research International. 2013 Mar 18;2013:462179. DOI: 10.1155/2013/462179

[98] Takahashi K, Yamanaka S. Induction of pluripotent stem cells from mouse embryonic and adult fibroblast cultures by defined factors. Cell. 2006 Aug 25;126(4):663–76. DOI: 10.1016/j.cell.2006.07.024

[99] Kirby GT, Mills SJ, Cowin AJ, Smith LE. Stem cells for cutaneous wound healing. BioMed Research International. 2015 Jun 2;2015. DOI: 10.1155/2015/285869

[100] Jarow JP, Baxley JH. Medical devices: US medical device regulation. Urologic Oncology: Seminars and Original Investigations, 2015 Mar 31; 33(3): 128–132. DOI: 10.1016/ j.urolonc.2014.10.004

[101] Alpert S. Cost Recovery and the Future of the Medical Device Regulation Program in Canada. Health Law Review. 2008 May 1;16(3):73–78.

9

Venous Leg Ulceration

Aslı Aksu Çerman, İlknur Kıvanç Altunay and
Ezgi Aktaş Karabay

Abstract

Venous leg ulcers are among the most common leg ulcerations. Advancing age, sex, race, phlebitis, family history, obesity, prolonged standing, and number of pregnancies are risk factors. Although the main pathogenetic mechanism is venous hypertension, leading to vein wall damage and thereby a cascade of events resulting in ulceration, there is no consensus about progression from venous hypertension to ulceration.

Diagnosis is based on a thorough patient history and physical examination. A typical venous ulcer is shallow and has irregular, well-defined borders with surrounding skin alterations. However, variable vascular and laboratory tests and skin biopsy may occasionally be necessary in differential diagnosis.

Although pain reduction, closure of the ulcers, and prevention of the recurrences are the main goals of the treatment, targeted therapy should be the reversal of deep venous insufficiency. Leg elevation and long-term compression therapy are essential in this context. Additionally, appropriate wound care including infection control, debridement, dressings, and antibiotics should be performed and, if needed, adjuvant therapies should be planned according to the patient.

Keywords: venous leg ulcers, lower extremity ulcers, venous insufficiency, diagnostic testing, management

1. Introduction

Venous ulcers are the most common form of leg ulcers and important medical problem, which causes significant morbidity and economic burden. Clinical findings and history are helpful in making the diagnosis, but additional diagnostic testing is helpful in confirming the diagnosis and excluding other causes of leg ulcerations. The main purpose of venous ulcer management includes healing of the ulcer and prevention of recurrence. This chapter highlights the epidemiology, pathophysiology, clinical presentation, diagnostic testing, differential diagnosis, and treatment of venous ulcers.

2. Epidemiology

Venous leg ulcers (VLUs) are the most common lower extremity ulceration and responsible for 70% of all leg ulcers, with overall prevalence ranging from 0.06 to 2% [1–4]. It occurs frequently between the ages of 60 and 80 years; however, most people have their first ulcer before the age of 60 years [5, 6]. VLUs have slight female predominance, with a female-to-male ratio ranging from 1.5:1 to 10:1 [7, 8].

Venous ulcers have a significant socioeconomic impact with reduced work productivity and quality of life. Long-term treatments are needed and recurrence is widely common, ranging from 54 to 78% of treated subjects [9]. The overall cost of VLU treatments was 1–2% of the healthcare budgets of European countries [10]. In the United States, approximately 2.5 billion dollars was expended for the treatment of VLUs per year [11].

Advancing age, sex, race, phlebitis, family history, obesity, occupation involving prolonged standing, and number of pregnancies are risk factors that have been described with chronic venous insufficiency and, subsequently, with venous ulcers [12, 13].

3. Pathogenesis

3.1. Normal venous anatomy and physiology

The venous system of the lower extremities includes the superficial veins, perforator veins, and the deep veins according to their relationship to the muscular fascia. The superficial veins comprises the reticular veins, the large (larger) and small (smaller) saphenous veins, and their tributaries. The great saphenous vein originates from where the dorsal vein of the first digit merges with the dorsal venous arch of the foot. After passing in front of the medial malleolus, it ascends the medial side of the leg. It joins the femoral vein just below the inguinal ligament. The small saphenous vein arises from the dorsal venous arch of the foot and ascends posterolaterally from behind the lateral malleolus. Usually, it drains into the popliteal vein near the popliteal fossa. The reticular veins, a network of veins parallel to the skin surface, communicate with either saphenous tributaries or the deep veins through perforators. The perforator veins connect the superficial and deep vein systems. The deep venous system is categorized as either intramuscular or intermuscular. Intermuscular veins are three paired tibial veins including, the posterior tibial vein, the anterior tibial vein, and the peroneal vein. These veins join to form the popliteal vein in the popliteal area. At the level of the adductor canal, the popliteal vein is renamed the superficial femoral vein. This vessel joins the deep femoral vein in the femoral triangle to form the common femoral vein. After passing beneath the inguinal ligament to enter the pelvis, the femoral vein is renamed the common iliac vein. The superficial veins are low-pressure systems, whereas the deep veins are high-pressure systems. All three venous systems have one-way bicuspid valves, which only open toward the deep venous system and, under normal conditions, prevent reflux of blood. Normally, ambulation and the pumping action of the calf muscles propel venous blood upward toward the heart, and the valves close when pressure rises in the deep venous system, which prevents retrograde flow [4, 14, 15].

3.2. Pathophysiology

In patients with venous disease or failure, venous pressure in deep system falls less than normal during ambulation and rises in orthostatic position, and this is termed venous hypertension. In conclusion, venous hypertension in the deep veins may be transmitted to the superficial veins [4, 16]. There is no general consensus about the transition from venous hypertension to venous ulceration. Several hypotheses have been proposed.

(a) Precapillary fibrin cuffs and fibrinolytic abnormalities hypotheses:

According to this theory of Browse and Burnand [17], venous hypertension leads to distention of capillary walls and leakage of macromolecules such as fibrinogen into the dermis and subcutaneous tissues of the calf. The leaked fibrinogen polymerizes to form precapillary fibrin cuffs in the extravascular space. These precapillary cuffs were assumed to act as a physical barrier, which impede the diffusion of oxygen and nutrients, resulting in ischemia, cell death, and ulceration [17–19]. In addition, local and systemic fibrinolytic/coagulation abnormalities such as prolonged euglobulin lysis time, elevated plasma fibrinogen levels, increased levels of protein C, fibrin-related antigens, D-dimer, D-monomer, fibrin monomer, and reduction in factor XIII activity may present in patients with venous disease [20–22]. However, it is unclear whether these abnormalities are primary or secondary to venous disease.

(b) Leukocyte trapping hypothesis:

As a result of venous hypertension, there is a decreased pressure in capillary bed perfusion and capillary flux. This gives rise to erythrocyte aggregation and leukocyte plugging in the capillaries, leading to local ischemia. Moreover, these leukocytes release cytokines, tumor necrosis factor α (TNF-α), proteolytic enzymes, and free radicals which can cause increased vascular permeability resulting in the leakage of fibrinogen into the pericapillary tissues and the decreased fibrinolytic activity [23–25].

(c) The growth factor trap hypothesis:

Falanga and Eaglstein [26] recommended that macromolecules such as fibrinogen and $\alpha_2$macroglobulin, which leak into the dermis as a result of venous hypertension, bind to or trap growth factors, which then become unavailable for the maintenance of tissue integrity and repair process. The precapillary fibrin cuff of the venous ulcer contains growth factors such as transforming growth factor β (TGF-β). Trapping of growth factors can impair activation of the cells that are needed for healing process [27].

4. Diagnosis

4.1. Clinical presentation

In general, the venous ulcer is an irregularly, well-defined border and typically non-painful [4, 8]. Nevertheless, deep ulcers or small venous ulcers surrounded by atrophie blanche are highly painful [28]. The size and site of ulcers are variable, but they usually located over the medial malleolus (**Figure 1**).

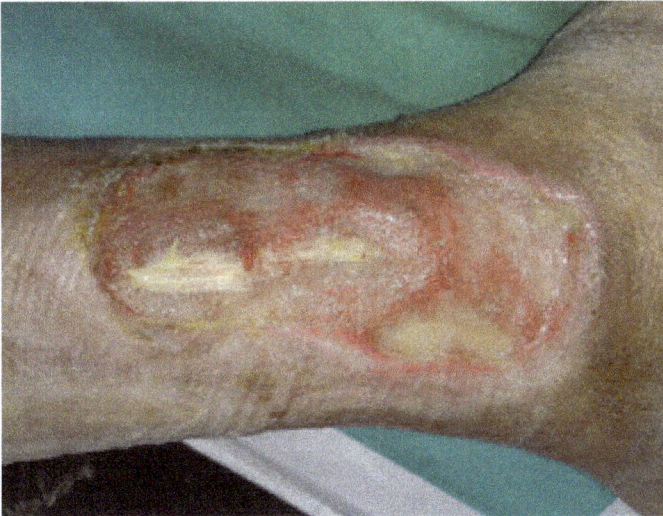

Figure 1. Typical venous ulcer over the medial malleolus.

There may be yellow fibrinous exudates on the ulcer bed. Varicose veins and ankle edema are common. The surrounding skin is erythematous or hyperpigmented with variable degrees of induration. Eczematous changes associated with venous dermatitis are commonly present. Long-standing venous disease can lead to loss of the subcutaneous fat and fibrotic changes in the skin called lipodermatosclerosis, giving the characteristic "inverted champagne-bottle" appearance of the leg [29]. The main complications of chronic venous ulcers are osteomyelitis and neoplastic transformation [4, 30]. Long-term ulcers may require biopsy at regular intervals for malignant change. If osteomyelitis is suspected, radiography, bone scanning, and bone biopsy should be considered.

4.2. Diagnostic testing

The diagnosis of venous ulcers is mainly based on patient history and clinical examination; however, there are diagnostic tests to evaluate venous anatomy and aid the diagnosis.

4.2.1. Venous duplex ultrasound

Duplex ultrasound is the first-line diagnostic test to evaluate the insufficiency in venous ulcers [31]. Continuous-wave Doppler provides information about superficial venous incompetence or obstruction; nonetheless, it can be difficult to differentiate deep from superficial venous incompetence [32, 33].

4.2.2. Venous plethysmography

Photoplethysmography and air plethysmography measure the degree of venous reflux and the calf muscle pump efficiency [8, 34, 35].

4.2.3. Venous imaging

In case of suspected venous obstruction, additional contrast imaging with computed tomography venography or magnetic resonance venography should be done; whereupon diagnosis should be confirmed by contrast venography and intravascular ultrasound [31].

4.2.4. Laboratory testing

Patients who have a history of venous thrombosis and thrombophilia should undergo a workup for inherited hypercoagulable factors including protein C and S, factor V Leiden, antiphospholipid antibodies, prothrombin gene mutation, homocysteine, cryoglobulins, and cryoagglutinins [8, 31].

4.2.5. Arterial testing—Ankle Brachial Pressure Index (ABI)

Patients with venous leg ulcers may have concomitant peripheral arterial disease component. Therefore, arterial pulse examination, Doppler ultrasound and ABI should be evaluated for the elimination of coexistent arterial disease. ABI is the ratio of the systolic blood pressure at the ankle compared with the systolic blood pressure in the arm. An ABI in the range of 0.9–1.1 is considered normal and 0.5–0.8 indicates moderate peripheral vascular disease and claudication, while less than 0.5 indicates more severe disease [4, 8, 36].

4.2.6. Wound biopsy

Most studies suggest wound biopsy for those that do not improve with standard wound and compression therapy after a period of 4–6 weeks of treatment. The biopsy specimen should be obtained from several sites, including the wound edge and central provisional matrix [31].

4.3. Classification

4.3.1. CEAP

Classification of venous ulcers, known as CEAP [clinical findings (C), etiology (E), anatomical distribution (A), and pathophysiology (P)] based on clinical findings was introduced in 1994 and revised in 2004 [37, 38] (**Table 1**).

CEAP	Definition
Clinical classification	
C0	No visible or palpable signs of venous disease
C1	Telangiectasies or reticular veins
C2	Varicose veins
C3	Edema
C4a	Pigmentation and/or eczema
C4b	Lipodermatosclerosis and/or atrophie blanche
C5	Healed venous ulcer
C6	Active venous ulcer
CS	Symptoms, including ache, pain, tightness, skin irritation, heaviness, muscle cramps, as well as other complaints attributable to venous dysfunction
CA	Asymptomatic
Etiologic classification	
Ec	Congenital
Ep	Primary
Es	Secondary (post-thrombotic)
En	No venous etiology identified
Anatomic classification	
As	Superficial veins
Ap	Perforator veins
Ad	Deep veins
An	No venous location identified
Pathophysiologic classification (basic)	
Pr	Reflux
Po	Obstruction
Pr,o	Reflux and obstruction
Pn	No venous pathophysiology identifiable

Modified from Eklöf et al. [38].

Table 1. Basic revised clinical, etiologic, anatomic, and pathophysiologic (CEAP) classification system.

The clinical findings are divided into six categories, where C_0 indicates no visible or palpable signs of venous disease; C1, the presence of telangiectasies or reticular veins; C2, varicose veins; C3, edema; C4, changes in skin and subcutaneous tissue secondary to venous disease (C4a, pigmentation or eczema; C4b, lipodermatosclerosis or atrophie blanche); C5, skin changes with healed venous ulcer; C6, active venous ulcer. Each clinical class is further supplemented by (A) for asymptomatic and (S) for symptomatic presentation. Symptoms include aching, pain, skin irritation, tightness, heaviness, muscle cramps, and other complaints. The etiologic classification is separated into three categories; Ec, congenital; Ep, primary; Es, secondary (post-traumatic or post-thrombotic); and En, no venous cause identified. The anatomical classification is divided into four categories: As, superficial veins; Ap, perforator veins; Ad, deep veins; and An, no venous location identified. The pathophysiologic classification is divided into four categories; Pr, reflux; Po, obstruction; Pr,o, combination of reflux and obstruction; and Pn, no venous pathophysiology identifiable.

The venous clinical severity score (VCSS) was developed because of subjective and inadequate definition of the categories in CEAP classification (**Table 2**).

	None: 0	Mild: 1	Moderate: 2	Severe: 3
Pain or other discomfort (i.e., aching, heaviness, fatigue, soreness, burning)		Occasional pain or other discomfort (i.e., not restricting regular daily activities)	Daily pain or other discomfort (i.e., interfering with but not preventing regular daily activities)	Daily pain or discomfort (i.e., limits most regular daily activities)
Presumes venous origin Varicose veins "Varicose" veins must be ≥3 mm in diameter to qualify in the standing position		Few: scattered (i.e., isolated branch varicosities or clusters) Also induces corona phlebectatica (ankle flare)	Confined to calf or thigh	Involves calf and thigh
Venous edema Presumes venous origin		Limited to foot and ankle area	Extends above ankle but below knee	Extends to knee and above
Skin pigmentation Presumes venous origin	None or focal	Limited to perimalleolar area	Diffuse over lower third of calf	Wider distribution above lower third of calf
Does not include focal pigmentation over varicose veins or pigmentation due to other chronic diseases				
Inflammation More than just recent pigmentation (i.e., erythema, cellulitis, venous eczema, dermatitis)		Limited to perimalleolar area	Diffuse over lower third of calf	Wider distribution above lower third of calf
Induration Presumes venous origin of secondary skin and subcutaneous changes (i.e., chronic edema with fibrosis,		Limited to perimalleolar area	Diffuse over lower third of calf	Wider distribution above lower third of calf

	None: 0	Mild: 1	Moderate: 2	Severe: 3
hypodermitis) Includes white atrophy and lipodermatosclerosis				
Active ulcer number	0	1	2	≥3
Active ulcer duration (longest active)	N/A	<3 months	>3 months but <1 year	Not healed for <1 year
Active ulcer size (largest active)	N/A	Diameter >2 cm	Diameter 2–6 cm	Diameter >6 cm
Use of compression therapy	0 Not used	1 Intermittent use of stockings	2 Wears stockings most days	3 Full compliance: stockings

Modified from Vasquez MA, Rabe E, McLafferty RB, Shortell CK, Marston WA, Gillespie D, et al. Revision of the venous clinical severity score: venous outcomes consensus statement: special communication of the American Venous Forum Ad Hoc Outcomes Working Group. J Vasc Surg 2010;52:1387–96.

Table 2. Revised venous clinical severity score (VCSS) system.

A VCSS may range from 0 to 30 [31, 33, 39]. A score of more than eight indicates the progression of venous problem. In addition, the VCSS has been shown to be useful to evaluate the response to treatment.

5. Differential diagnosis

5.1. Arterial ulcers

Arterial leg ulcers result from peripheral arterial occlusive disease. Arterial ulcers typically are round or punched out with a sharply demarcated border and extremely painful. A fibrous yellow base or necrotic eschar is commonly seen (**Figure 2**).

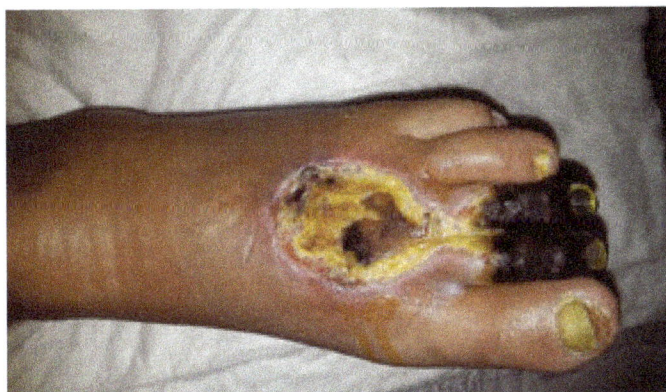

Figure 2. Arterial ulcer.

The surrounding skin is cool to the touch. These ulcers frequently occur at the tips of the toes and over the bony prominences. Associated findings are weak or nonexistent arteria dorsalis pedis pulse, hair loss, atrophic skin, dystrophic nails, the presence of claudication, or rest pain. The ABI of 0.5 or less indicates severe arterial disease [4, 40, 41].

5.2. Neuropathic ulcers

Neuropathic ulcers are more common in patients with diabetes mellitus (DM). Trauma and/or pressures can cause wounding and ulcer formation in patients with neuropathy [41–43]. These ulcers usually tend to be on the plantar surface of the foot. An abnormal, thickened callus develops at pressure areas, with ultimate disrupt of the tissue resulting in ulcer formation (**Figure 3**).

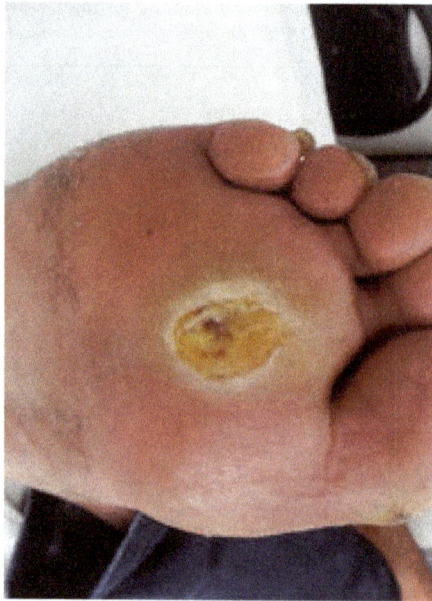

Figure 3. Diabetic neuropathic foot ulcer.

5.3. Pressure ulcers

Pressure ulcers mostly occur in patients with limited mobility. These ulcers can start to develop when soft tissue is compressed for a prolonged period of time. The main risky sites are the heel of the foot, malleoli, and sacral and trochanter areas [4, 44].

5.4. Hypertensive leg ulcer (Ulcus Cruris Hypertonicum Martorell)

Hypertensive leg ulcers are extremely painful and commonly located on the distal portion of the lower leg above the lateral malleolus. These ulcers are seen in patients with prolonged, severe, or poorly controlled hypertension [41, 42]. The ulceration is secondary to tissue ischemia caused by increased vascular resistance.

5.5. Mixed ulcer

Patients with mixed etiology ulcers have combined venous and arterial disease. Often further complicating factors such as DM, rheumatoid arthritis (RA), or lymphedema also exist [42].

5.6. Pyoderma gangrenosum

Pyoderma gangrenosum is a neutrophilic dermatosis. Clinically it starts with sterile pustules that rapidly progress and turn into painful ulcers with purplish-blue, undermined borders [42, 45]. It may be associated with inflammatory bowel disease, rheumatic, or myeloproliferative disorders [8, 12] (**Figure 4**).

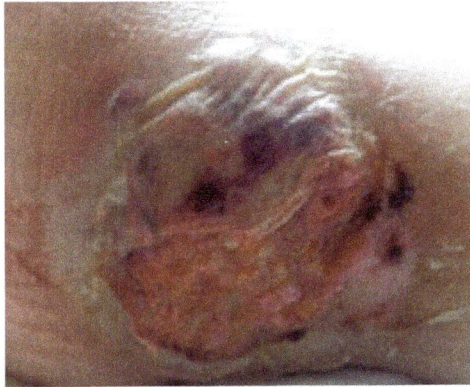

Figure 4. Pyoderma gangrenosum.

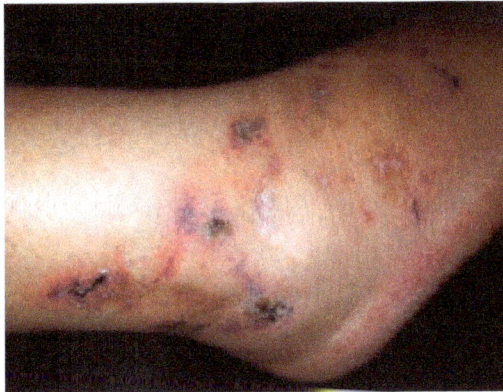

Figure 5. Livedoid vasculopathy and tiny ulcerations.

5.7. Vasculitis

Cutaneous vasculitis may present as palpable purpura, urticaria, nodule, bullae, livedo reticularis, necrotic areas, or skin ulceration. Vasculitic leg ulcers are often painful, multilocular and, surrounded by livid erythema and purpura (**Figure 5**). The different types of vasculitis that can cause cutaneous ulceration include small vessel vasculitis such as leukocytoclastic vasculitis, medium-sized vessel vasculitis such as polyarteritis nodosa, microscopic polyangiitis, and Wegener granulomatosis [41, 46]. Routine blood work, sedimentation, antineutrophil cytoplasmic antibody (ANCA), urinalysis, chest X-ray, and multiple skin biopsies should be done.

Livedoid vasculopathy (LV) is characterized by irregularly shaped, recurrent perimalleolar painful ulcers overlying areas of purpura. LV typically has three phases including livedo racemosa, ulcerations, and atrophie blanche [41, 42] (**Figure 5**).

5.8. Autoimmune diseases

5.8.1. Rheumatoid ulcers

Approximately 10% of individuals with RA develop leg ulcers [41] (**Figure 6**). The cause of leg ulcerations in RA is multifactorial, including vasculitis, venous insufficiency, paraproteinemias, medications, superficial ulcerating rheumatoid necrobiosis, pyoderma gangrenosum, and Felty's syndrome [45–48](**Figure 6**).

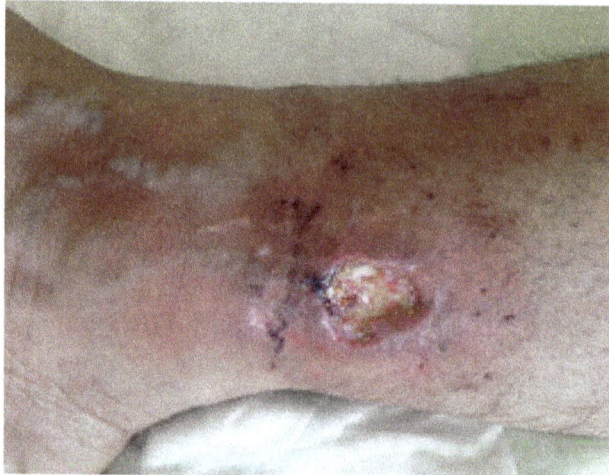

Figure 6. Rheumatoid ulcer.

5.8.2. Scleroderma

The prevalence of lower extremity ulcers in scleroderma is 3.6% and various parts of the leg can be affected [49]. These ulcers are painful and relatively refractory to standard treatment methods. Antiphospholipid antibody, fibrotic skin, vascular compromise, coagulation abnormalities, and tissue calcium deposition may have a role in their pathogenesis [45, 46, 48].

5.8.3. Systemic lupus erythematosus (SLE)

Leg ulcers of SLE are usually painful, sharply marginated, or punched out that located over the malleolar, supramalleolar, or pretibial areas [50]. Vasculitis, antiphospholipid antibody, thrombosis of vessels, venous insufficiency, lupus profundus, and drug-induced lupus syndrome have been associated with leg ulcerations.

5.8.4. Sjögren syndrome

Leg ulcerations of Sjögren syndrome have been associated with cryoglobulinemia, anticardio-lipin antibody, and vasculitis [46, 51].

5.8.5. Dermatomyositis

Leg ulcers of dermatomyositis have been reported to involve calcinosis cutis and vasculitis [46].

5.8.6. Mixed connective tissue disease (MCTD)

MCTD is an overlap syndrome combining features of SLE, RA, systemic sclerosis, and dermatomyositis together with the presence of antibodies to U1-RNP. Chronic leg ulcers are not rare in MCTD and they have been reported to be due to subcutaneous calcification, vasculitis, vasospasm (Raynoud's phenomenon), vascular thrombosis, and antiphospholipid antibodies [46, 52, 53].

5.9. Infections

Numerous infections can precipitate ulcerations on the lower legs. Ecthyma, atypical myco-bacterial infections, late syphilis, cutaneous leishmaniasis, actinomycoses, nocardioses, human immunodeficiency virus (HIV) infection, herpes simplex, and cytomegalovirus infections must be considered [41, 43, 54]. In addition, all chronic wounds may be secondarily contaminated with bacteria. Tissue culture will help elucidate the cause [4].

5.10. Metabolic diseases

Various metabolic factors such as diabetes mellitus, amyloidosis, hyperhomocysteinemia, prolidase deficiency, oxalosis, calciphylaxis, and gout can play a role for the lower leg ulcera-tions.

Necrobiosis lipoidica is a rare, chronic granulomatous disease of the skin. Clinical presentation characterized by atrophic, indurated plaques with a yellowish center and telangiectasies [42]. The lower legs, especially the shins, are the most common sites of involvement. During the course, ulcerations may occur. Necrobiosis lipoidica frequently occurs in association with diabetes mellitus (**Figure 7**).

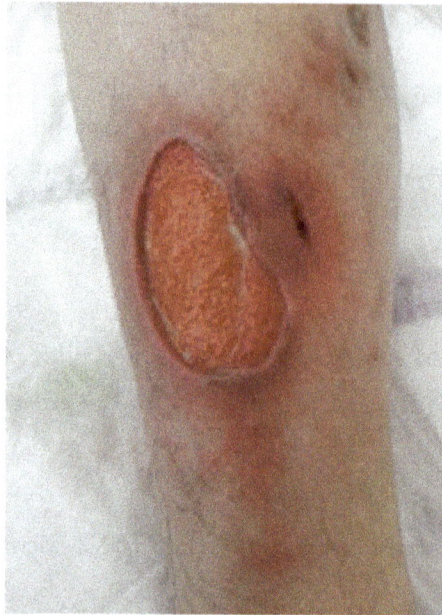

Figure 7. Necrobiosis lipoidica.

Calciphylaxis is an uncommon disorder, classically associated with renal disease and secondary parathyroidism [55]. Clinical presentation may begin as microlivedo that develop into painful ulcerations.

5.11. Hematologic diseases

Several forms of anemia (thalassemia, sickle cell anemia, hereditary spherocytosis, glucose 6 phosphate dehydrogenase deficiency), and hypercoagulable disorders (antiphospholipid antibody syndrome, antithrombin III, protein C or S deficiency, essential thrombocythemia, thrombotic thrombocytopenic purpura, polycythemia, or abnormal clotting factors such as factor V Leiden, factor II mutant) have been associated with lower leg ulceration [54].

5.12. Neoplasia

Many tumor types such as basal cell carcinoma, squamous cell carcinoma, and melanoma may present with skin ulceration. Basal cell carcinomas arising from venous ulcers appear as exuberant granulation tissue rolling onto the wound edges [4]. In addition, malignancy that presents as Marjolin's ulcers is most commonly associated with chronically inflamed, or scarred skin. Skin biopsy is necessary to identify ulcerated malignant tumors on the leg.

5.13. Medications

Hydroxyurea is a cytostatic drug used in various myeloproliferative disorders. A rare complication is the development of painful ulcers, usually localized on the malleoli or in neighboring regions [42, 54]. The coumarin derivatives, nifedipine, diltiazem, barbiturates, and erythropoietin in very rare cases, may trigger ulcer development [42].

6. Management

It is essential to treat the patients with multidisciplinary approach. The complete assessment of the chronic venous insufficiency should be evaluated together with vascular surgeons. The decision of the surgical treatment in appropriate cases should be considered with plastic surgeons. Knowledge of pathogenesis of venous ulcers and avoiding from its risk factors will be provided to choose the optimal treatment for patients with venous leg ulcers, which cause both impairment of life quality and socioeconomic burden. A multidisciplinary team of specialists will be helpful in the evaluation of venous leg ulcers and providing the most appropriate treatment.

Several treatment options are available for the management of venous ulcers. Pain reduction, closure of the ulcers, and prevention of the recurrences are the main goals of the treatment [56]. Reversing the effects of venous hypertension is the primary purpose of the treatment of venous leg ulcers. The easiest method is leg elevation [57]. Although it seems to be impractical to most of the patients, elevation of the legs above the heart level for 30 minutes, 3–4 times a day, provides the dissolution of the swelling and improves the microcirculation [58]. Leg elevation can also be performed at night by raising the foot 15–20 cm high [59]. Moreover, good nutrition and assessment with each dressing change are necessary to support the therapy. Initially and at each dressing change, the depth, width, and height of the wound bed should be measured to evaluate the improvement. Appropriate therapy of the wound must be selected patient centered. Infection control, debridement, antibiotics, dressings, compression, and adjuvant therapies will be described in this section.

6.1. Wound cleansers

Cleansers are the first and main step in preparing the wound bed. Wound cleansing with a neutral, nonirritating solution with a minimum chemical and mechanical trauma should be performed at each dressing change. Wound exudate and other debris around the wound area in venous leg ulcers must be cleansed with an appropriate solution. Although several cleansing solutions are in the market, the choice of the cleanser should have the purpose of avoiding toxicity to the viable tissue in the wound bed [31].

6.2. Debridement

Debridement during the initial evaluation is recommended to remove the necrotic tissue, excessive bacterial burden, and nonviable cells [31]. Although debridement of the wound is commonly performed to allow the formation of good granulation tissue and proper epitheli-alization by creating an appropriate environment to keratinocyte migration, there is a lack of evidence that routine wound debridement accelerates wound healing [31]. There are several ways of wound debridement, including autolytic, chemical, and mechanical [60].

6.2.1. Autolytic debridement

In venous ulcers, it is possible that wound occlusion itself promotes re-epithelialization, reduces associated pain, enhances autolytic debridement, and provides an additional barrier to bacteria [61, 62]. Hydrogels, alginates, hydrocolloids, foams, and films are the basic occlusive dressings. Wound features, exudate amount and cost of the material, and patient and physician preference affect the choice of dressing [63].

6.2.2. Chemical debridement

Several enzyme-debriding agents have been developed to promote the removal of the necrotic tissue and the formation of proper granulation tissue [64, 65]. Specific proteolytic enzyme therapies to the venous ulcers may accelerate the removal of fibrin cuffs [66]. Various enzyme-debriding agents are available, including collagenase, papain, trypsin, and tissue plasminogen activator [60, 67, 68]. Frequency of the application of the dressing may vary up to the manu-facturer's recommendations. Enzymatic debridement, which does not require a trained clinician for application, has been found in several studies to remove nonviable tissue from the wound beds of venous leg ulcers, but there is no evidence that this method provides a benefit over surgical debridement [69, 70].

6.2.3. Mechanical debridement

Application of wet-to-dry dressings, hydrotherapy, irrigation, and dextranomers are some of the methods of mechanical debridement [71]. The removal of the viable tissue along with the necrotic material is the major disadvantage of mechanical debridement [72]. Hydrosurgical debridement was showed to have a shorter procedure time but requires additional cost and a trained clinician [73, 74]. Furthermore, it may be associated with a significant periprocedural pain [69]. Dextranomer's hydrophilic structure that provides a high absorptive capacity makes it useful for wounds with heavy exudate. The possibility of dehydration of the wound bed demands caution [4]. Surgical debridement, which may be performed with a curette, forceps, scalpel, or sharp scissors, is another way to remove necrotic tissue. As venous ulcers do not comprise frank necrosis or eschar tissue, this method is rarely used in venous ulcers [75]. During surgical debridement, local infiltrative, regional block, or general anesthesia may be required according to the extensity of the wound [31].

6.3. Antibiotics

Antimicrobial therapy is suggested in venous ulcers with $>1 \times 10^6$ colony-forming unit (CFU)/g of bacteria on quantitative culture and clinical evidence of infection. Systemic antibiotic therapy, guided by sensitivities performed on wound culture, is recommended. Oral antibiotics are preferred in the beginning of the therapy duration and should be limited to 2 weeks [31]. Combination of mechanical debridement and antibiotic therapy is thought to be successful in eradicating infection in venous leg ulcer. In case of cellulitis, beta-lactam and non beta-lactam antibiotics may be treatment options. Trimethoprim-sulfamethoxazole and clindamycin are recommended as initial empiric therapy if methicillin-resistant Staphylococcus aureus is the suspected reason of cellulitis [76]. The use of topical silver for infected venous ulcers is controversial [31]. Recently, cadexomer iodine is reported to shorten the healing time of venous ulcers [77].

It is likely to be an increased risk of contact dermatitis in patients with chronic venous insufficiency, so in these patients any topical preparation must be used carefully [4]. There is a lack of evidence of the positive effects of topical antimicrobials in the healing of venous ulcers [31].

6.4. Periulcer skin management

It is important to keep the periulcer skin healthy to provide improvement in venous ulcers. Management of dermatitis and other abnormalities in periulcer skin accomplishes other therapy strategies in venous ulcers [31]. As mentioned above, contact dermatitis related to topical agents and dressings used in the treatment of venous ulcers are very common. In severe contact dermatitis, a short term of systemic steroids may be needed [4, 31]. Skin lubricants will be helpful in the terms of dermatitis in the calf and ankle due to venous hypertension [31]. Care of the periulcer skin will improve the venous wound healing; therefore, it is necessary to recognize the abnormalities in this area and start the appropriate treatment.

6.5. Dressing

Several types of wound dressings including gauzes, films, gels, foams, hydrocolloids, alginates, hydrogels, and other polymers are being used beneath compression bandages. Some of the dressings show biological activity on its own, while some provide the release of bioactive constituents. Different types of wound dressings such as hydrogels, hydrocolloids, foams, films, and wafers may comprise of antimicrobials, anti-inflammatory agents, analgesics, growth factors, and proteins, which would be useful in different problems of wound healing [78, 79]. During the choice of the wound dressing type, features of the ulcer should be considered and the mostly desired function of the dressing (such as cleaning, absorbing, regulating, creating a moist environment, and the possibility of adding medication, protecting the periulcer skin) should be decided [80]. Of course, the patient's needs and cost-effectiveness are other factors affecting the dressing choice [81]. The optimal wound dressing should absorb the exudate and also maintain a moist, warm wound bed and protect the periulcer skin [31, 76]. Routine use of topical antimicrobial dressings is not recommended [31]. While using wound dressings, risk of allergy should be kept in mind in venous ulcers. In conclusion, topical wound dressings are recommended as a part of the standard therapy in venous ulcers [31].

6.6. Compression

Compression therapy remains the mainstay treatment of venous leg ulcers [76]. Compression is a kind of mechanical therapy, which is simply based on applying pressure to the limb [31]. There is a significant improvement in ulcer healing and reduction in recurrence rates with an appropriate compression therapy [4, 82]. Compression therapy corrects the venous hypertension by improving venous pumping function and lymphatic drainage [83]. And as a result of compression, local hydrostatic pressure increases and superficial venous pressure decreases; thus, the edema dissolves resulting in cutaneous blood flow increase [83]. Other effects of compression therapy are clinical improvement in lipodermatosclerotic skin through lymph propulsion along with the increase in lymph transport and fibrinolysis [4]. Besides the mechanical effect, compression reduces the release of macromolecules into the extravascular space, some of which play role in wound healing [84].

Various types of devices have been used for compression therapy, such as different types of bandages, bandage systems, ready-to-use garments, and several pneumatic devices [31]. It is thought that an external pressure of 35–40 mm Hg at the ankle is necessary to overcome venous hypertension [85]. For acute disease, reducing edema and improving the healing process, inelastic or rigid bandages as well as elastic and multilayered bandages are suggested. The bandage system should have high pressures when the patient walks (working pressure) and low pressure when the patient is on rest (resting pressure). Traditional Unna boot, a moist zinc-impregnated paste bandage, is a prototype of this system [83, 86]. Modified Unna boots (short-stretch bandages) have the same properties. Their stable shape despite the volume changes in leg secondary to edema reduction, unpleasant odor due to wound exudate, and potential development of contact dermatitis are the limiting factors of Unna boots' use [76, 77]. After edema reduces, long-stretch bandages are beneficial as they provide appropriate working pressure and higher resting pressure. Its easy use and providing of frequent dressing changes make the elastic compression bandages practical. Covering the leg by overlapping the bandage between turns will produce a multilayer bandage. Different components of bandages may be applied at each layer. While this application increases the pressure and also makes the final multilayer bandage less elastic and more stiff due to the friction between the surfaces of each bandage [31], intermittent pneumatic compression (IPC) pumps are also used. These devices consist of plastic air chambers, encircling the lower leg. As the air chamber fills to a preset pressure then deflated. With this system, compression of the leg is provided periodically [87].

Although compression therapy is known to be effective in both healing of venous ulcers and prevention of recurrent ulcers, there is still no optimized compression method [31, 88].

6.7. Adjuvant therapies

Systemic pharmacotherapy may be useful as an adjuvant therapy in venous ulcers. Most of the systemic agents used as adjuvant therapy acts in mechanism of one or more points in the pathophysiology of venous leg ulceration.

6.7.1. Pentoxifylline

Pentoxifylline, an antifibrinolytic agent, is thought to promote wound healing as an adjunctive therapy. Pentoxifylline has been shown to play role in microcirculation by promoting leukocyte migration, reducing platelet aggregation and fibrinogen levels, decreasing plasma viscosity, stimulating collagenase production, and blocking the effects of tumor necrosis factor-alpha on fibroblasts [89, 90]. Pentoxifylline may act in venous ulcer healing through the effects of cytokine production [91]. The conventional dose of pentoxifylline in venous leg ulcers is 400 mg three times a day. But recently, it has been proposed that the use of pentoxifylline 800 mg three times a day is more effective in venous ulcer healing. The main side effects reported were gastrointestinal disturbances such as nausea, indigestion, and diarrhea [89, 92, 93]. In studies, pentoxifylline has shown to be an effective adjuvant to compression therapy in venous leg ulcers. According to a Cochrane review, pentoxifylline plus bandaging is more effective than compression plus placebo and pentoxifylline may even be effective in the absence of compression [93].

6.7.2. Aspirin

There is currently insufficient evidence for the effectiveness of aspirin in venous leg ulcers [94]. The use of acetylsalicylic acid as an adjunct for the treatment of venous ulcers has been evaluated in one pilot study and one randomized controlled trial to date. The effect of aspirin in venous ulcers is through its irreversible inhibition of cyclooxygenase, resulting in reduction in thromboxane A2 implicated in platelet aggregation [95].

6.7.3. Split-thickness skin grafting

There are no specific indications for skin grafting of the ulcers of lower extremities [4]. Surgical treatment should only be considered in patients with venous ulcers that do not heal with conservative therapies [96]. Autografts, allografts, or human skin equivalents can be used, with a resulting healing rate of 73% [97]. In venous ulcers, skin grafting can also be followed by additional treatment to accelerate healing. The outcomes of the split-thickness skin grafting in venous ulcers vary in different studies [31]. There is still lack of evidence in the routine use of split-skin thickness skin grafting.

6.7.4. Negative pressure therapy

Negative pressure wound therapy (NPWT) is currently used widely in wound care and is promoted for use on wounds. In this system, a wound dressing is applied to the wound, to which a machine is attached. The negative pressure (or vacuum) that the machine applies sucks any wound and tissue fluid away from the treated area into a canister.

The evidence is insufficient in clinical effectiveness of NPWT in the treatment of leg ulcers. It is thought to be effective in wound healing through providing excess drainage, promoting angiogenesis, and decreasing the bacterial load of the wound [98]. There is some positive evidence that the treatment may reduce time to healing as part of a treatment, tissue granulation, area and volume reduction have also been reported. NPWT is not suggested as a primary treatment for venous leg ulcers [31, 99].

6.7.5. Cellular therapy

In recent years, cellular and/or tissue-derived products (CTPs) such as extracellular matrix (ECM; OASIS®) [100], human skin equivalent (HSE; Apligraf®) [101–103], and living skin equivalent (LSE; Dermagraft®) [104–107] have been explored as alternative therapeutic options.

Studies investigating the effects of CTPs are applied to the wounds that have been stuck in the inflammatory phase. CTPs provide the healing by supplying various biological factors, reducing levels of unnecessary cytokines or enzymes (such as matrix metalloproteinases), and/ or forming a temporary ECM (which results in granulation) [108].

Recently, Apligraf, an allogeneic bilayer cellular therapy, has been approved by FDA for use in venous ulcers [31]. Before the application of cellular therapy, appropriate wound bed preparation, including the removal of debris and any necrotic tissue, should be done. The application of the graft is recommended to be done with a period of 1–3 weeks with observations of effectiveness before reapplication is considered. And reapplication is recommended as long as the venous ulcer continues to respond to the therapy [31]. In patients with venous leg ulcers who have failed with standard therapy for 4–6 weeks, cultured allogeneic bilayer skin replacements should be used [31].

Even though cellular treatments are initially more expensive, it may be more effective and less costly in the long term in chronic venous ulcers [109].

6.7.6. Tissue matrices, growth factors, human tissues, or other skin substitutes

In chronic wounds, human tissue (amniotic membrane, cryopreserved skin) or animal tissue (bladder, fetal bovine skin, others) constructs are being used. Growth factors or some other molecules, the tissues contain, may support healing process [110].

Granulocyte macrophage-colony stimulating factor (GMCSF) is a growth factor that has stimulatory effects on keratinocyte proliferation and endothelial cell and fibroblast differentiation [111]. In some studies, both intradermal injections of GM-CSF and topical application of GM-CSF have been shown to be effective in healing rates of venous ulcers [98]. But, injection site and bone pain can limit the intradermal use of GM-CSF [98].

Small intestine submucosa (SIS, Oasis®) is a biomaterial derived from porcine SIS that acts as an extracellular matrix. It is composed of Type I, III, IV, and V collagen, glycosaminogylcans, proteoglycans, proteoglycans, fibronectin, and growth factors [98, 112]. Successful results have only been reported in studies of using porcine small intestinal submucosa in venous leg ulcers [100]. It has been approved by FDA for use in wounds including venous leg ulcers. Use of porcine small intestinal submucosa tissue construct in addition to compression therapy for the treatment of venous leg ulcers is only suggested in patients who did not respond to the standard therapy for 4–6 weeks [31]. It was shown to be well tolerated and nontoxic and did not induce an adverse immunological reaction even in patients given repeated applications.

6.7.7. Therapeutic ultrasound

Ultrasound has been used as a therapeutic tool for nearly 50 years [113]. Recently, ultrasound therapy has been applied for the treatment of chronic wounds in some centers [114]. Although high-frequency ultrasound (HFU) (1–3 MHz) has been shown to promote healing of some injuries [115, 116], it has some disadvantages such as, burns or endothelial injury. However, in some studies low-dose application of ultrasound has been reported to be more successful than high-dose ultrasound in the treatment of skin wounds [117]. Thus, noncontact ultrasound therapy is among the newer modalities. Use of lower frequency (40 kHz) ultrasound in wound management was approved by the FDA in 2004 [118]. Low-frequency ultrasound therapy provides wound healing via the production, vibration, and movement of micron-sized bubbles in the coupling medium and tissue. The healing process improves by the reduced bioburden, increased angiogenesis, stimulated cellular activity, and the removal of necrotic tissues [119]. Additional studies are necessary to determine standardized protocols of therapeutic ultrasound in venous ulcers treatment. Routine use of ultrasound therapy in venous ulcer management is not suggested [31].

6.8. Surgical management

Surgical procedures are often applied when dressings and compression therapies fail in the venous ulcer treatment [76]. There are two approaches in surgical treatment of venous ulcers: ameliorating the cause of the ulcer and treating the ulcer itself by surgical procedures [4].

Superficial venous insufficiency is present in about forty to fifty percent of patients with venous ulcer [2]. Superficial vein surgery, simply comprised of ligation or sclerosis of the long and short saphenous systems, with or without communicating vein ligation or sclerosis, may be useful in patients with superficial venous insufficiency but only when deep veins are competent [120]. Although superficial vein surgery does not affect the success of improvement in venous ulcers, ulcer recurrence has shown to be reduced by the procedure [120]. Subfascial endoscopic perforating vein surgery, a new surgical technique, has proven to be effective in patients with perforator vein insufficiency [8]. In this technique, perforator veins are ligated by an endoscopic camera system through a small incision. This procedure has low complication rates and morbidity [121]. As mentioned above, it has been shown that venous surgery does not seem to improve the healing but delays or reduces the recurrences [76].

Radical excision of the diseased area including the whole ulcer bed, the fibrotic suprafascial tissues, and the abnormal superficial and perforating veins, and flapping this large soft tissue defect have been shown to be successful in a few cases. However, highly invasive character of this procedure limits its application [122].

Skin grafting has proven beneficial to heal large-size recalcitrant ulcers [120]. Contamination with microorganisms and risk of trauma are the main factors that should be kept in mind when grafting for ulcer [123]. Split-thickness skin grafts, punch grafting, and meshed grafts are some of the grafting methods used in venous leg ulcers. While pinched grafts are suitable for small ulcers, meshed grafts are useful for large highly exudative ulcers [4].

6.9. Prevention

In the period that patient has no venous ulcers, it is important to keep in cooperation with and offer some simple lifestyle changes to the patient. Leg elevation is thought to provide venous return, reduce edema, and improve cutaneous circulation [98]. Elevation of the legs above heart level for 30 minutes three or four times a day is a simple and effective method in reducing edema and improving the cutaneous microcirculation in patients with chronic venous insufficiency [87]. Calf muscle pump dysfunction is usually present in venous insufficiency and venous ulcers. Appropriate calf exercise regimes have shown to be useful to improve muscular endurance and may even provide proper functioning of the muscle pump [124]. Even in the first stages of chronic venous disease, starting the effective treatment of symptoms will help for preventing progression to ulcer. The most important step is to persuade the patient, with risk factors or early signs of venous insufficiency, to apply the appropriate compression. It is important to make the patients understand that compression therapy will be a lifelong therapy. The elastic bandages with the appropriate length and strength of compression must be worn daily. Moreover, weight management of obesity, regular exercise programs (with the aim of improving the efficiency of calf muscle pump), and treatment of varicosities (endovenous laser ablation, radiofrequency ablation, and other approaches to repair veins and valves) should be planned. Thrombophilia is increasingly recognized as a major risk factor for DVT, which is the most common identifiable risk factor for the development of chronic venous ulcer. More than 40% of patients with CVU have at least one thrombophilia and chronic venous ulcer patients with post-thrombotic disease are shown to have lower response rates to medical and surgical therapy. Thrombophilia screening is suggested to be performed in patients who have venous ulcer before the age of 50 to stratify the thrombotic risk and start the appropriate prophylactic and therapeutic management. Good nutrition is important in venous ulcer patients as protein deficiency is associated with impaired wound healing. Also smoking affects healing via decreasing the fibroblast proliferation [76]. All these factors together will help to prevent the progression of chronic venous disease to ulceration. Commitment to lifelong exercise programs, weight control, and protection against skin injury is necessary for the prevention of venous leg ulcers [31, 125].

Author details

Aslı Aksu Çerman*, İlknur Kıvanç Altunay and Ezgi Aktaş Karabay

*Address all correspondence to: aksuasli@hotmail.com

Dermatology Department, Sisli Hamidiye Etfal Training and Research Hospital, Istanbul, Turkey

References

[1] Baker SR, Stacey MC, Jopp-McKay AG, et al. Epidemiology of chronic venous ulcers. Br J Surg 1991;78:864–7. doi:10.1002/bjs.1800780729

[2] Nelzen O, Bergquist D, Lindhagen A. Venous and non-venous leg ulcers: clinical history and appearance in a population study. Br J Surg 1994;81:182–7. doi:10.1002/bjs.1800810206

[3] Goldman MP, Fronek A. The Alexander House Group: consensus paper on venous leg ulcer. J Dermatol Surg Oncol 1992;18:592–602. doi:10.1111/j.1524-4725.1992.tb03513.x

[4] Valencia IC, Falabella A, Kirsner R, et al. Chronic venous insufficiency and venous leg ulceration. J Am Acad Dermatol 2001;4:401–21. doi:10.1067/mjd.2001.111633

[5] Callam MJ, Ruckley CV, Harper DR, et al. Chronic ulceration of the leg: extent of the problem and provision of care. Br Med J 1985;290:1855–6.

[6] Callam MJ, Harper DR, Bale JJ, et al. Chronic ulcer of the leg: clinical history. Br Med J 1986;294:1389–91.

[7] Callam MJ. Epidemiology of varicose veins. Br J Surg 1994;81:167–73. doi:10.1002/bjs.1800810204

[8] Etufugh CN, Phillips TJ. Venous ulcers. Clin Dermatol 2007;25:121–30. doi:10.1016/j.clindermatol.2006.09.004

[9] Bergqvist D, Lindholm C, Nelzen O. Chronic leg ulcers: the impact of venous disease. J Vasc Surg 1999;29:752–5. doi:10.1016/S0741-5214(99)70330-7

[10] Ruckley C. Socioeconomic impact of chronic venous insufficiency and leg ulcers. Angiology 1997;46:67–9. doi:10.1177/000331979704800111

[11] Lazarus GS, Cooper DM, Knighton DR, et al. Definitions and guidelines for assessment of wounds and evaluation of healing. Arch Dermatol 1994;130:489–93. doi:10.1001/archderm.1994.01690040093015

[12] Abbade L, Lastoria S. Venous ulcer, epidemiology, physiopathology, diagnosis and treatment. Int J Dermatol 2005;44:449–56. doi:10.1111/j.1365-4632.2004.02456.x

[13] Scott TE, Lamarte WW, Gorin DR, et al. Risk factors for chronic venous insufficiency: a dual case control study. J Vasc Surg 1995;24:703–10. doi:10.1016/S0741-5214(95)70050-1

[14] Alguire PC, Mathes BM. Chronic venous insufficiency and venous ulceration. J Gen Intern Med 1997;12:374–83. doi:10.1046/j.1525-1497.1997.00063.x

[15] Meissner MH. Lower extremity venous anatomy. Semin Intervent Radiol 2005;22:147–56. doi:10.1055/s-2005-921948

[16] Gonsalves CF. Venous leg ulcers. Tech Vasc Interv Radiol 2003;6:132–6. doi:10.1053/S1089-2516(03)00055 6

[17] Browse NL, Burnand KG. The cause of venous ulceration. Lancet 1882;2:243–5. doi:10.1016/S0140-6736(82)90325-7

[18] Falanga V, Kirsner R, Katz MH, et al. Pericapillary fibrin cuffs in venous ulceration: Persistence with treatment and during ulcer healing. J Dermatol Surg Oncol 1992;18:409–13. doi:10.1111/j.1524-4725.1992.tb03694.x

[19] Burnand KG, Whimster I, Naidoo A, et al. Pericapillary fibrin in the ulcer-bearing skin of the lower leg: the cause of lipodermatosclerosis and venous ulceration. Br Med J (Clin Res Ed) 1982;285:1071–2.

[20] Falanga V, Bontempo FA, Eaglstein WH. Protein C and protein S plasma levels in patients with lipodermatosclerosis and venous ulceration. Arch Dermatol 1990;126:1195–7. doi:10.1001/archderm.1990.01670330075010

[21] Falanga V, Kruskal J, Franks JJ. Fibrin and fibrinogen-related antigens in patients with lipodermatosclerosis and venous ulceration. Arch Dermatol 1991;127:75–8.

[22] Paye M, Nusgens BV, Lapiere CM. Factor XIII of blood coagulation modulates collagen biosynthesis by fibroblasts in vitro. Haemostasis 1989;19:274–83.

[23] Dormandy JA, Nash A. Importance of red cell aggregation in venous pathology. Clin Hemorheol 1987;7:119–22.

[24] Thomas PR, Nash Gb, Dormandy JA. White cell accumulation in dependent legs of patients with venous hypertension: a possible mechanism for trophic changes in the skin. Br Med J (Clin Res Ed) 1988;296:1693–5.

[25] Dormandy JA. Pathophysiology of venous ulceration—an update. Angiology 1997;48:71–5. doi:10.1177/000331979704800112

[26] Falanga V, Eaglstein WH. The trap hypothesis of venous ulceration. Lancet 1993;341:1006–8.

[27] Higley HR, Ksander GA, Gerhardt CO, et al. Extravasation of macromolecules and possible trapping of transforming growth factor-β in venous ulceration. Br J Dermatol 1995;132:79–85. doi:10.1111/j.1365-2133.1995.tb08629.x

[28] Maessen-Visch MB, Koedam MI, Hamulyak K, et al. Atrophie blanche. Int J Dermatol 1999;38:161–72. doi:10.1046/j.1365-4362.1999.00581.x

[29] Kirsner RS, Pardes JB, Eaglstein WH, et al. The clinical spectrum of lipodermatosclerosis. J Am Acad Dermatol 1993;28:623–7.

[30] Baldursson B, Sigurgeirsson B, Lindelof B. Venous leg ulcers and squamous cell carcinoma: a large scale epidemiological study. Br J Dermatol 1995;133:571–4. doi: 10.1111/j.1365-2133.1995.tb02707.x

[31] O'Donnell TF Jr, Passman MA, Marston WA, et al. Management of venous leg ulcers: clinical practice guidelines of the Society for Vascular Surgery®and the American Venous Forum. J Vasc Surg 2014;60:3S–59S. doi:10.1016/j.jvs.2014.04.049

[32] McMullin GM, Smith C. An evaluation of Doppler ultrasound and photoplethysmography in the investigation of venous insufficiency. Aust N Z J Surg 1992;62:270–5. doi: 10.1111/j.1445-2197.1992.tb07554.x

[33] Sarin S, Sommerville K, Farrah J, et al. Duplex ultrasonography for assessment of venous valvular function of the lower limb. Br J Surg 1994;81:1591–5. doi:10.1002/bjs. 1800811108

[34] Criado E, Farber MA, Marston WA, et al. The role of air plethysmography in the diagnosis of chronic venous insufficiency. J Vasc Surg 1998;27:660–70. doi:10.1016/ S0741-5214(98)70231-9

[35] Lurie F, Rooke TW. Evaluation of venous function by indirect noninvasive testing (plethysmography). In: Gloviczki P, editor. Handbook of venous disorders: Guidelines of the American Venous Forum. 3rd ed. London: Hodder Arnold; 2009. p. 156–9. doi: 10.1201/b13654-17

[36] Barnes RW. Noninvasive diagnostic assessment of peripheral vascular disease. Circulation 1991;83:120–7.

[37] Porter JM, Moneta GL. International Consensus Committee on Chronic Venous Disease. Reporting standards in venous disease: an update. J Vasc Surg 1995;21:635–45.

[38] Eklöf B, Rutherford RB, Bergan JJ, et al. Revision of the CEAP classification for chronic venous disorders. Consensus statement. J Vasc Surg 2004;40:1248–52. doi:10.1016/j.jvs. 2004.09.027

[39] Marston WA, Vasquez MA, Lurie F, et al. Multicenter assessment of the repeatability and reproducibility of the revised venous clinical severity score (rVCSS). J Vasc Surg Venous Lymphat Disord 2013;1:219–24. doi:10.1016/j.jvsv.2012.10.059

[40] Falanga V. Venous ulceration: assessment, classification and management. In: Krasner D, Kane D, editors. Chronic wound care. 2nd ed. Wayne (PA): Health Management Publications; 1997. p. 165–71.

[41] Dissemond J, Körber A, Grabbe S. Differential diagnoses in leg ulcers. J Dtsch Dermatol Ges 2006;4:627–34. doi:10.1111/j.1610-0387.2006.06052.x

[42] Meyer V, Kerk N, Meyer S, et al. Differential diagnosis and therapy of leg ulcers. J Dtsch Dermatol Ges 2011;9:1035–51. doi:10.1111/j.1610-0387.2011.07814.x

[43] Kirsner RS, Vivas AC. Lower-extremity ulcers: diagnosis and management. Br J Dermatol 2015;173:379–90. doi:10.1111/bjd.13953

[44] Fukaya E, Margolis DJ. Approach to diagnosing lower extremity ulcers. Dermatol Therap 2013;26:181–6. doi:10.1111/dth.12054

[45] Goslen JB. Autoimmune ulceration of the leg. Clin Dermatol 1990;3:92–117. doi: 10.1016/0738-081X(90)90050-B

[46] Dabiri G, Falanga V. Connective tissue ulcers. J Tissue Viability 2013;22:92–102. doi: 10.1016/j.jtv.2013.04.003

[47] Oien RF, Hakansson A, Hansen BU. Leg ulcers in patients with rheumatoid arthritis—
      a prospective study of aeitology, wound healing, and pain reduction after pinch
      grafting. Rheumatology (Oxford) 2001;40:816–20. doi:10.1093/rheumatology/40.7.816

[48] Hafner J, Schneider E, Burg G, et al. Management of leg ulcers with rheumatoid arthritis
      or systemic sclerosis: the importance of concomitant arterial and venous disease. J Vasc
      Surg 2000;32:322–9. doi:10.1067/mva.2000.106942

[49] Shanmugam VK, Price P, Attinger CE, et al. Lower extremity ulcers in systemic sclerosis:
      features and response to therapy. Int J Rheumatol 2010:8, article ID 747946, doi:
      10.1155/2010/747946

[50] Reddy V, Dziadzio M, Hamdulay S, et al. Lupus and leg ulcers—a diagnostic quandary.
      Clin Rheumatol 2007;26:1173–5. doi:10.1007/s10067-006-0306-2

[51] Chapnick SL, Merkel PA. Skin ulcers in a patient with Sjögren's syndrome. Arthritis
      Care Res (Hoboken) 2010;62:1040–6. doi:10.1002/acr.20181

[52] Yamamura K, Takahara M, Masunaga K, et al. Subcutaneous calcification of the lower
      legs in a patient with mixed connective tissue disease. J Dermatol 2011;38:791–3. doi:
      10.1111/j.1346-8138.2010.01177.x

[53] Rozin AP, Braun-Moscovici Y, Bergman R, et al. Recalcitrant leg ulcer due to mixed
      connective tissue disease. J Med 2006;64:91–4.

[54] Mekkes JR, Loots MAM, Van Der Wal AC, et al. Causes, investigation and treatment of
      leg ulceration. Br J Dermatol 2003;148:388–401. doi:10.1046/j.1365-2133.2003.05222.x

[55] Harris RJ, Cropley TG. Possible role of hypercoagulability in calciphylaxis: review of
      the literature. J Am Acad Dermatol 2011;64:405–12. doi:10.1016/j.jaad.2009.12.007

[56] Alguire PC, Mathes BM. Chronic venous insufficiency and venous ulceration. J Gen
      Intern Med 1997;12:374–83. doi:10.1046/j.1525-1497.1997.00063.x

[57] Philips TJ, Dover JS. Leg ulcers. J Am Acad Dermatol 1991;25:965–87.

[58] Abu-Own A, Scurr JH, Coleridge Smith PD. Effect of leg elevation on the skin micro-
      circulation in chronic venous insufficiency. J Vasc Surg 1994;20:705–10.

[59] Cranley JJ, Krause RJ, Strasser ES. Chronic venous insufficiency of the lower extremity.
      Surgery 1961;49:48–58.

[60] Falabella AF. Debridement and management of exudative wounds. Dermatol Ther
      1999;9:36–43.

[61] Alvarez O, Rozint J, Wiseman D. Moist environment for healing: matching the dressing
      to the wound. Wounds 1989;1:35–51.

[62] Freidman S, Su WPD. Hydrocolloid occlusive dressing management of leg ulcers. Arch
      Dermatol 1984;120:1329–31.

[63] Phillips TJ. Successful methods of treating leg ulcers: the tried and true, plus the novel and new. Postgrad Med 1999;105:159–79.

[64] Durham DR, Fortney DZ, Nanney LB. Preliminary evaluation of vibriolysin, a novel proteolytic enzyme composition suitable for the debridement of burn wound eschar. J Burn Care Rehabil 1993;14:544–51.

[65] Falanga V. Occlusive wound dressings: why, when, which? Arch Dermatol 1988;124:544–51.

[66] Sinclair RD, Ryan TJ. Proteolytic enzymes in wound healing: the role of enzymtic debridement. Australas J Dermatol 1994;35:35–41. doi:10.1111/j.1440-0960.1994.tb01799.x

[67] Berger MM. Enzymatic debriding preparations. Ostomy Wound Management 1989;39:61–9.

[68] Falanga V, Carson P, Greenberg A, et al. Topically applied tPA for the treatment of venous ulcers. Dermatol Surg 1996;22:643–4. doi:10.1111/j.1524-4725.1996.tb00611.x

[69] Falanga V. Wound bed preparation and the role of enzymes: a case for multiple actions of the therapeutic agents. Wounds 2002;14:47–57.

[70] Mosher BA, Cuddigan J, Thomas DR, et al. Outcomes of 4 methods of debridement using a decision analysis methodology. Adv Wound Care 1999;12:81–8.

[71] Kennedy KL, Tritch DL. Debridement. In: Krasner D, Kane E, editors. Chronic wound care. 2nd ed. Wayne (PA): Health Management Publications; 1997. p. 227–34.

[72] Donati L, Magliano E, Colonna M, et al. Surgical versus enzymatic debridement. In: Westerhof W, Vanscheidt W, editors. Proteolytic enzymes and wound healing. New York: SpringerVerlag; 1994. p. 38–9. doi:10.1007/978-3-642-78891-8_4

[73] Dunn RM, Fudem GM, Walton RL, et al. Free flap valvular transplantation for refractory venous ulceration. J Vasc Surg 1994;19:525–31.

[74] Weinzweig N, Schuler J. Free tissue transfer in treatment of the recalcitrant chronic venous ulcer. Ann Plast Surg 1997;38:611–9.

[75] Falanga V. Overview of chronic wounds and recent advances. Dermatol Ther 1999;9:7–17.

[76] Tang JC, Marston WA, Kirsner RS. Wound Healing Society (WHS) venous ulcer treatment guidelines: what's new in five years? Wound Rep Reg 2012;20:619–37. doi: 10.1111/j.1524-475X.2012.00815.x

[77] Gilchrist B, on behalf of the European Tissue Repair Society. Should iodine be reconsidered in wound management? A report of a consensus meeting on the use of iodine in wound care. J Wound Care 1997;6:148–50.

[78] Maessen-Visch MB, van Montfrans C. Wound dressings, does it matter and why? Phlebology 2016;31:63–7. doi:10.1177/0268355516633383

[79] Boateng J, Catanzano O. Advanced therapeutic dressings for effective wound healing- a review. J Pharm Sciences 2015;104:3653–80.

[80] Heyer K, Augustin M, Protz K, et al. Effectiveness of advanced versus conventional wound dressings on healing of chronic wounds: systematic review and meta-analysis. Dermatology 2013;226:172–84. doi:10.1159/000348331

[81] Gottrup F, Apelqvist J, Price P. Outcomes in controlled and comparative studies on non-healing wounds: recommendations to improve the quality of evidence in wound management. J Woundcare 2010;19:239–68. doi:10.12968/jowc. 2010.19.6.48471

[82] Erickson CA, Lanza DJ, Karp DL, et al. Healing of venous ulcers in an ambulatory care program: the role of chronic venous insufficiency and patient compliance. J Vasc Surg 1995;22:629–36. doi:10.1016/S0741-5214(95)70051-X

[83] Partsch H. Compression therapy of the legs: a review. J Dermatol Surg Oncol 1991;17:799–808.

[84] Van de Scheur M, Falanga V. Pericapillary fibrin cuffs in venous disease. J Dermatol Surg Oncol 1997;23:955–9. doi:10.1111/j.1524-4725.1997.tb00759.x

[85] Stemmer R, Marescaux J, Furderer C. Compression treatment of the lower extremities, particularly with compression stockings. Dermatologist 1980;31:355–65.

[86] Dickey WJ Jr. Stasis ulcers: the role of compliance in healing. South Med J 1991;84:557–61.

[87] Alguire PC, Mathes BM. Chronic venous insufficiency and venous ulceration. J Gen Intern Med 1997;12:374–83. doi:10.1046/j.1525-1497.1997.00063.x

[88] Moffatt C, Kommala D, Dourdin N, et al. Venous leg ulcers: patient concordance with compression therapy and its impact on healing and prevention of recurrence. Int Wound J 2009;6:386–93. doi:10.1111/j.1742-481X.2009.00634.x

[89] Falanga V, Sabolinski M. A bilayered skin construct (Apligraf) accelerates complete closure of hard-to-heal venous ulcers. Wound Rep Reg 1999;7:201–7.

[90] Bertocchi F, Proserpio P, Lampugnai MG, et al. The effect of pentoxifylline on poly-morphonuclear cell adhesion to cultured endothelial cells. In: Mandell GL, Novicl WJ, editors. Pentoxifylline and leukocyte function. Sommerville (NJ): Hoechst Roussel Pharmaceuticals; 1988. p. 68–74.

[91] Zabel P, Wolter DT, Schonharting MM, et al. Oxpentifylline in endotoxaemia. Lancet 1998;2:1474–7. doi:10.1016/S0140-6736(89)92929-2

[92] Falanga V, For the Trental Collaborative Group: Pentoxifylline (Trental) accelerates the healing of venous ulcers in a double blind randomised study. In: Proceedings from the European Tissue Repair Society, Cologne, Germany, Aug 25, 1997.

[93] Jull AB, Arroll B, Parag V, et al. Pentoxifylline for treating venous leg ulcers. Cochrane Database Syst Rev 2012;12:CD001733. doi:10.1002/14651858.CD001733.pub3

[94] de Oliveira Carvalho P, Magolbo NG, De Aquino RF, et al. Oral aspirin for venous leg ulcers. Cochrane Database Syst Rev 2016 Feb 18;2:CD009432. doi: 10.1002/14651858.CD009432.pub2

[95] Cyrus T, Sung S, Zhao L, et al. Effect of low-dose aspirin on vascular inflammation, plaque stability, and atherogenesis in low-density lipoprotein receptor-deficient mice. Circulation 2002;106:1282–7. doi:10.1161/01.CIR.0000027816.54430.96

[96] Serra R, Rizzuto A, Rossi A, et al. Skin grafting for the treatment of chronic leg ulcers—a systematic review in evidence-based medicine. Int Wound J 2016 Mar 4. doi:10.1111/iwj.12575.

[97] Serra R, Buffone G, De Franciscis A, et al. Skin grafting followed by low-molecular-weight heparin long-term therapy in chronic venous leg ulcers. Ann Vasc Surg 2012;26:190–7. doi:10.1016/j.avsg.2011.04.008

[98] Richmond NA, Maderal AD, Vivas AC. Evidence-based management of common chronic lower extremity ulcers. Dermatol Ther 2013;26:187–96. doi:10.1111/dth.12051

[99] Dumville JC, Land L, Evans D, et al. Negative pressure wound therapy for treating leg ulcers. Cochrane Database Syst Rev 2015 Jul 14;7:CD011354. doi: 10.1002/14651858.CD011354.pub2

[100] Mostow EN, Haraway GD, Dalsing M, et al. OASIS Venus Ulcer Study Group. Effectiveness of an extracellular matrix graft (OASIS Wound Matrix) in the treatment of chronic leg ulcers: a randomized clinical trial. J Vasc Surg 2005;41:837–43.

[101] Ehrenreich M, Ruszczak Z. Update on tissue-engineered biological dressings. Tissue Eng 2006;12:2407–24. doi:10.1089/ten.2006.12.2407

[102] Cavorsi J, Vicari F, Wirthlin DJ, et al. Best-practice algorithms for the use of a bilayered living cell therapy (Apligraf) in the treatment of lower-extremity ulcers. Wound Repair Regen 2006;14:102–9. doi:10.1111/j.1743-6109.2006.00098.x

[103] Fivenson D, Scherschun L. Clinical and economic impact of Apligraf for the treatment of nonhealing venous leg ulcers. Int J Dermatol 2003;42:960–5. doi:10.1111/j.1365-4632.2003.02039.x

[104] Purdue GF. Dermagraft-tc pivotal efficacy and safety study. J Burn Care Rehabil 1997;18:13–4.

[105] Marston WA. Dermagraft, a bioengineered human dermal equivalent for the treatment of chronic nonhealing diabetic foot ulcer. Expert Rev Med Devices 2004;1:21–31. doi: 10.1586/17434440.1.1.21

[106] Marston WA, Hanft J, Norwood P, et al. The efficacy and safety of dermagraft in improving the healing of chronic diabetic foot ulcers: results of a prospective randomized trial. Diabetes Care 2003;26:1701–5. doi:10.2337/diacare.26.6.1701

[107] Hart CE, Loewen-Rodriguez A, Lessem J. Dermagraft: use in the treatment of chronic wounds. Adv Wound Care 2011;1:138–41. doi:10.1089/wound.2011.0282

[108] Lazic T, Falanga V. Bioengineered skin constructs and their use in wound healing. Plast Reconstr Surg 2011;127:75–90. doi:10.1097/PRS.0b013e3182009d9f

[109] Carter MJ, Waycaster C, Schaum K, et al. Cost-effectiveness of three adjunct cellular/tissue-derived products used in the management of chronic venous leg ulcers. Value Health 2014;17:801–13. doi:10.1016/j.jval.2014.08.001

[110] Hankin CS, Knispel J, Lopes M, et al. Clinical and cost efficacy of advanced wound care matrices for venous ulcers. J Manag Care Pharm 2012;18:375–84.

[111] Da Costa RM, Ribeiro Jesus FM, Aniceto C, et al. Randomized, double-blind, placebo-controlled, dose-ranging study of granulocyte-macrophage colony stimulating factor in patients with chronic venous leg ulcers. Wound Repair Regen 1999;7:17–25.

[112] Demling RH, Niezgoda JA, Haraway GD, et al. Small intestinal submucosa wound matrix and full-thickness venous ulcers: preliminary results. Wounds 2004;16:18–22.

[113] Hill OR. Ultrasound biophysics: a perspective. Br J Cancer 1982;82:46–51.

[114] Moffatt C, Martin R, Smithdale R. Leg ulcer management. Oxford: Blackwell Publishing Ltd.; 2007.

[115] Cameron MH. Thermal agents: cold and heat, ultrasound, and electrical currents. In: Cameron MH, editor. Physical agents in rehabilitation: from research to practice. St. Louis: WB Saunders; 2003, 2nd ed., p. 133–259.

[116] Busse JW, Bhandari M, Kulkarni AV, et al. The effect of low-intensity pulsed ultrasound therapy on time to fracture healing: a meta-analysis. CMAJ 2002;166:437–41.

[117] Ernst E. Ultrasound for cutaneous wound healing. Phlebology 1995;10:2–4.

[118] Unger PG. Low-frequency, noncontact, nonthermal ultrasound therapy: a review of the literature. Ostomy Wound Manage 2008;54:57–60.

[119] Beheshti A, Shafigh Y, Parsa H, et al. Comparison of high-frequency and MIST ultrasound therapy for the healing of venous leg ulcers. Adv Clin Exp Med 2014;23:969–75. doi:10.17219/acem/37353

[120] Douglas WS, Simpson NB. Guidelines for the management of chronic venous leg ulceration: report of a multidisciplinary workshop. Br J Dermatol 1995;132:446–52. doi: 10.1111/j.1365-2133.1995.tb08681.x

[121] Chong C. Subfascial endoscopic perforating vein surgery (SEPS) for the treatment of venous ulcers. Ostomy Wound Manage 2005;51:26–31.

[122] Weinzweig N, Schuler J. Free tissue transfer in treatment of the recalcitrant chronic venous ulcer. Ann Plast Surg 1997;38:611–9.

[123] Skouge JW. Techniques for split-thickness skin grafting. J Dermatol Surg Oncol 1987;13:841–9.

[124] Padberg FT, Johnston MV, Sisto SA. Structured exercise improves calf muscle pump function in chronic venous insufficiency: a randomized trial. J Vasc Surg 2004;39:79–87.

[125] Kelechi TJ, Johnson JJ. Chronic venous disease and venous leg ulcers: an evidence-based update. J Vasc Nurs 2015;33:36–46. doi:10.1016/j.jvn.2015.01.003

10

The Use of Amniotic Membrane in the Management of Complex Chronic Wounds

Gregorio Castellanos, Ángel Bernabé-García,

Carmen García Insausti, Antonio Piñero,

José M. Moraleda and Francisco J. Nicolás

Abstract

Chronic wounds do not follow the usual wound healing process; instead, they are stuck in the inflammatory or proliferative phase. This is particularly evident in large, massive wounds with considerable tissue loss, which become senescent and do not epithelialize. In these wounds, we need to remove all the factors that prevent or delay normal wound healing. After that, soft tissue granulation is stimulated by local negative pressure therapy. Lastly, after the granulation is completed, the epithelialization process must be activated. Although a plethora of wound dressings and devices are available, chronic wounds persist as a unresolved medical concern. We have been using frozen amniotic membrane (AM) to treat this type of wounds with good results. Our studies have shown that AM is able to induce epithelialization in large wounds that were unable to epithelialize. AM induces several signaling pathways involved in cell migration and/or proliferation. Among those, we can highlight the mitogen-activated protein kinase (MAPK) and Jun N-terminal kinase (JNK) signaling pathways. Additionally, AM is able to selectively antagonise the anti-proliferative effect of TGFß by modifying its genetic program on keratinocytes. The combined effect of AM on keratinocytes, promoting cell proliferation/migration and antagonising TGFß-effect, is the perfect combination allowing chronic wounds to progress into epithelialization.

Keywords: soft-tissue chronic wounds, amniotic membrane, TGF-β, epithelialization

1. Introduction

The evolution of knowledge about the biology of wound healing makes it possible to predict the sequence and prognosis of the events that occur in this complex process. However, there are wounds in which healing can be either prolonged over time or not fully achieved [1, 2].

Therefore, The keys to providing adequate and efficient treatment involve identifying, as soon as possible, the combination of either internal or external factors that contribute to the complexity of the wound and affect the healing process, and to detect at an early stage when it is likely that a wound would be slow or difficult to heal.

The actions undertaken should be aimed at reducing the aspects that lead to complexity, including factors related to the patient, the wound, relationships with healthcare personnel, and available resources. Only by assessing and understanding the interaction between these factors and their effect on healing will it be possible to develop efficient and appropriate strategies for improving results. Similarly, certain characteristics of the wound, such as its anatomical location, time duration, size, depth, and the state of the wound bed, are correlated with adequate healing [3–5].

The presence of necrotic tissue, crusts, slough, or foreign bodies in the wound bed, which are all obstacles for wound assessment, can lead to a delay in healing, and they can also be a focus of infection. Therefore, it is important to provide frequent, extensive, and efficient debridement until healthy tissue is found [6]. There are other situations that can have an influence and cause healing to fail, such as ischemia. Poor perfusion deprives tissue of an efficient oxygen and metabolic exchange, and causes an increase in vascular permeability, leukocyte retention, synthesis and the liberation of oxygen free radicals and proteolytic enzymes [7]. Inflammation in chronic wounds brings about a prolongation in healing time, resulting in an exacerbated inflammatory reaction, which in turn causes the hyperproduction of pro-inflammatory cytokines and proteolytic enzymes. This activity is combined with a decrease in the secretion of metalloproteinase tissue inhibitors, and it intensifies as the wound bed pH alters. As a consequence, we find that in the wound bed there is a sustained inflammation with matrix degradation, a limited bioavailability of growth factors and intense fibroblast aging, all of which reduce tissue repair, cell proliferation, and angiogenesis [8, 9].

In the same way, chronic wounds are characterized by the presence of one or more bacterial strains, with antibiotic-resistant microorganisms, and the presence of biofilms within which the bacteria are protected against the action of the silver-based antimicrobials [10–13].

The initial response to treatment is indicative of the viability of the tissue and its capacity to heal. When a patient's wound does not heal in the planned period of time using conventional treatment, it is essential to reassess the patient and modify the therapeutic guidelines [14, 15].

Thus, tissue wound healing usually follows a predictable sequence, although in some cases, it is prolonged over time or it is never achieved. The wound healing process is the result of a complex interaction between the patient and wound factors, the treatment adopted, and the skills and knowledge of healthcare professionals. Only by carrying out a detailed initial assessment and repeated treatment assessment will it be possible to identify the factors that contribute to the complexity of the wound and to assess its potential state. The challenge for professionals is to utilize the most efficient therapeutic strategies at the right time and in the most cost-effective way, in order to reduce the complex nature of wounds, to treat the symptoms, and whenever possible, to achieve wound healing.

2. How should chronic and complex soft-tissue wounds be managed?

2.1. Management and treatment strategies

Chronic and complex soft-tissue wounds usually involve difficult healing, which means that they require an appropriate management-treatment strategy using a comprehensive and dynamic approach, applying new therapies to confront this old problem: wound healing [16]. In order to carry out this comprehensive approach, we should take into account the complex nature of the wound and its healing, its relationship with psychosocial factors and delays in wound healing, together with the economic cost for the patient, family, community, and the healthcare system. The steps to follow in order to achieve this approach should take into account the complete assessment of the patient, the control of causal factors, general healthcare, and the preparation of the wound bed.

2.2. Preparation of the wound bed

The preparation of the wound bed is an essential and dynamic process that provides an appropriate framework for a structured approach to wound management. This notion stresses a comprehensive and systematic approach with the aim of assessing and eliminating barriers to the normal wound healing process. It develops the appropriate treatment strategies to be directed at the patient in general and for treating the underlying condition causing the wound. Its objective is to create an optimum healing setting, a well-vascularized wound, with a stable and balanced bed in terms of exudate production, aimed at reducing scar healing time and facilitating the efficiency of other therapeutic measures. The wound bed should be prepared in each phase of the wound healing process following an agreed-upon procedure.

The "Tissue, Inflammation-infection, Moisture, Edge" (T.I.M.E.) scheme, proposed by the European Wound Management Association (EWMA), is based on the research of the International Wound Bed Preparation Advisory Board (IWBPAB), which established an algorithm through the development of the acronym T.I.M.E., whose objective is to describe the characteristics of chronic wounds during wound bed preparation. Following on from this, the concept was updated by placing emphasis on the treatment of the cause of the wound and general patient factors during treatment, before dealing with local wound factors. This algorithm consists of four components that cover the different physiopathological alterations present in chronic wounds: the management and conditioning of non-viable tissue, the monitoring of inflammation and infection, the disequilibrium of moisture due to excess exudate, and the stimulation and progression of the wound edges. So we can see that the T.I.M.E. framework involves the overall strategies that can be applied to the management of different kinds of wound with the aim of maximizing the ability to heal wounds [16–18] (**Figure 1**).

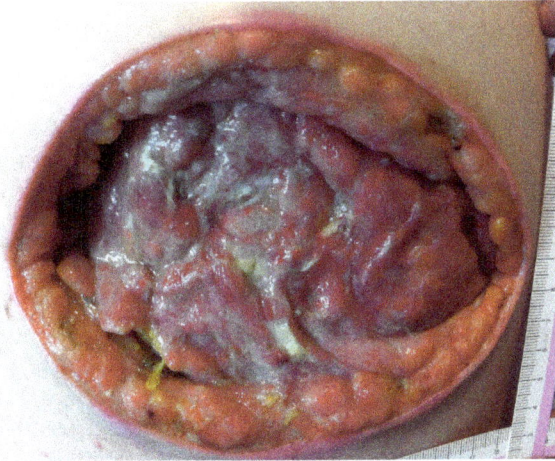

Figure 1. Complex and traumatic soft-tissue wound. Management and treatment of wound bed.

Wound treatment is initiated with a hydrodynamic washing using 0.9% saline solution at room temperature, with a 1–4 kg/cm effective washing pressure, without any damage being caused (a 20-ml syringe, with a 0.9-mm-diameter catheter), and the surrounding area is washed with a soapy antiseptic solution consisting of chlorhexidine digluconate.

For the monitoring of the non-viable tissues (necrotic tissue, crust, slough, and foreign bodies), episodic or continuous debridement is carried out until healthy tissue is found. It can be surgical, using tangential hydrodissection (Versajet™Plus, Smith & Nephew, London, United Kingdom); enzymatic, applying exogenous enzymes locally (collagenase, fibrolysine, trypsin, or chymotrypsin); chemical (cadexomer iodine); autolytic (due to the conjunction of three factors: hydration of the bed, fibrinolysis and the action of the endogenous enzymes on the devitalized tissue); or osmotic (hyperosmotic solutions). On occasions, an instillation therapy can also be used (VeraFlo™, KCI, Acelity LPI, San Antonio, TX) either in deep wounds with a viscous exudate or in uncontrolled infections on prosthetic materials, in order to eliminate the biofilm, reduce the pain, and reactivate healing. A noninvasive treatment option, for the debridement of chronic wounds, is low-frequency guided ultrasound [3].

In the management of the bacterial load (a contaminated or colonized lesion, with critical or infected colonization), foci of local and/or systemic infection have to be removed, which is why it is necessary to clean and debride the wound; take a wound culture; monitor the wound proteases; and use topical antimicrobials (silver, cadexomer iodine), systemic antibiotics according to the antibiogram data, anti-inflammatory drugs, and protease inhibitors if required.

It is important to monitor the exudate and achieve the equilibrium in the moisture, given that a dry wound makes it difficult for cell migration and exudate encourages infection and macerates the perilesional skin area. We should be aware that scarring is faster with wounds in an optimally moist environment in which the physiological and atmospheric conditions of the wound bed are maintained, thus fostering basal keratinocyte migration. A moist environment also prevents cell desiccation, encourages cell migration, promotes angiogenesis, stimulates collagen synthesis, and facilitates intercellular communication. A moist wound environment preserves a slightly acid pH and a low oxygen tension on the surface of the wound [18–20].

Thus, the edges of the wound do not advance because there are keratinocytes that do not migrate, senescent cells, and alterations in the extracellular matrix secondary to the disequilibrium in protease activity.

2.3. Clinical protocols

The preparation of the wound bed requires specific management protocols, which can be grouped into three sections following the T.I.M.E. procedure:

- Nonsurgical debridement with moisture monitoring and dressing every 48 h (**Table 1**).

- Local infection with moisture monitoring and dressing every 72 h (**Table 2**).

- A granulation phase with moisture monitoring and dressing every 72 h (**Table 3**).

Protocol 1: (T/M= Tissue and moisture)
-Non-viable tissue and moisture monitoring
-Non-surgical debridement
-Dressing every 48 h

-Type of wound	-Necrotic tissue -Low exudate	-Sloughy tissue -Moderate exudate	-Infected sloughy tissue -High exudate
-Debridement	-Collagenase + hydrogel	-Collagenase	-Cadexomer iodine + alginate
-Moist dressing	-Hydrocellular with acrylic adhesive or silicone adhesive	-Hydrocellular with acrylic adhesive or silicone adhesive	-Hydrocellular with acrylic adhesive or silicone adhesive

Table 1. Preparing the wound bed: management protocol (T/M).

Protocol 2: (I/M = Infection and moisture)
-Infection and moisture monitoring
-Wounds with local infection
-Dressing every 72 h

-Type of wound	-Infection -Low exudate	-Infection -Moderate exudate	-Infection -High exudate
-Decrease in bacterial load	-Nanocrystalline silver or -Silver-impregnated activated carbon+ hydrogel	-Nanocrystalline silver or -Silver-impregnated activated carbon	-Nanocrystalline silver or -Silver-impregnated activated carbon + alginate
-Moist dressing	-Hydrocellular with acrylic adhesive or silicone adhesive	-Hydrocellular with acrylic adhesive or silicone adhesive	-Hydrocellular with acrylic adhesive or silicone adhesive

Table 2. Preparing the wound bed: management protocol (I/M).

Protocol 3: (E/M = Edges and moisture)

-Epithelialization of edges and moisture monitoring

-Wounds in the granulation phase

-Dressing every 72 h

-Type of wound	-Granulation tissue	-Granulation tissue
	-Low or moderate exudate	-High exudate
-Granulation	-Collagen with silver protease modulator matrix or -Powder collagen	-Collagen with silver protease modulator matrix or -Powder collagen + alginate
-Moist dressing	-Hydrocellular with acrylic adhesive or silicone adhesive	-Hydrocellular with acrylic adhesive or silicone adhesive

Table 3. Preparing the wound bed: management protocol (E/M).

After finalizing the preparation of the wound bed, the wound remains open ready for its closure by secondary intention with granulation tissue and the re-establishment of the epidermis. At this point, the surgeon comes across two new problems: how to granulate the wound, and afterwards, how to epithelialize it.

2.4. Wound granulation using negative topical pressure therapy

For the granulation, we use a noninvasive topical negative pressure wound therapy (NPWT) (**Figure 2**), using aspirated drainage to eliminate the secretions, facilitate the closure and prevent complications. Its scientific fundamentals and physiopathology are based on the application of mechanical stress on the tissues, by creating a negative pressure on the surface of the wound [21]. The effect of the macrotension on the tissues is carried out using a sponge dressing (polyurethane-polyvinyl alcohol), with open pores, that contract under the negative pressure, bringing the edges closer together [22], eliminating the exudate, the non-viable tissue, and the soluble wound healing inhibitors (cytokines and matrix metalloproteinases) [23]. Other effects are a reduction in the edema, an increase in neutrophils and monocytes on the bacterial load and an improvement in local perfusion [24]. The effect of microtension, at the cell level, triggers cell stretching, which increases fibroblasts, the formation and division of new cells and the rapid growth of granulation tissue [25], the migration of fibroblasts to the area of the wound (displacing new cells to its surface), the formation of new blood vessels [26], and the formation of granulation tissue through mitosis stimulation. In this way, moist healing of the wound helps wound debridement (**Figure 3**).

The NPWT is contraindicated when either the wound has not been well explored, it has necrotic tissue with eschar or it has weakened blood vessels due to irradiation or suture. Also, NPWT is contraindicated in case of intestinal anastomosis, exposed nerves, the presence of tumors or untreated osteomyelitis. Equally, it is not advisable for either enterocutaneous or enteroatmospheric fistulas. Finally, active bleeding wounds and/or patients treated with anticoagulants are not suitable for NPWT treatment.

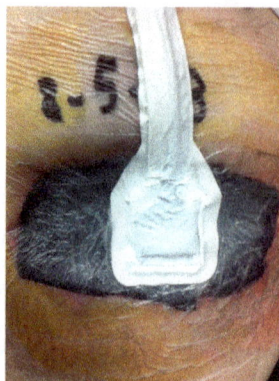

Figure 2. Complex and traumatic soft-tissue wound. Treatment with TNP therapy.

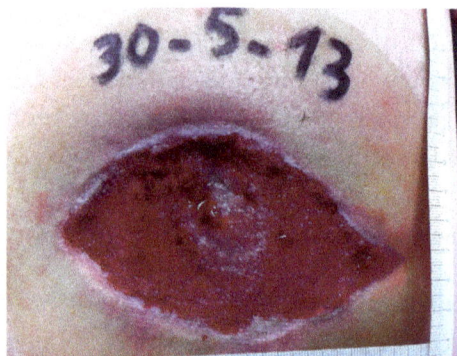

Figure 3. Complex and traumatic soft-tissue wound. Completed granulation after TNP therapy.

2.5. Epithelialization of the chronic and complex soft-tissue wounds

A large variety of wound coverings and procedures have become available over the past two decades, including several types of synthetic dressings and allo-skin or auto-skin substitutes, although their cost is too high for routine clinical practice [27, 28]. New technologies involving growth factors and bioengineered tissues are relatively new and have produced relatively good results; however, they are quite expensive.

2.6. Amniotic membrane and wound healing

Amniotic membrane (AM), the innermost layer of the placenta, has a fetal origin and can easily be separated from the placenta by blunt dissection. AM, due to its special structure, biological properties and immunological characteristics, is a tissue of particular interest as a biological dressing. AM exhibits low immunogenicity and well-documented reepithelialization effects. Moreover, AM shows anti-inflammatory, antifibrotic, antimicrobial, analgesic and nontumori-genic properties. This diversity of its effects is related to its capacity to synthesize and release biologically active molecules including cytokines and signaling factors such as tumor necrosis factor (TNF)-α, transforming growth factor (TGF)-α, TGF-β, basic fibroblast growth factor (b-FGF), epidermal growth factor (EGF), keratinocyte growth factor (KGF), hepatic growth factor (HGF), interleukin-4 (IL-4), IL-6, IL-8, natural inhibitors of metalloproteases, β-defensins, and prostaglandins among others [29–31]. Moreover, AM is a biomaterial that can be easily obtained, processed, and transported. On the other hand, AM may function as a substrate where cells can easily proliferate and differentiate [32]. When compared to skin transplantation, AM treatment offers considerable advantages. Its application does not produce rejection because it has low immunogenicity and does not induce uncontrolled proliferation [33]. All these effects are related to its capacity for the production and release of biologically active substances (see above).

AM has been applied in medicine for more than 100 years. In 1910, Davis [34] reported a comprehensive review of 550 cases of skin transplantation to various types of burns and wounds using natural AM obtained from labor and delivery at the Johns Hopkins University. In 1913, Sabella [35] and Stern [36] separately reported on the use of preserved AM in skin grafting for burns and ulcers. Since then, there have been several reports of the uses of AM in the treatment of wounds of different etiologies and other applications: first, in the reconstructive surgery of different tissues and organs including the mouth, tongue, nasal mucosa, larynx, eardrum, vestibule, bladder, urethra, vagina, and tendons [37–43]; second, as a peritoneum substitute in reconstruction procedures of pelvic exenteration surgery; third, in adherence prevention in the abdomen and pelvic surgery; and finally, as a covering of onphaloceles and the like [34–37, 44].

In ophthalmology, the use of AM was reported for the first time in 1940 by De Rötth, who used fresh fetal membranes, namely amnion and chorion, at the ocular surface as a biological dressing in the management of conjunctival alterations [45]. Later, Sorsby et al. [46] used preserved AM as a temporary coating in the treatment of acute caustic ocular lesions. Even though the results were favorable, its use was abandoned for almost four decades. In 1995, with the reconstitution assays of rabbit corneas with limbic disorder using human preserved AM, by Kim and Tseng [47], there was a renewed widespread interest in the use of AM in ophthalmology. Several publications appeared related to the efficacy of the AM in various ocular surface conditions and in diseases like epidermolysis bullosa [44, 48, 49]. Nowadays, AM is a resource widely used in ophthalmology [49–51] and to a lesser degree in the treatment of wounds, burns lesions, and chronic ulcers of the legs [48, 52–54] and in other surgical and nonsurgical procedures [38–43, 55–59].

3. Using AM in chronic wound healing

Once granulation of the wound is finalized, the process of epithelialization by using AM can be initiated. The source of AM for wound healing is donated placenta. AM has been used for wound healing either as intact AM without epithelium removal or as denuded AM, without the epithelium, [60, 61]. In some cases, AM was used fresh, and in others AM was preserved. Nowadays, it is known that the use of fresh AM is not practical for clinical use [62]. Methods

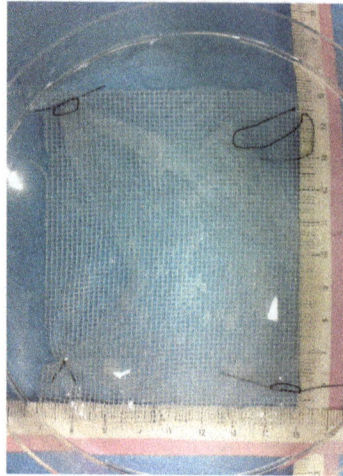

Figure 4. Amniotic membrane fixed to sterile petrolatum gauze (Tulgrasum®) ready for its application.

to remove the epithelium or preserve AM are very diverse and exceed the scope of this chapter. In our case, the placenta is obtained from an uncomplicated elective cesarean of a healthy mother, excluding patients with positive human immunodeficiency virus (HIV), hepatitis B virus (HBV), and hepatitis C virus (HCV) serology. Using an aseptic technique, AM is separated from the subjacent chorion by blunt dissection and stored in saline solution or phosphate buffered saline with antibiotics (cotrimoxazol, tobramycin, vancomycin, and amphotericin B). In this solution, AM is taken to the clean room [55]. Then, its processing, under sterile conditions, is carried out in a type II vertical laminar flow cabinet (HEPA filter). Then it is cut up into fragments measuring 10 × 10cm, which are then placed on a sterile scaffold of sterile petrolatum gauze (Tulgrasum®) and fixed with silk points at their ends (**Figure 4**). Finally, individual fragments are introduced into a bag with cryopreservative solution to freeze them in liquid nitrogen. These fragments cannot be used in the clinical practice until 3 months have passed, when there is a certainty that their donor has not been seroconverted to HIV, HBV, or HCV. After its defrosting in a 37°C bath, they are taken back to the surgical area and are applied on the wounds of the selected patient [55] (**Figures 5** and **6**).

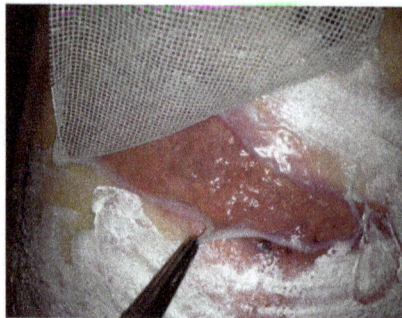

Figure 5. Complex and traumatic soft-tissue wound. Application of the amniotic membrane.

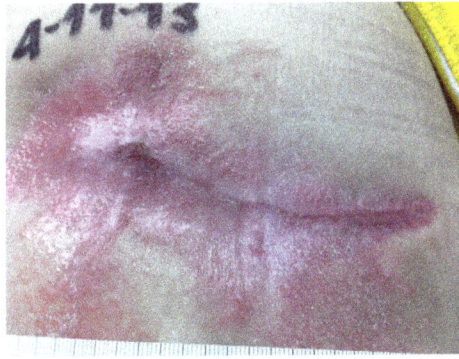

Figure 6. Complex and traumatic soft-tissue wound. Complete epithelialization after amniotic membrane treatment.

3.1. Molecular mechanisms underlying AM-induced skin reepithelialization

The molecular mechanisms underlying AM-induced skin reepithelialization are largely unknown. AM might have a wound healing effect by improving keratinocyte migration from the wound edge and stimulating its differentiation, thereby generating an intact epithelium [63]. Niknejad et al. [64] reflected that the stimulatory effect on epithelialization from the wound bed and/or the wound edge is facilitated by growth factors and progenitor cells released by AM. In addition, it has been described that the preservation of the integrity of the basement membrane and stromal matrix increases the healing potency of AM and is crucial in promoting a fast reepithelialization [65].

Insausti et al. [55] had previously worked on HaCaT cells, a spontaneously immortalized human keratinocyte cell line, as a model to comprehend the molecular consequences of AM application on human wounds [66]. This research showed that HaCaT cells exhibited different molecular reactions upon stimulation with AM that were attributed to the effects of soluble AM-released factors on HaCaT cells [55]. The application of AM to keratinocytes induced the activation of the phosphorylation of ERK1/2, JNK1/2, and p38 [55]. Also, AM-conditioned medium induced similar responses, suggesting a trans-effect of AM on the triggering of these events. Additionally, the authors reported that HaCaT cells stimulated with AM showed an increased expression of *c-JUN*. Members of the AP1 family had been involved in keratinocyte migration and the wound healing process [67–70]. AM induced the phosphorylation of Jun N-terminal kinase (JNK)1 and two kinases in HaCaT cells [55]; JNK1 is a positive regulator of c-JUN, contributing to its phosphorylation and stabilization [71, 72]. Finally, the expression of c-Jun in the wounds treated with AM was very strong, and particularly evident at the basal epithelium near the leading edge and at the dermal leading edge or keratinocyte tongue, indicating that c-Jun expression might be an important event for epithelialization occurring at the AM-stimulated wound borders [55].

3.2. Chronic wound healing, AM, and TGF-β

Wound fluid derived from chronic venous leg ulcers is rich in pro-inflammatory cytokines such as TNF-α, interleukin-1β (IL-1β), and TGF-β1 [73]. In addition, the quantities of these cytokines drop as the chronic wound commences to heal, denoting a strong correlation between non-healing wounds and an increased level of pro-inflammatory cytokines [74]. TGF-β has a critical role in regulating multiple cellular responses that occur in all phases of wound healing [75]. Of the many cytokines shown to influence the wound healing process, TGF-β has the broadest spectrum of action because it affects the behavior of a wide variety of cell types and mediates a diverse range of cellular functions [76]. Platelets are thought to be the primary source of TGF-β at the wound site; also, activation of latent TGF-β occurs immediately after wounding [75]. The TGF-β signaling pathway is considered as a promising target for the treatment of many pathological skin conditions including chronic non-healing wounds [75]. Keratinocytes, fibroblasts, and monocytes are among the targeted cells in the TGF-β management of the wound [76]. Monocytes/macrophages and fibroblasts then contribute to autocrine-perpetuated high concentrations of TGF-β at the wound site [76].

TGF-β exerts its effect on cells by increasing the phosphorylation of members of the receptor activated (R-)Smad family (Smad2 and 3). Additionally, non-Smad pathways are also activated, including the extracellular-signal-regulated kinase (ERK), JNK, and p38 mitogen-activated protein (MAP) kinase pathways, the tyrosine kinase Src, and phosphatidylinositol 3-kinase (PI3K) [77, 78]. Once receptor-induced phosphorylation has taken place, R-Smads form complexes with the common-mediator (Co-) Smad4, which are translocated to the nucleus [79] where they, in cooperation with other transcription factors, co-activators, and corepressors, regulate the transcription of specific genes [80].

The effects of TGF-β on full-thickness wound reepithelialization have been studied in a transgenic mouse. The study in the ear mouse model suggests that TGF-β has an inhibitory effect on epithelialization when the wound involves all the layers of the skin [81]. Also, the overexpression of TGF-β, at the epidermis level, causes a decrease in reepithelialization [82, 83]. Abolishing part of the TGF-β signaling pathway has been suggested as a way to improve wound healing, so abolishing part of the TGF-β-stimulated Smad pathways may enhance wound healing and benefit the effect of TGF-β signaling over matrix synthesis by fibroblasts, for instance [76]. TGF-β causes the growth arrest of epithelial cells. The mechanisms, which differ somewhat between different cell types, involve the inhibition of the expression of the transcription factor Myc and members of the Id family, and the transcriptional induction of the cell cycle inhibitors CDKN2B (p15) and CDKN1A (p21) [84].

In order to further unravel the molecular mechanism by which AM may contribute to the epithelialization and wound border proliferation in chronic post-traumatic wounds, Alcaraz et al. [85] analyzed the association between TGF-β signaling and AM regulation in wound healing using keratinocytes. Strikingly, AM was capable of attenuating the TGF-β-induced phosphorylation of Smad2 and Smad3 in HaCaT cells. Both the strength and duration of TGF-β signaling, expressed as sustained phosphorylation of Smads, are essential to achieve proper cell responses to TGF-β; the impossibility to do so produces a loss of the cell cycle arrest in response to TGF-β [86]. AM attenuates TGF-β-induced Smad2 and Smad3 phosphorylation and hence attenuates CDKN2B (p15) and CDKN1A (p21) expression [85], which has been connected to cell cycle regulation [86]. Therefore, the presence of AM counteracts the cell cycle arrest induced by TGF-β on keratinocytes, releasing them from the restrain imposed by TGFß [85]. The effect of AM on TGF-β-regulated genes is not indiscriminate, and not all genes are affected by the presence of AM. Interestingly, genes that positively participate in wound healing such as *SNAI-2* and *PAI-1* were synergistically up-regulated by the presence of AM and TGF-β [85]. Finally, the expression of c-Jun was maximal when both TGF-β and AM were present in either HaCaT or primary keratinocyte cells [85].

It has been suggested that AM might exert its wound healing effect by increasing keratinocyte migration speed from the wound edge [63]. Growth factors and progenitor cells released by AM [64] are supposed to mediate the epithelialization stimulatory effect. AM induces cell migration in a wound healing assay in keratinocytes and mesenchymal cells [85]. Furthermore, in keratinocytes, inhibition of cell proliferation with mitomycin C, affected the migrating properties of AM. In the same study, the use of JNK1 inhibitors prevented AM-induced cell migration in both cell types. Moreover, a closer inspection of the margins of the scratch wound healing assays showed a high expression of c-JUN in the AM-stimulated cells engaged in the migratory wave. The AM-induced high expression of c-JUN at the wound border was prevented by inhibitors SP600125 and PD98059, which is consistent with the fact that AM induces the activation of a signaling cascade that produces the phosphorylation of ERK1/2 and JNK1/2. A local increase of c-JUN was observed in the patient wound border when the wound had been treated with AM. This is coherent with the AM effect on cell migration. In fact, in the examination of patient wound borders a few days after AM application, a clear proliferation/migration was observed [85]. This correlates well with the robust expression of c-Jun at the wound border, which is particularly robust at the *stratum basale* of the epidermis that overlaps the keratinocyte tongue, the area where the migration of keratinocytes happens to epithelialize the wound [85]. Additionally, in that investigation, the authors revealed that the application of AM promotes healing in chronic wounds by refashioning the TGF-β-induced genetic program, stimulating keratinocyte migration and proliferation [85]. Additionally, there might be a synergy of AM and TGF-β signaling for the resolution of chronic wounds [85, 87]. Thus, stimulation of keratinocytes with both AM and TGF-β was synergistic when compared to both stimulus being added separately [85]. Moreover, the treatment of cells with TGF-β signaling inhibitors hampered the effect of AM, indicating that both AM and TGF-β signaling positively contribute to cell migration [87]. The down-regulation of Smad3 has been suggested as a possible way of improving wound healing [76]. In this sense, the effect of R-Smads, Smad2 or 3, seems to be different given that the overexpression of Smad2 increased AM-induced cell migration while the overexpression of Smad3 prevented it [87]. Notably, the ability of keratinocytes to sense TGF-β through Smad3 prevents the cell proliferation of keratinocytes and consequently prevents wound healing resolution when the levels of TGF-β are high [88].

Presently, in order to evaluate the effect of AM on chronic post-traumatic wounds, a clinical trial is being conducted in our hospital, with exceptional results. The TGF-β-stimulated Smad pathway has also been involved in the production of fibrosis and inflammation in response to TGF-β. Thus, interfering with TGF-β signaling may be a good way of interfering with fibrosis and improving the evolution of wound healing [76]. In different experimental models, the application of AM is able to ameliorate fibrosis [89–92]. Currently, we are exploring whether the application of AM is able to reduce fibrosis and inflammation in chronic wounds.

4. Summary

To summarize, AM is a biological dressing that stimulates proper epithelialization in chronic wounds. It has several advantages; among them, it is economical, easy to obtain, and in endless supply. Additionally, AM can be cryopreserved at a low temperature while preserving all its biological functions. Finally, it can be used as a treatment in the outpatient clinic, which reduces costs even more. Thus, AM must be taken into account as a consolidated treatment option for chronic wounds.

Acknowledgements

We would like to thank other members of the different laboratories who contribute in our daily task of increasing our knowledge of AM and chronic wound healing. Ana M García, María D. López and Mónica Rodríguez working in the clean room and providing AM. Paola Romencín, José E. Millán, David García and Noemi Marín, working on AM and animal models, and Miguel Blanquer, working in the cell therapy group. Antonia Alcaraz, Catalina Ruiz-Cañada, Ania Mrowiec, Eva M. García, and Sergio Liarte working on molecular aspects of AM and wound healing using cell models. This work was supported by a grant from the Fundación Séneca de la Región de Murcia and a grant from the Instituto de Salud Carlos III, Fondo de Investigaciones Sanitarias. Plan Estatal I+D+i and the Instituto de Salud Carlos III-Subdirección General de Evaluación y Fomento de la Investigación (Grant no.: PI13/00794) http://www.isciii.es/Fondos FEDER (ERDF funds) http://ec.europa.eu/regional_policy/es/funding/erdf/. We are indebted to the Hospital Clínico Universitario Virgen de la Arrixaca for strongly supporting this research.

Author details

Gregorio Castellanos[1], Ángel Bernabé-García[2], Carmen García Insausti[3], Antonio Piñero[1], José M. Moraleda[3] and Francisco J. Nicolás[2*]

*Address all correspondence to: Franciscoj.nicolas2@carm.es

1 Surgery Service, Virgen de la Arrixaca University Clinical Hospital, El Palmar, Murcia, Spain

2 Molecular Oncology and TGFβ, Research Unit, Virgen de la Arrixaca University Hospital, El Palmar, Murcia, Spain

3 Cell Therapy Unit, Virgen de la Arrixaca University Clinical Hospital, El Palmar, Murcia, Spain

References

[1] Troxler M, Vowden K, Vowden P. Integrating adjunctive therapy into practice: the importance of recognising 'hard-to-heal' wounds. World Wide Wounds (online) 2006; available from URL: http://www.worldwidewounds.com/2006/december/Troxler/Integrating-Adjunctive-Therapy-Into-Practice.html.

[2] Falanga V, Saap LJ, Ozonoff A. Wound bed score and its correlation with healing of chronic wounds. Dermatol Ther. 2006;19(6):383–90.

[3] Doerler M, Reich-Schupke S, Altmeyer P, Stucker M. Impact on wound healing and efficacy of various leg ulcer debridement techniques. J Dtsch Dermatol Ges. 2012;10(9):624–32.

[4] Margolis DJ, Berlin JA, Strom BL. Risk factors associated with the failure of a venous leg ulcer to heal. Arch Dermatol. 1999;135(8):920–6.

[5] Henderson EA. The potential effect of fibroblast senescence on wound healing and the chronic wound environment. J Wound Care. 2006;15(7):315–8.

[6] Steed DL. Clinical evaluation of recombinant human platelet-derived growth factor for the treatment of lower extremity diabetic ulcers. Diabetic Ulcer Study Group. J Vasc Surg. 1995;21(1):71–8; discussion 9–81.

[7] Mogford J., Mustoe T. Experimental models of wound healing.In: Falanga V., editor. Cutaneous Wound Healing. London: Martin Dunitz Ltd.; 2001. p. 109–22.

[8] Medina A, Scott PG, Ghahary A, Tredget EE. Pathophysiology of chronic nonhealing wounds. J Burn Care Rehabil. 2005;26(4):306–19.

[9] Shukla VK, Shukla D, Tiwary SK, Agrawal S, Rastogi A. Evaluation of pH measurement as a method of wound assessment. J Wound Care. 2007;16(7):291–4.

[10] Bowler PG, Duerden BI, Armstrong DG. Wound microbiology and associated approaches to wound management. Clin Microbiol Rev. 2001;14(2):244–69.

[11] Ngo Q, Vickery K, Deva AK. PR21 Role of Bacterial Biofilms in Chronic Wounds. ANZ Journal of Surgery. 2007;77:A66.

[12] Percival SL, Bowler PG, Dolman J. Antimicrobial activity of silver-containing dressings on wound microorganisms using an in vitro biofilm model. Int Wound J. 2007;4(2):186–91.

[13] Bjarnsholt T, Kirketerp-Moller K, Kristiansen S, Phipps R, Nielsen AK, Jensen PO, et al. Silver against Pseudomonas aeruginosa biofilms. APMIS. 2007;115(8):921–8.

[14] Attinger CE, Janis JE, Steinberg J, Schwartz J, Al-Attar A, Couch K. Clinical approach to wounds: débridement and wound bed preparation including the use of dressings and wound-healing adjuvants. Plast Reconstr Surg. 2006;117(7 Suppl):72S–109S.

[15] Baharestani M, de Leon J, Mendez-Eastman S, et al. Consensus statement: a practical guide for managing pressure ulcers with negative pressure wound therapy utilizing vacuum-assisted closure-understanding the treatment algorithm. Adv Skin Wound Care. 2008(21(Suppl 1)):1–20.

[16] EWMA, editor. Position Document: Wound Bed Preparation in Practice. (EWMA). London: MEP Ltd.; 2004.

[17] Falanga V. Classifications for wound bed preparation and stimulation of chronic wounds. Wound Repair Regen. 2000;8(5):347–52.

[18] Sibbald RG, Williamson D, Orsted HL, Campbell K, Keast D, Krasner D, et al. Preparing the wound bed--debridement, bacterial balance, and moisture balance. Ostomy Wound Manage. 2000;46(11):14–22, 4–8, 30–5; quiz 6–7.

[19] Falanga V. Wound bed preparation: science applied to practice. In: (EWMA). EWMA, editor. Position Document: Wound Bed Preparation in Practice. London: MEP Ltd.; 2004. p. 2–5.

[20] Halim AS, Khoo TL, Saad AZ. Wound bed preparation from a clinical perspective. Indian J Plast Surg. 2012;45(2):193–202.

[21] Morykwas MJ, Argenta LC, Shelton-Brown EI, McGuirt W. Vacuum-assisted closure: a new method for wound control and treatment: animal studies and basic foundation. Ann Plast Surg. 1997;38(6):553–62.

[22] Banwell PE, Musgrave M. Topical negative pressure therapy: mechanisms and indications. Int Wound J. 2004;1(2):95–106.

[23] Stechmiller JK, Kilpadi DV, Childress B, Schultz GS. Effect of vacuum-assisted closure therapy on the expression of cytokines and proteases in wound fluid of adults with pressure ulcers. Wound Repair Regen. 2006;14(3):371–4.

[24] Timmers MS, Le Cessie S, Banwell P, Jukema GN. The effects of varying degrees of pressure delivered by negative-pressure wound therapy on skin perfusion. Ann Plast Surg. 2005;55(6):665–71.

[25] Saxena V, Hwang CW, Huang S, Eichbaum Q, Ingber D, Orgill DP. Vacuum-assisted closure: microdeformations of wounds and cell proliferation. Plast Reconstr Surg. 2004;114(5):1086–96; discussion 97–8.

[26] Greene AK, Puder M, Roy R, Arsenault D, Kwei S, Moses MA, et al. Microdeformational wound therapy: effects on angiogenesis and matrix metalloproteinases in chronic wounds of 3 debilitated patients. Ann Plast Surg. 2006;56(4):418–22.

[27] Greaves NS, Iqbal SA, Baguneid M, Bayat A. The role of skin substitutes in the management of chronic cutaneous wounds. Wound Repair Regen. 2013;21(2):194–210.

[28] Lorenz HP, Longaker M. Wounds: biology, pathology, and management. Essential practice of surgery. New York: Springer; 2003. p. 77–88.

[29] Yang L, Shirakata Y, Shudou M, Dai X, Tokumaru S, Hirakawa S, et al. New skin-equivalent model from de-epithelialized amnion membrane. Cell Tissue Res. 2006;326(1):69–77.

[30] Parolini O, Soncini M. Human placenta: a source of progenitor/stem cells? J Reproduktionsmed Endokrinol. 2006;3(2):117–126.

[31] Parolini O, Alviano F, Bagnara GP, Bilic G, Buhring HJ, Evangelista M, et al. Concise review: isolation and characterization of cells from human term placenta: outcome of the first International Workshop on Placenta Derived Stem Cells. Stem Cells. 2008;26(2):300–11.

[32] Miki T, Strom SC. Amnion-derived pluripotent/multipotent stem cells. Stem Cell Rev. 2006;2(2):133–42.

[33] Insausti CL, Blanquer M, Bleda P, Iniesta P, Majado MJ, Castellanos G, et al. The amniotic membrane as a source of stem cells. Histol Histopathol. 2010;25(1):91–8.

[34] Davis JS. A method of splinting skin grafts. Skin transplantation. 1910; 21:44.

[35] Sabella N. Use of fetal membranes in skin grafting. Med Records NY. 1913;83:478–80.

[36] Stern M. The grafting of preserved amniotic membrane to burned and ulcerated surfaces, substituing skin grafts: a preliminary report. J Am Med Assoc. 1913;60(13):973–4.

[37] Ganatra MA. Amniotic membrane in surgery. J Pak Med Assoc. 2003;53(1):29–32.

[38] Tolhurst DE, van der Helm TW. The treatment of vaginal atresia. Surg Gynecol Obstet. 1991;172(5):407–14.

[39] Georgy M, Aziz N. Vaginoplasty using amnion graft: new surgical technique using the laparoscopic transillumination light. J Obstet Gynecol. 1996;16(4):262–4.

[40] Morton KE, Dewhurst CJ. Human amnion in the treatment of vaginal malformations. Br J Obstet Gynaecol. 1986;93(1):50–4.

[41] Fishman IJ, Flores FN, Scott FB, Spjut HJ, Morrow B. Use of fresh placental membranes for bladder reconstruction. J Urol. 1987;138(5):1291–4.

[42] Brandt FT, Albuquerque CD, Lorenzato FR. Female urethral reconstruction with amnion grafts. Int J Surg Investig. 2000;1(5):409–14.

[43] Zohar Y, Talmi YP, Finkelstein Y, Shvili Y, Sadov R, Laurian N. Use of human amniotic membrane in otolaryngologic practice. Laryngoscope. 1987;97(8 Pt 1):978–80.

[44] Trelford JD, Trelford-Sauder M. The amnion in surgery, past and present. Am J Obstet Gynecol. 1979;134(7):833–45.

[45] de Rötth A. Plastic repair of conjunctival defects with fetal membranes. Arch Ophthalmol. 1940;23(3):522–5.

[46] Sorsby A, Symons HM. Amniotic membrane grafts in caustic burns of the eye: (burns of the second degree). Br J Ophthalmol. 1946;30(6):337–45.

[47] Kim JC, Tseng SC. Transplantation of preserved human amniotic membrane for surface reconstruction in severely damaged rabbit corneas. Cornea. 1995;14(5):473-84.

[48] Mermet I, Pottier N, Sainthillier JM, Malugani C, Cairey-Remonnay S, Maddens S, et al. Use of amniotic membrane transplantation in the treatment of venous leg ulcers. Wound Repair Regen. 2007;15(4):459–64.

[49] Gomes JA, Romano A, Santos MS, Dua HS. Amniotic membrane use in ophthalmology. Curr Opin Ophthalmol. 2005;16(4):233–40.

[50] Dua HS, Gomes JAP, King AJ, Maharajan VS. The amniotic membrane in ophthalmology. Surv Ophthalmol. 2004;49(1):51–77.

[51] Baradaran-Rafii A, Aghayan HR, Arjmand B, Javadi MA. Amniotic membrane transplantation. Iranian J Ophthalmic Res. 2007;2(1):58–75.

[52] Colocho G, Graham WP, Iii, Greene AE, Matheson DW, Lynch D. Human amniotic membrane as a physiologic wound dressing. Arch Surg. 1974;109(3):370–3.

[53] Singh R, Chouhan US, Purohit S, Gupta P, Kumar P, Kumar A, et al. Radiation processed amniotic membranes in the treatment of non-healing ulcers of different etiologies. Cell Tissue Bank. 2004;5(2):129–34.

[54] Hasegawa T, Mizoguchi M, Haruna K, Mizuno Y, Muramatsu S, Suga Y, et al. Amnia for intractable skin ulcers with recessive dystrophic epidermolysis bullosa: report of three cases. J Dermatol. 2007;34(5):328–32.

[55] Insausti CL, Alcaraz A, Garcia-Vizcaino EM, Mrowiec A, Lopez-Martinez MC, Blanquer M, et al. Amniotic membrane induces epithelialization in massive posttraumatic wounds. Wound Repair Regen. 2010;18(4):368–77.

[56] Sangwan VS, Matalia HP, Vemuganti GK, Fatima A, Ifthekar G, Singh S, et al. Clinical outcome of autologous cultivated limbal epithelium transplantation. Indian J Ophthalmol. 2006;54(1):29–34.

[57] Díaz-Prado S, Rendal-Vázquez ME, Muiños-López E, Hermida-Gómez T, Rodríguez-Cabarcos M, Fuentes-Boquete I, et al. Potential use of the human amniotic membrane as a scaffold in human articular cartilage repair. Cell Tissue Bank. 2010;11(2):183–95.

[58] Yeager AM, Singer HS, Buck JR, Matalon R, Brennan S, O'Toole SO, et al. A therapeutic trial of amniotic epithelial cell implantation in patients with lysosomal storage diseases. Am J Med Genet. 1985;22(2):347–55.

[59] Redondo P, Giménez de Azcarate A, Marqués L, García-Guzman M, Andreu E, Prósper F. Amniotic membrane as a scaffold for melanocyte transplantation in patients with stable vitiligo. Dermatol Res Pract. 2011;2011:6.

[60] Akle C, McColl I, Dean M, Adinolfi M, Brown S, Fensom AH, et al. Transplantation of amniotic epithelial membranes in patients with mucopolysaccharidoses. Exp Clin Immunogenet. 1985;2(1):43–8.

[61] Wilshaw SP, Kearney JN, Fisher J, Ingham E. Production of an acellular amniotic membrane matrix for use in tissue engineering. Tissue Eng. 2006;12(8):2117–29.

[62] Zelen CM, Snyder RJ, Serena TE, Li WW. The use of human amnion/chorion membrane in the clinical setting for lower extremity repair: a review. Clin Podiatr Med Surg. 2015;32(1):135–46.

[63] Lee SH, Tseng SC. Amniotic membrane transplantation for persistent epithelial defects with ulceration. Am J Ophthalmol. 1997;123(3):303–12.

[64] Niknejad H, Peirovi H, Jorjani M, Ahmadiani A, Ghanavi J, Seifalian AM. Properties of the amniotic membrane for potential use in tissue engineering. Eur Cell Mater. 2008;15:88–99.

[65] Kubo M, Sonoda Y, Muramatsu R, Usui M. Immunogenicity of human amniotic membrane in experimental xenotransplantation. Invest Ophthalmol Vis Sci. 2001;42(7): 1539–46.

[66] Boukamp P, Petrussevska RT, Breitkreutz D, Hornung J, Markham A, Fusenig NE. Normal keratinization in a spontaneously immortalized aneuploid human keratino-cyte cell line. J Cell Biol. 1988;106(3):761–71.

[67] Angel P, Szabowski A, Schorpp-Kistner M. Function and regulation of AP-1 subunits in skin physiology and pathology. Oncogene. 2001;20(19):2413–23.

[68] Yates S, Rayner TE. Transcription factor activation in response to cutaneous injury: role of AP-1 in reepithelialization. Wound Repair Regen. 2002;10(1):5–15.

[69] Gangnuss S, Cowin AJ, Daehn IS, Hatzirodos N, Rothnagel JA, Varelias A, et al. Regulation of MAPK activation, AP-1 transcription factor expression and keratinocyte differentiation in wounded fetal skin. J Invest Dermatol. 2004;122(3):791–804.

[70] Li G, Gustafson-Brown C, Hanks SK, Nason K, Arbeit JM, Pogliano K, et al. c-Jun is essential for organization of the epidermal leading edge. Dev Cell. 2003;4(6):865–77.

[71] Ronai Z. JNKing Revealed. Mol Cell. 2004;15(6):843–4.

[72] Sabapathy K, Hochedlinger K, Nam SY, Bauer A, Karin M, Wagner EF. Distinct roles for JNK1 and JNK2 in regulating JNK activity and c-Jun-dependent cell proliferation. Mol Cell. 2004;15(5):713–25.

[73] Harris IR, Yee KC, Walters CE, Cunliffe WJ, Kearney JN, Wood EJ, et al. Cytokine and protease levels in healing and non-healing chronic venous leg ulcers. Exp Dermatol. 1995;4(6):342–9.

[74] Trengove NJ, Bielefeldt-Ohmann H, Stacey MC. Mitogenic activity and cytokine levels in non-healing and healing chronic leg ulcers. Wound Repair Regen. 2000;8(1):13–25.

[75] Finnson KW, McLean S, Di Guglielmo GM, Philip A. Dynamics of transforming growth factor beta signaling in wound healing and scarring. Advances Wound Care. 2013;2(5): 195–214.

[76] Ashcroft GS, Roberts AB. Loss of Smad3 modulates wound healing. Cytokine Growth Factor Rev. 2000;11(1–2):125–31.

[77] Moustakas A, Heldin CH. Non-Smad TGF-beta signals. J Cell Sci. 2005;118(Pt 16):3573–84.

[78] Mu Y, Gudey SK, Landstrom M. Non-Smad signaling pathways. Cell Tissue Res. 2012;347(1):11–20.

[79] Pierreux CE, Nicolas FJ, Hill CS. Transforming growth factor beta-independent shuttling of Smad4 between the cytoplasm and nucleus. Mol Cell Biol. 2000;20(23): 9041–54.

[80] Heldin CH, Moustakas A. Role of Smads in TGFbeta signaling. Cell Tissue Res. 2012;347(1):21–36.

[81] Tredget EB, Demare J, Chandran G, Tredget EE, Yang L, Ghahary A. Transforming growth factor-beta and its effect on reepithelialization of partial-thickness ear wounds in transgenic mice. Wound Repair Regen. 2005;13(1):61–7.

[82] Chan T, Ghahary A, Demare J, Yang L, Iwashina T, Scott PG, et al. Development, characterization, and wound healing of the keratin 14 promoted transforming growth factor-beta1 transgenic mouse. Wound Repair Regen. 2002;10(3):177–87.

[83] Yang L, Chan T, Demare J, Iwashina T, Ghahary A, Scott PG, et al. Healing of burn wounds in transgenic mice overexpressing transforming growth factor-beta 1 in the epidermis. Am J Pathol. 2001;159(6):2147–57.

[84] Heldin CH, Landstrom M, Moustakas A. Mechanism of TGF-beta signaling to growth arrest, apoptosis, and epithelial-mesenchymal transition. Curr Opin Cell Biol. 2009;21(2):166–76.

[85] Alcaraz A, Mrowiec A, Insausti CL, Bernabe-Garcia A, Garcia-Vizcaino EM, Lopez-Martinez MC, et al. Amniotic membrane modifies the genetic program induced by TGFss, stimulating keratinocyte proliferation and migration in chronic wounds. PLoS One. 2015;10(8):e0135324.

[86] Nicolas FJ, Hill CS. Attenuation of the TGF-beta-Smad signaling pathway in pancreatic tumor cells confers resistance to TGF-beta-induced growth arrest. Oncogene. 2003;22(24):3698–711.

[87] Ruiz-Canada C, Bernabé-García A, Angosto D, Castellanos G, Insausti CL, Moraleda JM, et al. Amniotic membrane stimulates migration by modulating TFG-β signaling. (In press).

[88] Ashcroft GS, Yang X, Glick AB, Weinstein M, Letterio JL, Mizel DE, et al. Mice lacking Smad3 show accelerated wound healing and an impaired local inflammatory response. Nat Cell Biol. 1999;1(5):260–6.

[89] Hodge A, Lourensz D, Vaghjiani V, Nguyen H, Tchongue J, Wang B, et al. Soluble factors derived from human amniotic epithelial cells suppress collagen production in human hepatic stellate cells. Cytotherapy. 2014;16(8):1132–44.

[90] Cargnoni A, Gibelli L, Tosini A, Signoroni PB, Nassuato C, Arienti D, et al. Transplantation of allogeneic and xenogeneic placenta-derived cells reduces bleomycin-induced lung fibrosis. Cell Transplant. 2009;18(4):405–22.

[91] Cargnoni A, Piccinelli EC, Ressel L, Rossi D, Magatti M, Toschi I, et al. Conditioned medium from amniotic membrane-derived cells prevents lung fibrosis and preserves blood gas exchanges in bleomycin-injured mice-specificity of the effects and insights into possible mechanisms. Cytotherapy. 2014;16(1):17–32.

[92] Cargnoni A, Ressel L, Rossi D, Poli A, Arienti D, Lombardi G, et al. Conditioned medium from amniotic mesenchymal tissue cells reduces progression of bleomycin-induced lung fibrosis. Cytotherapy. 2012;14(2):153–61.

Permissions

The contributors of this book come from diverse backgrounds, making this book a truly international effort. This book will bring forth new frontiers with its revolutionizing research information and detailed analysis of the nascent developments around the world.

We would like to thank all the contributing authors for lending their expertise to make the book truly unique. They have played a crucial role in the development of this book. Without their invaluable contributions this book wouldn't have been possible. They have made vital efforts to compile up to date information on the varied aspects of this subject to make this book a valuable addition to the collection of many professionals and students.

This book was conceptualized with the vision of imparting up-to-date information and advanced data in this field. To ensure the same, a matchless editorial board was set up. Every individual on the board went through rigorous rounds of assessment to prove their worth. After which they invested a large part of their time researching and compiling the most relevant data for our readers.

The editorial board has been involved in producing this book since its inception. They have spent rigorous hours researching and exploring the diverse topics which have resulted in the successful publishing of this book. They have passed on their knowledge of decades through this book. To expedite this challenging task, the publisher supported the team at every step. A small team of assistant editors was also appointed to further simplify the editing procedure and attain best results for the readers.

Apart from the editorial board, the designing team has also invested a significant amount of their time in understanding the subject and creating the most relevant covers. They scrutinized every image to scout for the most suitable representation of the subject and create an appropriate cover for the book.

The publishing team has been an ardent support to the editorial, designing and production team. Their endless efforts to recruit the best for this project, has resulted in the accomplishment of this book. They are a veteran in the field of academics and their pool of knowledge is as vast as their experience in printing. Their expertise and guidance has proved useful at every step. Their uncompromising quality standards have made this book an exceptional effort. Their encouragement from time to time has been an inspiration for everyone.

The publisher and the editorial board hope that this book will prove to be a valuable piece of knowledge for researchers, students, practitioners and scholars across the globe.

List of Contributors

Junna Ye, Yiwen Niu, Liang Qiao, Ming Tian, Chun Qing and Shuliang Lu
Institute of Burns, Ruijin Hospital, Shanghai Jiao Tong University, Shanghai, China

Ting Xie
Department of Wound Healing, Shanghai Ninth Hospital, Shanghai Jiao Tong University, Shanghai, China

Mohammad Bayat
Cellular and Molecular Biology Research Center, and Department of Biology and Anatomical Sciences, School of Medicine, Shahid Beheshti University of Medical Sciences, Tehran, Iran

Jill M. Monfre
University Hospital, University of Wisconsin, Madison, Wisconsin, USA

Vlad-Adrian Alexandrescu and François Triffaux
Department of General, Thoracic and Vascular Surgery, Princess Paola Hospital, IFAC/ Vivalia, Marche-en-Famenne, Belgium

Vlad-Adrian Alexandrescu
Department of Cardio-Vascular and Thoracic Surgery, CHU Sart-Tilmant, University of Liège, Liège, Belgium

Amir Feily and Fatemeh Moeineddin
Skin and Stem Cell Research Center, Tehran University of Medical Sciences, Tehran, Iran

Shadi Mehraban
Jahrom University of Medical Sciences, Jahrom, Iran

Sherif Sultan and Wael Tawfick
Department of Vascular and Endovascular Surgery, Western Vascular Institute, University College Hospital Galway, Galway, Ireland

Sherif Sultan, Edel P Kavanagh and Niamh Hynes
Department of Vascular and Endovascular Surgery, Galway Clinic, Doughiska, Galway, Ireland

Omar Sarheed and Douha Shouqair
RAK College of Pharmaceutical Sciences, RAK Medical and Health Sciences University, Ras Al Khaiamah, United Arab Emirates

Asif Ahmed and Joshua Boateng
Department of Pharmaceutical, Chemical and Environmental Sciences, Faculty of Engineering and Science, University of Greenwich, Kent, UK

Lina Fu
Department of Chemical and Biochemical Engineering, Western University, London, Ontario, Canada
Fordham Centre for Biomedical Engineering, London, Ontario, Canada

Aslı Aksu Çerman, İlknur Kıvanç Altunay and Ezgi Aktaş Karabay
Dermatology Department, Sisli Hamidiye Etfal Training and Research Hospital, Istanbul, Turkey

Gregorio Castellanos and Antonio Piñero
Surgery Service, Virgen de la Arrixaca University Clinical Hospital, El Palmar, Murcia, Spain

Ángel Bernabé-García and Francisco J. Nicolás
Molecular Oncology and TGFβ, Research Unit, Virgen de la Arrixaca University Hospital, El Palmar, Murcia, Spain

Carmen García Insausti and José M. Moraleda
Cell Therapy Unit, Virgen de la Arrixaca University Clinical Hospital, El Palmar, Murcia, Spain

Index

www.ingramcontent.com/pod-product-compliance
Lightning Source LLC
Chambersburg PA
CBHW061956190326

41458CB00009B/2883